WITHDRAWN 11/06/24
RM

OXFORD MEDICAL PUBLICATIONS

Oxford Handbook of
Clinical Diagnosis

SECOND EDITION

Oxford Handbook of
Clinical
Diagnosis

SECOND EDITION

Huw Llewelyn

Consultant Physician, Kettering General Hospital,
Kettering, Northamptonshire, UK

Hock Aun Ang

Honorary Senior Lecturer in Medicine, Penang Medical
College, Consultant Physician and Endocrinologist,
Seberang Jaya Hospital,
Penang, Malaysia

Keir Lewis

Senior Lecturer in Medicine, Swansea University,
Honorary Consultant Physician, Prince Philip Hospital,
Llanelli, Carmarthenshire, UK

Anees Al-Abdullah

General Practitioner, Meddygfa Minafon, Kidwelly,
Carmarthenshire, UK

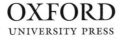
OXFORD
UNIVERSITY PRESS

OXFORD

UNIVERSITY PRESS

Great Clarendon Street, Oxford OX2 6DP

Oxford University Press is a department of the University of Oxford.
It furthers the University's objective of excellence in research, scholarship,
and education by publishing worldwide in

Oxford New York

Auckland Cape Town Dar es Salaam Hong Kong Karachi
Kuala Lumpur Madrid Melbourne Mexico City Nairobi
New Delhi Shanghai Taipei Toronto

With offices in

Argentina Austria Brazil Chile Czech Republic France Greece
Guatemala Hungary Italy Japan Poland Portugal Singapore
South Korea Switzerland Thailand Turkey Ukraine Vietnam

Oxford is a registered trade mark of Oxford University Press
in the UK and in certain other countries

Published in the United States
by Oxford University Press Inc., New York

British Library Cataloguing in Publication Data
Data available

Library of Congress Cataloging-in-Publication-Data
Data available

Typeset by Cepha Imaging Private Ltd., Bangalore, India
Printed in Italy
on acid-free paper by
L.E.G.O. S.p.A–Lavis TN

ISBN 978–0–19–923296–3

10 9 8 7 6 5 4 3 2 1

Contents

For Angela

Foreword

All healthcare involves decisions made by patients and those providing their care[1].

No decision is more important than coming to the appropriate diagnosis (or diagnoses) and no topic is shrouded in more mystery. Although many volumes have been written on differential diagnosis, few have attempted to provide a reasoned approach to a process that inevitably underpins all clinical practice. Lists of possible conditions associated with specific symptoms, physical signs and laboratory results become ever more complex without providing any reasoned approach to the diagnostic process. Clinicians appreciate that they must learn to live with uncertainty. Yet patients and clinicians alike have a common interest in reducing the areas of uncertainty to a minimum and being able to plan future management in partnership.

This is the second edition of a book that helps approach the diagnostic process in a reasoned way. The fact that experienced practitioners use 'intuitive' reasoning is explained and contrasted with 'transparent' reasoning using the concept of a particularly significant finding—the diagnostic lead. How to evaluate and then confirm the likely diagnosis is also described. This basic methodology is then applied to clinical conditions affecting the major systems of the body in a way that both makes the diagnostic process logical and mitigates against serious errors.

Working in partnership with patients, clinicians must be sufficiently skilled and confident in their diagnostic abilities to help plan future management. Concise and lucid, this book is of real value to all involved in patient care whatever their level of experience.

Sir Graeme Catto
President
The General Medical Council

1. General Medical Council (2008). *Consent: patients and doctors making decisions together.* http://www.gmc-uk.org/guidance/ethical_guidance/consent_guidance/part1_principles.asp

Preface

This book helps doctors and students to arrive at a diagnosis and to explain and to justify their reasoning, especially when seeing patients with new problems that lie outside their personal range of experience. This will happen very frequently to students, frequently to house officers but will still happen regularly to very experienced senior hospital doctors and general practitioners. This second edition also provides details of the initial clinical management once the diagnosis has been made.

The book adopts the approach used by experienced diagnosticians, by focusing on the finding with the shortest differential diagnosis (i.e. the best diagnostic lead). The book describes the differential diagnoses of such findings that may be encountered by a reader in the history, examination and usual preliminary tests and how the diagnoses can be confirmed and treated initially. It describes what tactics to adopt in order to find better leads while not losing sight of the patient's original concern.

The entries on each page of the book resemble a traditional past medical history with multiple diagnoses. The reader scans down the page to see which of the diagnoses with its findings and initial management match the patient's findings so far. The compatible findings can then be used as evidence for the diagnosis and initial treatment, to be shared with the patient and other members of the multidisciplinary team such as nurses, pharmacists, physiotherapists and other professionals allied to medicine. It can be used to create high-quality discharge or handover summaries.

Patients or their carers may wish to share in the diagnostic and decision making process. In order to do this, they need to know what problems have been identified and the tests and treatments being proposed. They will need to know which of these diagnoses explain each problem and treatment. They may also need to know which findings are being used to confirm each diagnosis and to choose its treatments and to mark the outcome. The book describes how this information can be provided in writing. The patient or carer will then be in a position to explain all this to another doctor if necessary.

Huw Llewelyn
2008

Acknowledgements

This book is based on ideas and teaching methods developed by Dr Huw Llewelyn originally at King's College Hospital, London. We thank staff and students at Luton and Dunstable Hospital, Eastbourne District General Hospital, Newham University Hospital and the Whittington Hospital in London for their helpful advice. We also thank Dr Arthur Miller, formerly Head of the Department of Chemical Pathology at the University College and Middlesex Hospitals London for his helpful advice.

The second edition was prepared with the support of students and staff at Kettering General Hospital. It was influenced by the experience of using a software system in Kettering called 'Easy-Note' that allows doctors in all medical and surgical specialties to write discharge summaries by using the 'problem-structuring' approach described in chapter 2. This 'Easy-Note' system was designed by Dr James Findlay and Dr Anwar Hussain; it was written for hospital networks in Microsoft Office Access by Glenn Lennie with the support of Mike Smeeton. The 'Easy-Note' system was applied to patient care by using the principles and information in the second edition of this book with the support of Dr Brendan O'Malley, Dr Naeem Shaukat and Graham Bell.

We are grateful to the staff at Oxford University Press for their support and patience, particularly Kate Wanwimolruk, Anna Winstanley, Elizabeth Reeve, Beth Womack, and Selby Marshall.

Advisors

Symbols and abbreviations

OHCD	Oxford Handbook of Clinical Diagnosis
OHCS	Oxford Handbook of Clinical Surgery
📖	cross reference
↑	increased
↓	decreased
→	leading to
+ve	positive
−ve	negative
±	with or without
>	greater than
<	less than
≥	equal to or greater than
≤	equal to or less than
α	alpha
β	beta
γ	gamma
®	registered
1°	primary
2°	secondary
ABG	arterial blood gas
AC	acromioclavicular
ACE	angiotensin-converting enzyme
ACL	anterior cruciate ligament
ACTH	adrenocorticotropin
ADH	antidiuretic hormone
AER	albumin excretion rate
AF	atrial fibrillation
AFB	acid-fast bacilli
ALT	alanine transaminase
ANA	anti-nuclear antibody
ANCA	anti-neutrophil cytoplasmic antibody
A–P	antero-posterior
ARB	angiotensin receptor blocker
ARDS	acute respiratory distress syndrome
5-ASA	5-aminosalicylic acid
ASOT	anti-streptolysin O titre
AST	aspartate transaminase

ATLS	advanced trauma life support
AXR	abdominal X-ray
bd	twice daily
BMI	body mass index
BP	blood pressure
bpm	beats per minute
Ca^{2+}	calcium
CCU	coronary care unit
CIN	cervical intraepithelial neoplasia
cm	centimeter
CNS	central nervous system
CO_2	carbon dioxide
COPD	chronic obstructive pulmonary disease
CPK	creatinine phosphokinase
CRF	chronic renal failure
CRP	C-reactive protein
CSF	cerebrospinal fluid
CT	computer tomography
CVP	central venous pressure
CXR	chest X-ray
d	day
DC	direct current
dL	decilitre
DH	drug history
DIC	disseminated intravascular coagulation
DMARD	disease-modifying anti-rheumatic drug
DNA	deoxyribonucleic acid
DOB	date of birth
DU	duodenal ulcer
DVT	deep vein thrombosis
ECG	electrocardiogram
ECT	electroconvulsive therapy
EEG	electroencephalogram
EMG	electromyography
e.g	for example
ELISA	enzyme-linked immunosorbent assay
ERCP	endoscopic retrograde cholangiopancreatography
ESR	erythrocyte sedimentation rate
FBC	full blood count
FEV_1	forced expiratory volume in 1 second

FFP	fresh frozen plasma
FH	family history
FSH	follicular stimulating hormone
FT3	free T3
FT4	free T4
FVC	forced vital capacity
g	gram
GALS	gait, arms, legs, spine
GCS	Glasgow Coma Score
γGT	gamma glutamyl transpeptidase
GI	gastrointestinal
G6PD	glucose-6-pyruvate dehydrogenase
GnRH	gonadotropin-releasing hormone
GTN	glyceryl trinitrate
GTT	glucose tolerance test
GU	gastric ulcer
h	hour
Hb	haemoglobin
HBsAg	hepatitis B surface antigen
hCG	human chorionic gonadotropin
HCV	hepatitis C virus
HDU	high dependency unit
Hg	mercury
5-HIAA	5-hydroxyindole acetic acid
HIV	human immunodeficiency virus
HMMA	4 hydroxy-3-methoxymadelic acid
HPC	history of presenting complaint
HOCM	hypertrophic cardiomyopathy
HRT	hormone replacement therapy
IC	intercostals
IgM	immunoglobulin M
IHD	ischaemic heart disease
IM	intramuscular
IP	interphalangeal
ITU	intensive treatment unit
IUCD	intrauterine contraceptive device
IV	intravenous
IVC	inferior vena cava
IVU	intravenous urography
JVP	jugular venous pressure

K	potassium
kg	kilogram
L	litre
LCL	lateral collateral ligament
LFT	liver function test
LH	luteinizing hormone
LIF	left iliac fossa
LMW	low molecular weight
LP	lumbar puncture
LVF	left ventricular failure
mcg	microgram
MCL	medial collateral ligament
MCP	metacarpophalangeal
mg	milligram
MI	myocardial infarction
min	minute
mL	millilitre
mm	millimeter
mmHg	millimeter of mercury
mmol	milllimole
MMSE	mini-mental state examination
mo	month
MR	magnetic resonance
MRCP	magnetic resonance cholangiopancreatography
MRI	magnetic resonance imaging
MS	multiple sclerosis
MSU	midstream urine
MTP	metatarsophalangeal
Na	sodium
NB	*nota* bene
NG	nasogastric
NIV	non-invasive ventilation
NNT	number needed to treat
NSAID	non-steroidal anti-inflammatory drug
NSAP	non-specific abdominal pain
O_2	oxygen
OBAS	observation, bracing, and surgery
od	*omni die* (once daily)
OGD	oesophagogastroduodenoscopy
p	page

P2	pulmonary component of 2nd heart sound
P–A	postero-anterior
PC	presenting complaint
PCL	posterior cruciate ligament
PCR	polymerase chain reaction
PE	pulmonary embolism
PEFR	peak expiratory flow rate
PEG	percutaneous endoscopic gastrostomy
PET	positron emission tomography
PMH	past medical history
PN	perussion note
PND	paroxysmal nocturnal dyspnoea
PO	*per os* (by mouth)
PPI	proton pump inhibitor
PR	*per rectum* (by rectum)
prn	as required
PSA	prostatic-specific antigen
PUO	pyrexia of unknown origin
PUVA	psoralen UVA
qds	*quater die sumendus* (four times daily)
RA	rheumatoid arthritis
RBC	red blood cell
RF	rheumatoid factor
RICE	rest, ice, compression, and elevation
RICER	rest, ice, compression, elevation, and referral
RIF	right iliac fossa
RLQ	right lower quadrant
RNA	ribonucleic acid
RUQ	right upper quadrant
S2	2nd heart sound
SALT	speech and language therapy
SH	social history
SHBG	sex hormone-binding globulin
SLE	systemic lupus erythematosus
SSRI	selective serotonin reuptake inhibitor
STEMI	ST elevated myocardial infarction
SVC	superior vena cava
SVT	supraventricular tachycardia
T3	triiodothyronine
T4	thyroxine

TB	tuberculosis
tds	*ter die sumendus* (three times daily)
TNF	tumour necrosis factor
TSH	thyroid stimulating hormone
TFT	thyroid function test
TURP	transurethral resection of prostate
TVF	tactile vocal fremitus
U&E	urea and electrolytes
UTI	urinary tract infection
URTI	upper respiratory tract infection
US	ultrasound
UV	ultraviolet
V/Q	ventilation/perfusion
VSD	ventriculoseptal defect
VMA	vanillylmandelic acid
WBC	white blood cell
WCC	white cell count
wk	week
y	year
ZN	Ziehl–Neelsen

Detailed contents

3 General and endocrine symptoms and physical signs

6 Respiratory symptoms and physical signs   **285**

7 Gastrointestinal symptoms and physical signs 347

8 Urological and gynaecological symptoms

and physical signs   **497**

11 Laboratory tests   685

The diagnostic process

The purpose of this book

This book explains how to interpret symptoms, physical signs and test results during the differential diagnostic process. There are many books that provide lists of differential diagnoses. However, this book also explains how you should use them. Each page describes

- The main differential diagnoses of a single diagnostic 'lead'
- How to 'differentiate' between these differential diagnoses
- How to confirm the diagnosis and to begin treatment

Making diagnostic reasoning and decisions transparent

The book explains how to outline your diagnostic reasoning on paper. It does this by showing you how to write a list of differential diagnoses and established diagnoses, each with its supportive evidence so far and proposed management (see 📖 p.13). This can be used as a draft management plan and later as a hospital discharge summary. The differential diagnoses in the pages of this book with their evidence and initial management are described in the same format and can be used as example entries when writing out an outline of the diagnoses, evidence and management for a patient.

Understanding the reasoning of others

This book helps you to understand the diagnostic reasoning and decisions of others. In order to do so, you (and patients, carers, nurses and other health professionals) have to ask:

- What problem findings have been identified (including the presenting complaint)?
- What diagnoses are being considered (provisional and final)?
- What is the evidence for each diagnosis (how it presented, how it was confirmed and how its progress or outcome is being assessed)?
- What is the management of each diagnosis (the treatments, the tests being requested and plan)?

Look up the 'problem findings' and diagnoses in this book so that you know what type of answers to expect to the above questions. You can write them out in a similar format (see 📖 p.13). After hearing these answers, you may wish to add new information to the pages of this book. You will learn more quickly by doing this.

Checking a clinical impression and explicit reasoning

It is important to check all diagnoses and decisions. Reasoning alone using knowledge from a book of this kind is not enough. Such reasoning should be checked by discussing it with someone who is familiar with the situation from past experience and who can recognize if the reasoning makes sense. However, it is equally important to check that diagnoses and decisions made 'intuitively' make sense when checked with transparent reasoning of the type described in this book.

When and how to use it

This book can be used:

- When assessing a patient, e.g. after the history of presenting complaint, after completing the full history, after completing the examination, and when the test results come back
- In the same way during problem-based learning with case histories
- During private study to allow you to solve clinical problems later without having to refer to the book
- When asking someone else to explain a diagnosis and decision to you

If the presenting complaint is severe (e.g. pain or breathlessness), disabling (e.g. inability to move a limb or speak), or unusual (e.g. coughing or vomiting blood), then it will tend to be good lead with a shorter differential diagnosis. The most useful diagnostic leads are described in this book—look at the 'Contents' page of each section and the title of every page so that you can recognize them.

If the presenting complaint is not a good lead, then consider what systems (e.g. cardiovascular or respiratory) it came from and ask 'direct questions' directed at this system to try to find better leads. Also, focus on that system first in your examination. Note the speed of onset; this will suggest the underlying disease process. Onset within seconds suggests an 'electrical' cause, e.g. a fit or rhythm abnormality; onset over seconds to minutes suggests an embolus, a trauma, or rupture; onset over minutes to hours suggests a thrombotic process, over hours to days an acute infection, over days to weeks a chronic infection, weeks to months a tumour, and months to years a degenerative process.

Read the book during private study by covering the column of diagnoses on the left of the page with a bookmark and testing your ability to recognize the diagnoses when you read the nature of the diagnostic lead on top of the page, the suggestive and confirmatory findings. If you are able to do this successfully, you will soon learn to take a history and examine a patient without having to use this book. Do it first with the symptoms and physical signs that are common in your current (and next) clinical attachment so that you are prepared.

'Intuitive' reasoning

It is important to bear in mind that most of the time, experienced doctors use a non-transparent reasoning process. This seems to involve recognizing combinations or patterns of findings consciously or subconsciously which suggest or confirm a diagnosis, or indicate that some treatment should be given. This is a skill that is improved by experience. This book will encourage you to do this sooner. However, all doctors specialize and the information in this book will be of help to experienced doctors with patients outside their specialty.

If you were told that a patient had suffered sudden onset of sharp chest pain over seconds to minutes, then this lead will make you think consciously or subconsciously of a pneumothorax, pulmonary infarction, etc. If another patient has suddenly started coughing up blood, then this lead would suggest acute bronchitis, pulmonary infarction, bronchial carcinoma, pulmonary tuberculosis, etc. However, if both happened in the same patient, your mental links would 'intersect' mentally on pulmonary infarction and it would surface to consciousness.

If you were to come across this combination of features and had read in this book during private study that they 'suggested' pulmonary infarction, then you might think of this diagnosis directly. If you came across these findings many times and a diagnosis of pulmonary infarction was usually confirmed on CT-pulmonary angiogram, then you would soon recognize that the combination of findings as suggesting pulmonary infarction (like recognizing someone's face).

If a diagnosis or small number of differential diagnoses do not come to mind readily in one of these ways, then it is important to use a 'transparent' reasoning process. You will always come across unfamiliar situations, however experienced you become, so the 'transparent' approach will always be important.

'Transparent' reasoning

'Transparent' reasoning involves assembling a combination of features that identifies a group of patients within which the frequency of those with a diagnosis would be high. This can be done by first selecting a diagnostic lead. It can be a symptom, sign, or any test result (e.g. acute abdominal tenderness in the right lower quadrant, see 📖p.480).

One of the lead's differential diagnoses is then chosen (e.g. appendicitis on p.480), and a finding is looked for that occurs often in the chosen diagnosis (e.g. guarding occurs often in appendicitis), but less often in others (e.g. guarding occurs less often in non-specific abdominal pain or NSAP). Appendicitis will thus occur more frequently (and NSAP less frequently) in a group of patients with right lower quadrant pain and guarding.

If a new finding becomes available which is a better lead with fewer differential diagnoses (e.g. a CT scan result), then this can be seized upon instead. You can select any finding as a lead from the total evidence. It does not have to be the first finding you come across such as the presenting complaint. But this does not mean that you can ignore other findings.

A single diagnosis will only become final if it can explain all the patient's findings. For example, in some cases, a CT scan might also show an absent kidney shadow on the left side. None of the differential diagnoses of this finding would explain acute right sided abdominal tenderness. Therefore, it would be wrong to focus on the lead of an absent renal outline and ignore the other findings, so at least two diagnoses will be needed.

Differentiating between diagnoses

Eddy and Clanton analyzed the thoughts processes of senior doctors participating in the Clinico-Pathological Conferences at the Massachusetts General Hospital[1]. They pointed out that choosing a diagnostic lead, e.g. right lower quadrant pain (which they called a 'pivot') was central to these experienced doctors' explanations when solving diagnostic problems. They also noted that during diagnostic reasoning, other findings (e.g. guarding) were used to 'prune' some of the differential diagnoses (e.g. pruning away NSAP).

If a finding (e.g. being male) occurs often in a diagnosis being pursued (e.g. appendicitis) but cannot happen in a differential diagnosis (e.g. ectopic pregnancy), then that diagnosis can be ruled out. However, if a finding such as guarding occurs commonly in the diagnosis being chased (e.g. appendicitis) and less frequently in another diagnosis (e.g. NSAP), the other diagnosis will become less probable, not ruled out. That is, the diagnostic lead together with the new finding will form a combination within which the frequency of the diagnosis being chased becomes more frequent; the diagnosis in which the finding occurs less often thus becomes less frequent.

The frequency with which a finding occurs in a diagnosis is often described as its 'sensitivity' by epidemiologists, i.e. the frequency with which the finding 'detects' the diagnosis when screening a population. Statisticians also call the 'sensitivity' the 'likelihood' of the finding being discovered when the patient is known to have the diagnosis. If the finding is 'likely' to occur in a diagnosis being chased and is 'unlikely' to occur in one of its differential diagnoses, then the ratio of the two likelihoods represents the finding's ability to differentiate between those two diagnoses. This makes one more probable and the other less probable. This book describes such findings under the headings of 'Suggested by' and 'Confirmed by'.

Changing diagnostic leads

A patient presenting with breathlessness will have a long list of differential diagnoses. A circular shadow on a chest X-ray (CXR) will have a much shorter list of differential diagnoses and a CT scan showing a lesion contiguous with a bronchus an even shorter one. A biopsy might provide a diagnostic criterion for a bronchial carcinoma. However, this may only be a working diagnosis. All the diagnoses applicable to that patient will not become final until the patient's symptoms have been cured, stabilized, or predicted correctly.

So if we come across a powerful finding or combination of findings (e.g. a dense round shadow within an organ on a CXR), this will form a stronger lead with a shorter list of differential diagnoses. It is easier to make a fresh start with such a powerful new finding than to try to work out which of the original diagnostic possibilities are being made more probable or less probable. Therefore, another measure of a powerful finding is the number of differential diagnoses required to explain, say 99% of patients with that finding. The better the lead the fewer the differential diagnoses.

Confirming a diagnosis

A diagnosis can be confirmed in different ways, the different confirming (or 'sufficient') findings taken together form the 'definitive criteria' of the diagnosis. The definitive criteria thus identify all those and only those with the diagnosis. Such criteria can be based on symptoms, signs, and test results (and in some cases, on the result of treatment). Ideally, the 'pre-treatment' criteria should identify all those who respond to the various treatments available for patients with that diagnosis or those for whom such a label is of practical value in other ways (e.g. prognosis alone). In some cases, the diagnostic criteria are proposed by experts set up by official bodies.

In many cases, a diagnostician will start treatment when a diagnosis is probable or suspected strongly without waiting for formal criteria to be fulfilled (e.g. a treatment given on suspicion of meningitis or of inhalation pneumonia). In such a situation, the diagnostician might imagine the existence of a large number of identical patients who were randomized into different treatment limbs of a randomized clinical trial. The treatment chosen would be the one imagined to produce the best outcome, bearing in mind the benefits and adverse effects. If the patient responds to treatment, then this may also be regarded as confirmation of the diagnosis in some circumstances.

There may be no formal criteria that are suitable for use in day-to-day clinical care and it is up to the individual doctor to use what he or she considers reasonable. One such subjective approach is to provide a trial of therapy, and if the patient improves, to regard this as a confirmatory result. If the treatment is successful, then no other explanation is looked for. The confirmatory findings in this book are based on all of the above approaches. They reflect typical approaches used by doctors in the authors' experience. However, none of these approaches are ideal; future medical research may improve matters.

Looking at the situation in a different way, the group of patients with a probable or confirmed diagnosis encloses other subgroups of patients for which different actions are indicated. For example, some patients with a diagnosis have mild conditions so that treatment is not necessary, others may be so severe that it is too late to treat while others are treatable ('triage' in emergency situations is a special case of this principle). The group with a diagnosis may also contain subgroups with causes and complications that also require treatment. Therefore, diagnoses (probable or confirmed) may be thought as 'envelopes' that enclose subgroups of patients for which different actions are indicated. The way in which symptoms, signs, and test results can be chosen as diagnostic gold standard criteria is described in the Appendix (see 🕮p.751).

Evidence that 'suggests' a diagnosis

It is important to remember what 'evidence' means. Evidence is made up of facts, which are records of observations and actions that took place at a place and time. A fact becomes evidence when it is used to persuade someone else to accept an opinion—a diagnosis and what should be done in the context of this book. A diagnosis is the title to what we picture is happening to a patient. This will include causes and complications. This may be pictured with certainty or with a degree of probability, depending on the available evidence.

Evidence may be based on facts such as symptoms, signs, and test results recorded in a particular patient. This is 'particular' evidence by analogy with a 'particular' proposition in logic. In contrast to this, 'general' evidence will be based on facts related to groups of patients such as the result of a clinical trial, which is analogous to a 'general' proposition in logic. In order to practice evidence-based medicine, we have to relate the 'particular' evidence from a particular patient to 'general' evidence about groups of similar patients published in the medical literature.

The opinions supported by 'particular' evidence are diagnoses with different degrees of probability about what is wrong with patients and what to do. If the listener is going to accept such an opinion on the basis of the evidence, there has to be agreement as to what is acceptable as evidence. This book contains typical evidence that is used to 'suggest' and 'confirm' diagnoses as accepted at present by most doctors in their day-to-day work. These conventions will no doubt change as more 'general' scientific evidence is published.

Each differential diagnosis on every page is followed by the evidence that 'suggests' the presence of the diagnosis, the diagnosis being considered to be present when the 'confirmatory' findings is present. The confirmatory evidence for each diagnosis is provided under another subheading, followed by the initial management.

For example, acute abdominal tenderness localized to the right lower quadrant in combination with guarding 'suggests' that the diagnosis will probably be appendicitis (see □p.446). The diagnosis of appendicitis is 'confirmed' by the appearances at laparotomy and by histological examination. It is important to note that not all the findings have to be used in the reasoning process at one time; this is discussed in more detail later in this chapter.

Confirmatory findings based on general evidence

A confirmatory finding identifies a group of patients that envelops all those with indications for treatment explained by the diagnosis. If new treatment indications are discovered that are explained by the diagnostic theory, then 'the envelope' may need to be expanded. For example, it was discovered some years ago that many patients with features of diabetic retinopathy requiring treatment had blood sugars outside the criteria for diabetes mellitus. Because of this, meetings were convened by the World Health Organization and the American Diabetes Association, and the 'envelope' for diabetes was expanded by lowering the diagnostic cut-off point of fasting blood glucose.

It is also possible that new tests may be discovered in future that select patients more efficiently for treatment. If these new treatable patients lie outside the diagnostic group that was previously considered for treatment, then it might be appropriate to use the new test to identify patients who should be deemed to have the diagnosis. So if 'confirmatory' tests are to be chosen in an evidence-based way, then they should be shown to be superior to rival tests by including more patients who respond to the treatments directed at the diagnosis and/or excluding more patients with no prospect of responding.

Many diagnoses are based on test results that are 'abnormal', i.e. above or below two standard deviations of the test result in the general population. This means that the 2.5% of patients above and 2.5% of those below these two standard deviations could be regarded as 'abnormal'. The use of two standard deviations is arbitrary and not 'evidence-based'. For example, patients with diabetes mellitus are 'diagnosed' as having 'diabetic microalbuminuria' if their albumin excretion rates (AER) are above two standard deviations of the mean (i.e. >20mcg/min).

In a clinical trial on patients with type 2 diabetes mellitus where their blood pressures had been controlled, there was no difference between those on treatment and placebo in the proportion of patients developing nephropathy within two years if they had an AER between 20 and 40mcg/min.[2] This suggests that the cut-off point should be 40mcg/min. However, before changing the definition, it would be important to ensure that the patients inside the envelope with an AER between 20 and 40mcg/min might not benefit in other ways.

Ruling diagnoses in and out

A diagnosis is ruled in if at least one of its confirming (or sufficient) criteria is present. A diagnosis is ruled out if it can be shown that the patient lies outside the diagnostic envelope. One way of doing this is to show that not one of the possible confirming (or sufficient) features is present. Another way is to show that a single feature is absent which must occur in those with the diagnosis, e.g. that the patient is not female and therefore, cannot have an ectopic pregnancy. Such a constant diagnostic finding is called a 'necessary' criterion.

Findings that suggest diagnoses based on general evidence

The best findings for 'suggesting' probable diagnoses are those which, when used alone or in combination with others, predict the presence of 'confirmatory' test results with the highest frequency of success. The general evidence for the ability of findings to do this during population screening is usually offered in the form of indices such as sensitivity, specificity, and likelihood ratios. However, in order to assess the usefulness of tests during the differential diagnostic process, other indices have to be used. One index is the number of diagnoses required to explain most (e.g. 99%) of the differential diagnoses of a diagnostic lead—the fewer the better.

Another index is the ability of a test to differentiate between pairs of diagnoses in such a lead. If a test result occurs commonly in patients with confirmatory findings of one diagnosis and uncommonly in patients with another diagnosis, then that test will help to differentiate between them. The difference in these frequencies of occurrence can be measured by their ratio.

Statisticians describe the frequency of a finding that occurs in those known to have a diagnosis as the 'likelihood' of it occurring (the 'likelihood' is also known to epidemiologists as the 'sensitivity'). The difference between these 'likelihoods' for two different diagnoses can be represented by the ratio of the two likelihoods. As this ratio refers to a pair of differential diagnoses, we can call it a 'differential likelihood ratio'. This is different to the plain 'likelihood ratio' which is the frequency of a finding in patients with a confirmed diagnosis divided by the frequency of the same finding in ALL those confirmed NOT to have that diagnosis. This 'non-differential' likelihood ratio is more useful when screening populations by using one test to detect one diagnosis.

Explaining a diagnostic thought process

You may well have arrived at differential diagnoses by using intuitive, non-transparent, pattern recognition and not considered in an explicit way how it was done. Alternatively, you may have recorded your team's consensus opinion. However, you may be asked by a patient, student, nurse or doctor to explain your thinking. In fairness, the way that your own mind (let alone someone else's mind) has actually worked subconsciously may be impossible to explain.

The first step is to write a summary of the positive findings, diagnoses, evidence, and management as shown on p.13. The original evidence for established diagnoses (e.g. type 2 diabetes) may not be available. However, for new diagnoses, choose from the evidence the best lead with the shortest differential diagnosis. Use the other findings to show that the one (or some) diagnoses are more probable or confirmed, and others less probable or ruled out.

If these conclusions of the non-transparent and transparent thought processes are not the same, you may wish to revise your opinion and list of differential diagnoses. By doing this, you will be checking diagnoses by using a different mental process in the same way as you would check the answer to arithmetic addition by adding up the list of numbers in a different order.

In order to avoid overlooking diagnoses, jog your memory by using 'sieves' to use 'recognition' to and help 'recall' by listing the possible broad anatomical and physiological explanations (see 📖p.14).

An evidence-based diagnosis and plan

Positive findings summary
Central chest pain for 4h with jaw discomfort, sweating, and nausea (1/10/08). PMH of hypertension for 10y. History of mild jaundice during febrile illnesses for years. BP 146/88 on admission (1/10/08). ECG: T wave inversion S2, AvF, V4, and V5. Latest HbA1c=8.7% (5/8/08).

Assessment and plan

?Unstable angina
?Non-ST elevated myocardial infarction (NSTEMI)
Outline evidence: central chest pain for 4h with jaw discomfort, sweating and nausea (1/10/08). ECG: T wave inversion S2, AvF, V4 and V5.
Plan: for troponin I 12h after onset of pain. Aspirin 300mg stat, bisoprolol 5mg od, isosorbide mononitrate 10mg bd.

?Gilbert's disease
?Cholelithiasis
Outline evidence: jaundiced sclera, history of mild jaundice during febrile illnesses for years, none of liver disease (1/10/08).
Plan: check bilirubin, urobilinogen, AST, γGT.

Other active diagnoses
Essential hypertension
Outline evidence: history of raised BP for 10y. Current BP 146/88 on admission (1/10/08).
Plan: continue bendroflumethiazide 2.5mg od, perindopril 2mg od.

Type 2 diabetes mellitus
Outline evidence: latest HbA1c = 8.7% (5/8/08).
Plan: stop gliclazide 160mg bd. Start insulin sliding scale.

Medical and surgical sieves

Check that you have not forgotten something by using the following 'medical sieve'. Under each heading, think of the structures involved in flow (air, blood, food, etc.). Think of function in terms of feedback cycles (sugar, blood pressure (BP), etc.):

- Social system and environment
- Locomotor system
- Nervous system
- Cardiovascular system
- Respiratory system
- Alimentary system
- Renal and urinary tract
- Reproductive system
- Endocrine and autonomic system
- Haematological and immune system

Consider each of these systems by using the 'surgical sieve'. Is there a problem which is congenital, infective, traumatic, neoplastic, or degenerative?

The information in the pages of the OHCD is also set out in the same format as the Assessment and Plan (compare diagnoses of 'unstable angina' and 'NSTEMI' with those on p.216). The page on chest pain gives some dif-ferential diagnoses with typical suggestive and confirmatory evidence that could also be added to those opposite. You may refer to these as examples when writing your own assessments and plans.

Diagnoses, hypotheses, and theories

Although the findings used to confirm a diagnosis can be observed, all things pictured or imagined under the title of the diagnosis cannot be confirmed by observation, e.g. molecular changes in damaged tissue or what would have happened in a particular patient if a treatment had not been given. Not only does this apply to hypotheses for individual patients, it also applies to what is imagined about populations of patients in scientific hypotheses and theories. It is thus possible that something else will be imagined or pictured in future which is also compatible with findings previously explained by another theory.

This is why the philosopher of science, Karl Popper, argued that general hypotheses and theories cannot be proven or confirmed in their entirety. However, if a new observation is inconsistent with one aspect of the hypothesis, it will have been 'falsified'. It will thus have to be changed to some degree (perhaps completely or slightly) to take the new observation into account.

Raised ST segments on an ECG in someone with severe central chest pain were formerly part of the criterion for confirming MI, which suggested that a part of the myocardium was dead. However, one aspect of this theory has been 'falsified' because it has been discovered that some (or all) of the 'infarcted' myocardium is salvageable. With our new understanding, we use the same findings to 'confirm' an 'ST Elevated Myocardial 'Infarction'. We have modified the theory and now think that the process of infarction is not complete and can be stopped with treatment with reversal of many changes.

However, it is important to assess the reliability of the 'falsifying' fact. This is done by estimating the probability of the 'falsifying' observation being replicated by other scientists (or another doctor if the hypothesis is a diagnosis about an individual patient based on particular evidence). If the probability of replication of the evidence is high about a 'general' observation, then the observation may be accepted by the scientific community (but many may go to the trouble of repeating the study to make sure). If the P value is low or the 95% confidence intervals are narrow, then the probability of non-replication due to chance observations alone will be low.

Imagining an ideal clinical trial

The findings used to define a 'diagnostic envelope' should enclose the best treatment indication criteria. These criteria should be chosen ideally from a number of candidate criteria. The chosen treatment criterion should be the one that produces the clearest outcome difference between the treatment and control in a comparative trial. For example, method A for measuring microalbumin in urine chose patients for a trial; 24% developed nephropathy on placebo and 12% developed nephropathy on treatment. However, with method B, 12% developed nephropathy on placebo and 12% developed it on treatment. This would suggest that method B was not identifying patients who benefited and would be inferior to method A.

In the absence of detailed trial data, a doctor may have to guess whether a patient's findings would identify a group of patients who would benefit from the treatment more than a placebo, bearing in mind side effects, costs, etc. If on balance, this would be the case, the doctor could apply a diagnostic term that would summarize his theoretical explanation as to why giving that treatment to a patient with that combination of findings would be better than not doing so.

Decision analysis

Decision analysis is a discipline that models mathematically what would happen if a detailed clinical trial were performed to compare the treatment options being considered for a particular patient. A 'decision tree' is constructed first to show all the possible diagnoses. The tree is extended to show the possible interventional limbs into which the patient could be randomized, followed by all the possible outcomes of each treatment. The branches would end with the effect that each outcome would have on the overall well-being of the patient.

An estimate is then made of the proportions of patients with each diagnosis, the proportions opting for each treatment and the proportions of those experiencing various degrees of well-being. These proportions are then multiplied together to estimate the average degree of well-being experienced by patients sharing each treatment outcome. Each of these average degrees of benefit are regarded as the 'expected' degree of well-being that would be experienced by an individual patient with each outcome. This is regarded as a representation of what an experienced doctor would do when he or she estimates the effect on the patient of the different interventions available.[3, 4]

Medical science aims to provide diagnostic criteria, treatment indication criteria, and treatments that when used together will predict with a high degree of certainty which treatment will work best for each patient (or would not help at all). Such well designed diagnostic systems would make it easier to choose the best option and to justify it using evidence in the form of data. This will not be possible without a clear understanding of the diagnostic process and criteria for confirming diagnoses that also indicate the best treatment for that patient.

Diagnostic classifications, pathways and tables

A diagnostic pathway or algorithm is a way representing diagnostic reasoning processes or a diagnostic classification (see opposite 📖p.19). The same reasoning processes can be displayed using a table of the kind shown below. This is also how information in this book is displayed. It is flexible and also allows findings to be shown which do not form part of the diagnostic criteria. The reader can scan down such a table to find the diagnoses that are compatible with the findings so far. The entry can then be copied into a table in the patient's records as a draft entry for that diagnostic possibility.

Diagnostic table for the differential diagnoses of jaundice

Carotinaemia (not 'real' jaundice)
Suggested by: onset over months. Skin yellow with white sclerae, normal stools, and normal urine. Diet rich in yellow vegetables/fruits).
Confirmed by: no bilirubin, no **urobilinogen** in the urine, and normal **serum bilirubin.** Normal **liver function tests (LFT)**. Response to diet change.

'Pre-hepatic' jaundice due to haemolysis
Suggested by: jaundice and anaemia (the combination seen as 'lemon' or pale yellow). Normal dark stools and normal-looking urine.
Confirmed by: ↑(unconjugated and thus insoluble) **serum bilirubin**, but normal (conjugated and soluble) bilirubin and thus no ↑bilirubin in urine. **↑urobilinogen in urine** and **↓serum haptoglobin**. Normal LFT. **↑reticulocyte count**.

'Hepatic' jaundice due to congenital enzyme defect
Suggested by: jaundice. Normal-looking stools and normal-looking urine. Jaundice worse during febrile illnesses.
Confirmed by: ↑serum bilirubin (unconjugated), but no (conjugated) bilirubin in urine. No **urobilinogen in urine** and **normal haptoglobin**. Normal **LFT**.

'Hepatocellular' jaundice ('hepatic' with some 'obstructive' jaundice)
Suggested by: onset of jaundice over days or weeks, pale or stools but <u>dark</u> urine.
Confirmed by: ↑serum (conjugated) **bilirubin** and thus ↑**urine bilirubin**. Normal **urine urobilinogen**. **LFT** all abnormal, especially ↑↑**ALT**.

'Obstructive' jaundice
Suggested by: onset of jaundice over days or weeks with <u>pale</u> stools and <u>dark</u> urine. Bilirubin (i.e. conjugated and thus soluble) in urine.
Confirmed by: ↑**serum conjugated bilirubin** and **urine bilirubin**, but no ↑**urobilinogen** in urine. Markedly (↑↑) **alkaline phosphatase**, but less abnormal (↑) **LFT** and ↑γ**GT**.

A diagnostic pathway for jaundice

Skin yellow with white sclera or normal bilirubin→→→→→→→→

OR

Sclera yellow or ↑ bilirubin

↓

No ↑serum bilirubin AND no bilirubin nor urobilinogen in the urine. Response to diet change.

→

Carotinaemia (not 'real' jaundice)

Status of unconjugated bilirubin? → → →

↑unconjugated serum bilirubin

↓   ↓   ↓

↓

↓

Unconjugated bilirubin NOT ↑?

↓

↑unconjugated serum bilirubin OR ↑urobilinogen in urine OR ↓serum haptoglobin OR ↑reticulocyte count

→

'Pre-hepatic' jaundice due to haemolysis

↓

↓

↓

↓

↓

↓

↓

↓

↓

↓

↑unconjugated serum bilirubin AND Normal urobilinogen in urine AND Normal serum haptoglobin AND Normal liver function tests AND Normal reticulocyte count

→

'Hepatic' jaundice due to congenital enzyme defect, e.g. Gilbert's syndrome

↑CONJUGATED serum bilirubin OR urine bilirubin

→ → → ↓

↓

↑**CONJUGATED serum bilirubin** OR ↑urine bilirubin AND ↑↑**ALT** AND/OR **Non-dilated bile ducts on ultrasound scan**

→

'Hepatocellular' jaundice ('hepatic' with element of 'obstructive' jaundice)

↑**CONJUGATED serum bilirubin** OR ↑urine bilirubin AND ↑↑**alkaline phosphatase** AND/OR **Dilated bile ducts on ultrasound scan**

→

'Obstructive' jaundice

Dynamic diagnoses

It is important to understand that clinical diagnosis is not a static classification system based on diagnostic criteria or their probable presence. It is a dynamic process. Diagnostic algorithms 'classify' patients by following a logical pathway based mainly on diagnostic criteria. Other systems predict the probable presence of diagnostic criteria. All these methods can be regarded as 'diagnosing' a snapshot of what is happening at a particular time.

The diagnostician has to imagine the presence of a dynamic process that changes with time. There may be several processes taking place at the same time, some progressing over years (e.g. atheromatous changes), some over minutes to hours (e.g. a thrombosis in a coronary artery), some over minutes or seconds (e.g. ventricular tachycardia), and others instantaneously (e.g. a cardiac arrest).

A diagnostic process leading to treatment may have to happen repeatedly and for a number of diagnoses at the same time. It might be more appropriate to think of the process as one of 'feedback' control. In this way, the doctor would be acting as an external control mechanism to assist those of the patient who are failing. After the initial history and examination, the feedback information may come from electronic monitoring, nursing observations, ward rounds, hospital clinic, or primary care follow-up.

There are three types of mechanisms of interest to the diagnostician.

• Those that control the 'internal milieu' by keeping temperature, tissue perfusion, blood gases, and biochemistry constant.
• Those that control the body's structure by effecting repair in response to any damage.
• Those that control the 'external milieu' of day-to-day living.

These are all interdependent. If one mechanism fails, then it may unmask other weaknesses by causing other failures. It may not be enough to treat the main failure. It is often necessary also to treat the causes and consequences as they may be unable to recover on their own. For example, a coronary thrombosis may be treated with thrombolysis, but any resulting rhythm abnormalities may need to be treated and also the causative risk factors (e.g. smoking) that could result in recurrence. So when we explain our diagnostic thought processes, it helps to think of each diagnosis as a subheading with its own evidence and decision.

The whole patient

A 'diagnosis' does not imply that only one solution needs to be discovered. The complete diagnosis (or diagnostic formulation) may have to include various causes, consequences, interactions, and other independent processes. As well as internal medical processes, it has to include external factors such as circumstances at home and the effects on selfcare, employment, and leisure.

There may be many diagnoses which have been confirmed previously and for which the patient is on established treatment. Therefore, the diagnostician must imagine what is happening to the 'whole patient'. This requires a broad medical education that allows a range of phenomena to be pictured, from molecular events to events in the home and outside world.

Explaining diagnoses to patients

The patient may already be imagining with some trepidation what might be happening. It is important to find out what the patient is imagining and to use this as a starting point for your own explanation. The patient's own views are usually sought and documented at the end of the history of the presenting complaint.

Although patients may understand explanations at the time they are given them, even the most intelligent may forget unfamiliar technical terms and their meaning within a short time. Therefore, it is important to provide a written reminder of such terms and how they are related. This can be done by giving the patient a printed summary similar to that on page 12. This can also allow the patient to ask questions at his or her own pace.

Patients and relatives usually ask questions spontaneously or request an appointment for time to be set aside to do this. Some may be too shy and need encouragement to do so, in which case this important aspect of care will be omitted. Informed consent is also based on similar questions and discussion. The process is more effective if the patient is able to ask the questions (i.e. if the process is 'patient-centred'). Such a process may be facilitated if they refer to a summary such as that shown on p.13.

Ideally, patients should know the presenting complaint for their latest problems, the primary diagnosis or differential diagnoses, and what actions are being taken in terms of tests and treatments. They should also be aware of their past medical history: the various diagnoses, how they presented and were confirmed, their treatments, follow-up arrangements, and markers of progress. Again, the relevant technical terms and how they are linked can be summarized for them as shown on p.13.

Informed consent

In order for a patient to consent to treatment, he or she must understand what has been said and be able to retain that explanation. A basic understanding means the patient must know what actions have been agreed and the possible diagnoses in each case. In order to understand each diagnosis, it is essential to know which symptoms it explains and how these symptoms or some other markers are progressing. Few patients are able to retain all of this, especially if there are many technical terms that are unfamiliar to them. Therefore, it would be a sensible policy to provide the patient with a typed explanation setting out these basic relationships as shown on p.13. This would then become the next 'past medical history' when the patient is asked to provide it by another doctor or nurse. It would thus allow patients to ask a doctor or nurse to remind them of the meanings of the various terms.

Minimizing diagnostic errors

The diagnostic and decision-making process usually takes place in busy clinics, wards, operating theatres, and emergency rooms. Therefore, most diagnoses have to take place by some rapid conscious or subconscious pattern recognition, and there is usually little time for reflection. Mistakes are kept to a minimum by good training, especially listening carefully and writing out what has been observed, thought, and done.

Another important principle to bear in mind is that even the most expert and well-founded diagnoses and decisions can only be successful in a proportion of cases. Therefore, there must be a strategy to monitor their outcome and to change diagnoses and decisions, if possible.

Diagnostic errors can be classified in terms of cognitive psychology[5] into:

- Faulty triggering
- Faulty context information
- Faulty verification
- No fault errors
- Faulty information gathering and processing

Faulty triggering

This is a failure to consider appropriate diagnostic possibilities, often attributed to a weakness of medical education, which focuses on disease processes instead of the diagnostic processes. This type of error can be kept to a minimum by using the suggestions on pp.5–13, and by referring to the differential diagnoses on the other pages. Finally, this error can be reduced by not only writing down the differential diagnoses, but also by writing down the findings from which were chosen the leads that 'triggered' them as shown on p.13. This can be given to the patient to be shown to other doctors who might also spot any omissions.

Faulty context information

This is focusing on one diagnosis and failing to consider others that may also be present. It involves jumping to conclusions. This can be avoided by using the sieves on p.14, referring to the appropriate page in this book and writing out an overall plan as shown on p.13 so that other doctors might spot any errors. Again, this can be given to the patient (to show to other doctors who might spot any errors).

Faulty verification

This is failure to ensure that the patient's presenting symptom and other markers of poor health have been controlled or stabilized as well as possible. This is discussed on p.8. It also helps to set out each diagnosis with its evidence as shown on p.13, which includes the markers being followed and their latest results. Again, this summary can be given to the patient to be shown to other doctors who might spot such omissions.

No fault errors

Even the most expert and well-founded diagnoses and decisions can only be successful in a proportion of cases. This is why diagnoses and decisions are qualified with probabilities. Therefore, there must be a strategy to monitor the outcome of all diagnoses and decisions and to change them, if possible. If a summary of the kind shown on p.13 is given to the patient to be shown to other doctors, they will be able to understand the basis of previous decisions and take appropriate action.

Faulty information gathering and processing

This is poor use of leads and differentiators in appropriate settings. This book focuses on this process. It is important to know the differential diagnoses of leads and the frequency with which they occur in different clinical settings. It is also important to know the frequency with which findings occur in pairs of diagnoses. At present, this is gained from personal experience. Little research is done into leads and differential likelihood ratios because the main focus of research is currently on sensitivity, specificity, and overall likelihood ratios.

References

1. Eddy DM, Clanton CH (1982). The art of diagnosis: solving the clinico-pathological conference. N Engl J Med 306, 1263–8.

2. Llewelyn DEH, Garcia-Puig J (2004) How different urinary albumin excretion rates can predict progression to nephropathy and the effect of treatment in hypertensive diabetics. J Renin Angiotensin Aldosterone Syst 5, 141–5.

3. Llewelyn H., Hopkins A. eds. (1993). Analysing how we reach clinical decisions. Royal College of Physicians of London, London.

4. Dowie J, Elstein A. eds. Professional judgement: a reader in clinical decision making. Cambridge University Press, Cambridge.

5. Kassirer JP. Kopleman RI (1999). Cognitive errors in diagnosis: instantiation, classification and consequences. *Acad Med* 1999; 74: S138–43.

Interpreting the history and examination

Thoughtful history taking

The aim of the diagnostic process is to build up a picture of what is happening to the patient. 'Diagnosis' is derived from the Greek 'to know through' (i.e. the history, examination, etc. to what is beyond).

The diagnosis (or diagnostic formulation) may have to include various causes, consequences, interactions, and other independent processes. As well as internal medical processes, it has to include external factors such as circumstances at home and the effects on self-care, employment, and leisure.

It is important to establish very clearly why the patient has sought help. This is known as the presenting complaint. Ask about its severity and duration. Be prepared to act immediately to give symptomatic relief (e.g. for pain) if the patient is distressed.

In some cases, the presenting complaint may not explain the decision to seek help. The patient may be too ill, shy, guilty, or embarrassed to describe what is happening accurately. In other cases, it may be someone else who is unduly worried. Be alert to the real reason.

Having established the presenting complaint(s), establish the factual details of 'place and time'. It is the ability to give a place and time that establishes the complaints as 'facts'.

Listen without prompting first, but if necessary, ask where they were and what they were doing when the problem was first noticed. This will help the patient's recall and help your diagnostic thought process.

Establish the speed of initial onset and subsequent change in severity with time. Onset within seconds suggests a fit or heart rhythm abnormality, over minutes a bleed or clotting process, hours to days an acute infection, days to weeks a chronic infection, weeks to months a tumour, and months to years a degenerative process.

If there are other complaints, note the same details. Ask about other associated, aggravating, and relieving factors, especially as a result of the patient's own actions and other professional care.

Ask what the patient thinks is going on and is afraid of. This will be the starting point for your own explanation and suggestions to the patient later about what is to be done.

The history also allows patients and supporters to identify the issues that they want addressed in terms of discomfort, loss of function, and difficulties with day-to-day existence. Final diagnoses are based on the initial history because they have to explain it completely. If the diagnoses arrived at cannot explain the entire history, then the diagnosis or diagnoses will be incomplete and others will have to be considered.

Write out your history in a systematic way, e.g. as shown in the next section and go over it with the patient, if possible, to check that it is right.

This is a lot to remember, especially if you are trying to put it into practice in a busy, noisy environment. However, writing out your findings according to a plan each time will help you to remember.

The plan on the next page is an example—make up your own.

A plan for writing out the history

History taker's name: *Date of assessment:*

Patient's name: *DOB:* *Age* *Occupation*
Patient's address:

Admitted as an emergency/from the waiting list on (date) at (time)

Presenting complaints (PC)
1st symptom—duration
2nd symptom—duration
etc.

History of each presenting complaint (HPC)
1. *Nature of complaint (e.g. pain in chest), circumstances, and speed of onset, progression (change with time—picture a graph), aggravating and relieving factors, associated symptoms (describe under 2, etc.)*
2. *Next associated symptom, etc. described as in (1).*

Add response to direct questions from chasing up some diagnostic possibilities that come to mind as the history is taken. Add the patient's opinion or fear about what may be happening.

Past medical history (PMH)
1st diagnosis and when—evidence—treatment—name of doctor
2nd

Drug history (DH)
Name, dose, and frequency—diagnostic indication—evidence—prescriber
Next drug etc.
Alcohol and tobacco consumption, other 'recreational' drugs
Drug sensitivities and allergies

Developmental history
(in paediatrics and psychiatry): pregnancy, infancy, childhood, puberty, adulthood

Family history (FH)
Age Illnesses
(Arrange around 'family tree', if preferred)
Mention especially:

Parents	Tuberculosis?
Siblings	Asthma? Eczema?
Children	Diabetes? Epilepsy?
Spouse	Hypertension?

Social history (SH)
Home and domestic activity support—job and financial security—travel and leisure. (Consider the effect of all these on the illness and the effect of the illness on these.)

Interpreting the case history

History by A N Other   3.00 p.m 18 October 2008
Miss AM (DOB: 28/2/79) Aged 29 Secretary
23, Smith Square, Old Town
Emergency admission 18 October 2008 at 2.00 p.m

PC: 1. Severe sore throat, sweats, and malaise for 2 days

2. Sudden loss of consciousness in A&E at 2.00 p.m

*HPC: The patient was well until last Friday afternoon 17 October when she developed a **sore throat** at work. It was relieved that day by warm drinks and paracetamol, but when she woke this Saturday morning, it was very severe. She remembered that she had been told to report sore throats because she was taking carbimazole and to get a white cell count. She was worried that she might have developed a low white cell count because of this drug. She came to A&E because it was a Saturday. When she got up from her seat in the waiting room after being called, she felt dizzy, blacked out, and fell to the floor, striking her head. She recovered consciousness within a minute.*

There are two striking symptoms: (1) a severe sore throat that is getting worse and (2) the sudden loss of consciousness. Both are examples of findings with short lists of causes: good diagnostic 'leads' or 'pivots'.

Most readers will have experienced a sore throat and will be aware that it is usually due to a viral pharyngitis, bacterial tonsillitis (e.g. due to a haemo-lytic *streptococcus*), or glandular fever. It could also be due to bone marrow dysfunction (e.g. due to drug effect) or something else in a small proportion of cases (see 📖p.30). The onset over days is compatible with all these possibilities. A white cell count might give results (in bold, see problem-solving note on p.29) that would differentiate between these possible causes.

The sudden loss of consciousness with rapid recovery is known as 'syncope'. It is also a good lead with a well-defined differential diagnosis. It can be due to a vasovagal attack, cough, micturition or carotid sinus syncope, postural hypotension, transient cerebral ischaemia, a Stokes-Adams attack, aortic stenosis, hypertrophic cardiomyopathy (HOCM), hypoglycaemia, or epilepsy (see 📖p.29). The fact that it happened after the patient got up from a chair suggests postural hypotension (because this always occurs in this condition, but rarely, if ever, in the others). Postural hypotension may be due to fever and dehydration so although the two leads have common causes, postural hypotension could be a consequence of any infection. Therefore, the syncope does not differentiate between any of the causes of a sore throat. The patient has expressed a fear that the sore throat could be drug-induced because she has been warned about this.

These thoughts can be summarised in the 'problem-structuring note' on the opposite page. Such thoughts only usually take place mentally without writing them down, which is why the diagnostic thought process can be difficult to learn from others.

These thoughts can be summarized in the problem-structuring note opposite. You can write this on a sheet of paper, perhaps in pencil for easy editing, on a computer, or on a black or white board when discussing a case with colleagues. Such thoughts are usually considered mentally without writing them down, which is why the diagnostic thought process can be difficult to learn from senior colleagues.

Problem-structuring note (version 1)

Outline findings

After outlining your thoughts in the problem-structuring note as shown below, turn to the appropriate page in this book by looking up 'sore throat'. Check that you have not forgotten to include something. The entry in this book for 'sore throat' is shown on p.30 and on p.386. You may wish to read this before moving on to the next step.

Female. Aged 29. Severe sore throat for 2 days, getting worse. Taking carbimazole for 6 months. Sudden loss of consciousness after getting up from chair, recovery within a minute.

Diagnoses	Outline evidence	Management
Viral pharyngitis?	Severe sore throat for 2 days, getting worse (18/10/08)	Paracetamol 500mg 6 hourly PRN. Examine throat. Request **WCC**: ↓neutrophils, ↑lymphocytes?
Acute bacterial (or follicular) tonsillitis (mainly streptococcal)?	Severe sore throat for 2 days, getting worse (18/10/08)	Paracetamol 500mg 6 hourly PRN. Examine throat. Request **WCC**: ↑neutrophils?
Glandular fever (infectious mononucleosis due to Epstein–Barr virus)?	Severe sore throat for 2 days, getting worse (18/10/08)	Paracetamol 500mg 6 hourly PRN. Examine throat. Request **WCC**: lymphocytes atypical? Paul–Bunnell or Monospot® +ve?
Drug-induced agranulocytosis? (this is what the patient fears)	Severe sore throat for 2 days, getting worse (18/10/08). Taking carbimazole	Paracetamol 500mg 6 hourly PRN. Examine throat. Request **WCC**: ↓granulocytes (neutrophils, eosinphils, basophils)?
Postural hypotension syncope? Due to dehydration?	Sudden loss of consciousness after getting up from chair, recovery within a minute (18/10/08). Evidence of acute infection	Look for fall in BP when standing. Request U&E. Consider fluids IV to rehydrate
Thyrotoxicosis now controlled?	Taking carbimazole	Examine for tremor, etc. Carbimazole 5mg od. FT4 and TSH normal?

Sore throat

Initial investigations (other tests in bold below): FBC, U&E, throat swab, Paul–Bunnell test.

Main differential diagnoses and typical outline evidence, etc.	
Viral pharyngitis	*Suggested by:* sore throat, pain on swallowing, fever, cervical lymphadenopathy, and injected fauces. WCC: ↑lymphocytes, leucocytes normal.
	Confirmed by: negative **throat swab** for bacterial culture, self-limiting: resolution within days.
	Initial management: analgesics, e.g. paracetamol.
Acute follicular tonsillitis (streptococcal)	*Suggested by:* severe sore throat, pain on swallowing, fever, enlarged tonsils with white patches (like strawberries and creamy lines). Cervical lymphadenopathy, especially in angle of jaw. Fever, WCC: ↑leucocytes.
	Confirmed by: **throat swab** for culture and sensitivities of organisms.
	Initial management: analgesics, antibiotics, e.g. penicillin; if no allergy, good fluid intake.
Infectious mono-nucleosis (glandular fever) due to Epstein–Barr virus	*Suggested by:* very severe throat pain with enlarged tonsils covered with grey mucoid membrane. Petechiae on palate. Profound malaise. Generalized lymphadenopathy, splenomegaly. **WCC:** ↑atypical lymphocytes.
	Confirmed by: **Paul–Bunnell or Monospot ® test** +ve. **Viral titres:** ↑Epstein–Barr.
	Initial management: analgesia, no antibiotics (amoxicillin may cause skin rash).
Candidiasis of buccal or oesophageal mucosa	*Suggested by:* painful dysphagia, white plaque, history of immunosuppression/diabetes/recent antibiotics.
	Confirmed by: **oesophagoscopy** showing erythema and plaques, **brush cytology:** spores and hyphae.
	Initial management: local antifungal agents, e.g. Daktarin® oral gel or nystatin oral suspension. Parenteral administration if systemic involvement.
Agranulocytosis	*Suggested by:* sore throat, background history of taking a drug, or contact with noxious substance.
	Confirmed by: ↓ or absent neutrophil count.
	Initial management: stop potential causative drugs, antibiotic cover until resolved.

The systems enquiry

The systems enquiry may take place at various points in the history. The questions below are detailed. They can also be asked as broad prompts (e.g. do you have any chest, abdominal, bladder symptoms, etc?). Some may prefer to perform the systems enquiry immediately after the history of presenting complaint because they would not have enough knowledge to ask the questions to differentiate between the initial differential diagnoses (e.g. asking about generalized lymph node enlargement that might differentiate between glandular fever and the other causes of a sore throat). If the patient said 'yes' to a question during the systems enquiry, it could be added to the problem-structuring note and looked up later in this book.

If a direct question turns up a positive response, it has to be treated with caution. It may be a 'false positive' response to a leading question. A positive response has to be treated as an extra presenting complaint, added to the original list and explored carefully with the history of presenting complaint. They can also be looked up in the pages of this book.

If there is a negative response to a direct question, this is more reliable (unless the patient is very forgetful or is purposely withholding information). The absence of all symptoms under a heading indicates that it is less probable that there is an abnormality in that system.

Systems enquiry

Locomotor symptoms
No pain and stiffness in the neck, shoulder, elbow, wrist, hand, or back
No pain and stiffness in the hip, knee, or foot
No pain or stiffness in any joints and muscles
Negative responses make locomotor abnormalities less probable. If any are positive, then a 'GALS' examination screen is performed under the headings of Gait, Arms, Legs, Spine. Care can be taken with painfully inflamed or damaged joints.

Skin, lymph nodes and endocrine
No heat or cold intolerance (e.g. wanting to open or close windows when others are comfortable)
Sweats and shivering for 2d
No drenching night sweats
No episodes of rigors
No rashes and itching
No skin lumps or lumps elsewhere
No heat or cold intolerance makes an abnormality of thyroid metabolism less probable (suggesting that the carbimazole is probably controlling the thyrotoxicosis). Positive findings (e.g. sweats and shivering for 2 days) can be looked up in this book—they will be found to be poor leads and differentiators (because they occur often in each condition), and not very helpful in differentiating between the causes of a sore throat.

No further information is gained with the following responses. However, they provide an opportunity to reflect on the function of each system.

Cardiovascular symptoms

No tiredness and breathlessness on exertion (non-specific)
Syncope after rising from chair in A&E—see HPC
No leg pain on walking

Negative responses make cardiac output and peripheral vascular disease less probable.

No ankle swelling

A negative response makes a right-sided venous return abnormality less probable.

No exertional dyspnoea
No orthopnoea
No paroxysmal nocturnal dyspnoea

Negative responses make a left-sided venous return abnormality less probable.

No palpitations
No central chest pain on exertion or at rest

Negative responses make a cardiac abnormality less likely.

Respiratory symptoms

No chronic breathlessness
No acute breathlessness

Negative responses make abnormality of overall respiratory and blood gas abnormality less probable.

No hoarseness
No cough, sputum, haemoptysis
No wheeze

Negative responses make airway disease less probable.

No pleuritic chest pain

A negative response makes pleural reactions and chest wall disease less probable.

Alimentary symptoms

No loss of appetite (non-specific)
No weight loss (non-specific)
No jaundice, dark urine, pale stools
Negative responses make metabolic gut and liver disease less probable.
No nausea or vomiting (non-specific)
No haematemesis or melaena
No dysphagia but **sore throat—see HPC**
No indigestion
No abdominal pain
No diarrhoea or constipation
No recent change in bowel habit
No rectal bleeding ± mucus

Negative responses make gastrointestinal disease less probable.

Genitourinary symptoms

Menstrual history—date of menarche, duration of cycle, and flow normal
Volume of flow and associated pain normal
Any pregnancy outcomes normal
No dyspareunia and vaginal bleeding
No vaginal discharge

Negative responses make gynaecological disease less probable.

No haematuria or other odd colour
No urgency or incontinence
No dysuria
No polyuria or nocturia
No loin pain or lower abdominal pain

Negative responses make urological disease less probable.

No impotence or loss of libido
No urethral discharge

Negative responses make male urological disease less probable.

Nervous system symptoms

No vision loss, blurring, or double vision
No hearing loss or tinnitus
No loss of smell and taste
No numbness, pins and needles, or other disturbance of sensation
No disturbance of speech
No weakness of limbs
No imbalance
No headache
No sudden headache and loss of consciousness
Dizziness and blackouts in A&E—see HPC
No vertigo
No 'fit'
No transient neurological deficit

Negative responses make neurological disease less probable.

Psychiatric symptoms

No fatigue, not tired all the time
No mood change
No odd voices or odd visual effects
No anxiety and sleep disturbance
No loss of self-confidence
No new strong beliefs
No phobias, no compulsions, or avoidance of actions
No use of recreational drugs

Patients may hide or forget many symptoms. There is a school of thought that regards symptom reviews as being of little value, and that only symptoms that are volunteered are worthwhile investigating. Many doctors do not conduct systemic reviews and only ask these questions if other symptoms have been volunteered already in that system.

The past medical history

The past medical history (PMH) in this case has three components: the diagnosis, the evidence, and the management. The management may be omitted if it is mentioned elsewhere, e.g. if carbimazole is in the drug history together with its indication of thyrotoxicosis.

PMH

> **Thyrotoxicosis discovered 6 months ago**
>
> Outline evidence: anxiety, weight loss, abnormal thyroid function tests in Osler Hospital by Dr Miller.
>
> Management: taking carbimazole, 5mg daily.

'Anxiety, weight loss, abnormal thyroid function tests' outlines the evidence for the thyrotoxicosis. Knowing the doctor responsible and the institution would allow the details to be checked, if necessary. In many cases, patients are not able to provide these details and they would have to be extracted from the records, in which case it is helpful to name the hospital or primary care centre or doctor responsible.

A comprehensive past medical history in this format could be written immediately after any consultation, in hospital or primary care with results and dates given to the patient. This would be more reliable than the next doctor having to do so, but this is not customary. This information can be added to the problem-structuring note version 2. This can be set out in different formats; in this case, it is set out in subheading style, which is in effect a draft of the 'next' past medical history. This problem-structuring approach can also be used to draft discharge summaries on a hospital computer network, which can be updated during the patient's stay and printed out when the patient leaves hospital.[1]

The family history

FH:

Father		Aged 56—hypertension
Mother		Aged 55—diabetes (onset at 50)
Siblings	male	Aged 34—alive and well
		Aged 26—alive and well
	female	Aged 30—alive and well
Children		None

The family history (FH) rarely contains features that form powerful leads. In general, there will be risk factors in the FH. For example, the fact that the patient's mother had type 2 diabetes means that there is an increased risk of the patient developing type 2 diabetes mellitus. This may have no immediate bearing on the current problems (but she should be checked for diabetes if only to exclude its presence so far). The patient could also be advised to adopt a healthy diet and lifestyle.

The new additions to the problem-structuring note are in **bold**.

Problem-structuring note (version 2)

Outline findings: female. Aged 29. Severe sore throat for 2 days, getting worse. Taking carbimazole for 6 months. Sudden loss of consciousness after getting up from chair, recovery within a minute. PMH of thyrotoxicosis (anxiety, weight loss, abnormal thyroid function tests in Osler Hospital) treated with carbimazole. **FH of type 2 diabetes mellitus**.

Viral pharyngitis?

Outline evidence: severe sore throat for 2 days, getting worse (18/10/08).

Management: paracetamol 500mg 6 hourly PRN. Examine throat. Request WCC: ↓neutrophils, ↑lymphocytes?

Acute bacterial (or follicular) tonsillitis? (mainly streptococcal)

Outline evidence: severe sore throat for 2 days, getting worse (18/10/08).

Management: paracetamol 500mg 6 hourly PRN. Examine throat. Request WCC: ↑neutrophils?

Glandular fever (infectious mononucleosis due to Epstein–Barr virus)?

Outline evidence: severe sore throat for 2 days, getting worse (18/10/08). No skin lumps or lumps elsewhere.

Management: paracetamol 500mg 6 hourly PRN. Examine throat. Request WCC: lymphocytes atypical? Paul–Bunnell or Monospot® +ve?

Drug-induced agranulocytosis? (this is what the patient fears)

Outline evidence: severe sore throat for 2 days, getting worse (18/10/08). Taking carbimazole. Bruising on forehead.

Management: paracetamol 500mg 6 hourly PRN. Examine throat. Request WCC: ↓granulocytes (neutrophils, eosinophils, basophils)?

Postural hypotension syncope? Due to dehydration from infection?

Outline evidence: sudden loss of consciousness after getting up from chair, recovery within a minute (18/10/08). Evidence of acute infection.

Management: look for fall in BP when standing. Request U&E. Consider fluids IV to rehydrate.

Thyrotoxicosis now controlled?

Outline evidence: **anxiety, weight loss, abnormal thyroid function tests in April 2008**. No heat or cold intolerance currently.

Management: examine for tremor, etc. Carbimazole 5mg od. FT4 and TSH normal?

Increased risk of type 2 diabetes mellitus

Outline evidence: FH of type 2 diabetes mellitus
Management: test urine for sugar. **Fasting glucose.**

The above version of the problem-structuring note is in the same format as the 'textbook' page on 'Sore throat' (see 📖 pp.30 and 110). This makes comparison easier and allows the 'textbook' entries to be used as templates that can be copied into the problem-structuring note.

The drug history

The drug history (DH) is often placed near the end of the history. If the patient is on medication, then it indicates that this is for an active medical condition as opposed to a PMH. Therefore, there is something to be said for documenting the drug history immediately after the PMH so and current conditions can be thought about together.

> **Drug history:**
> *Paracetamol 1g 6 hourly (for ?viral pharyngitis, etc.)*
>
> *Carbimazole 5mg daily for thyrotoxicosis (see PMH for evidence)*
> *Alcohol 10 units per week*
> *Non-smoker*
> *No other recreational drugs*

There is nothing to add to the problem-structuring note from the drug history.

The social history

The social history (SH) is always relevant. The activities of daily living can be considered under the heading of domestic, work, and leisure. Imagine what any person has to do from waking up in the morning to going to sleep at night, and consider whether the patient needs support with any of these activities. Fit young adults who are expected to recover completely may miss school, college, or work and the timing of their return will have to be considered. Patients, who are more dependent on others such as children and the elderly, may need special provisions. Patients with permanent disabilities may need help with most, if not all, activities of daily living.

> **SH:**
> *Alone in a flat at present (flatmate on holiday for another week)*
> *Parents live 200 miles away*
> *Works as secretary for insurance firm*

The patient has little domestic support and it would be sensible to admit her to be rehydrated until she is in no danger of fainting on discharge. This has been added to the problem-structuring note.

When the history is complete

The findings that will differentiate between the causes of a sore throat (see 📖 p.30) are the appearance of the throat and the white cell count. Generalized lymphadenopathy, splenomegaly, and petechiae on the palate would also occur commonly in glandular fever and uncommonly in the other differential diagnoses.

Page 230 shows that a fall in BP on standing would support postural hypotension because it occurs commonly in patients with this diagnosis and rarely in the other causes of syncope. A raised creatinine and urea would support dehydration because this happens often in dehydration, but infrequently in the other causes of postural hypotension.

The diagnostic thoughts so far are represented in the problem-structuring note on p.39.

Problem-structuring note (version 3)

Outline findings: female. Aged 29. Severe sore throat for 2 days, getting worse. Taking carbimazole for 6 months. Sudden loss of consciousness after getting up from chair, recovery within a minute. PMH of thyrotoxicosis (anxiety, weight loss, abnormal thyroid function tests). FH of type 2 diabetes mellitus.

Viral pharyngitis?	Severe sore throat for 2 days, getting worse (18/10/08)	Paracetamol 500mg 6 hourly PRN. Examine throat. Request WCC: ↓neutrophils, ↑lymphocytes?
Acute bacterial (or follicular) tonsillitis? (mainly streptococcal)	Severe sore throat for 2 days, getting worse (18/10/08)	Paracetamol 500mg 6 hourly PRN. Examine throat. Request WCC: ↑neutrophils?
Glandular fever (infectious mononucleosis due to Epstein–Barr virus)?	Severe sore throat for 2 days, getting worse (18/10/08)	Paracetamol 500mg 6 hourly PRN. Examine throat. Request WCC: lymphocytes atypical? Paul–Bunnell or Monospot® +ve?
Drug-induced agranulocytosis? (this is what the patient fears)	Severe sore throat for 2 days, getting worse (18/10/08). Taking carbimazole	Paracetamol 500mg 6 hourly PRN. Examine throat. Request WCC: ↓granulocytes (neutrophils, eosinophils, basophils)?
Postural hypotension syncope? Due to dehydration from infection?	Sudden loss of consciousness after getting up from chair, recovery within a minute (18/10/08). Evidence of acute infection	Look for fall in BP when standing. Request U&E. Consider fluids IV to rehydrate.
Thyrotoxicosis now controlled?	Anxiety, weight loss, abnormal thyroid function tests in April 2008. No heat or cold intolerance currently	Examine for tremor etc. Carbimazole 5mg od. FT4 and TSH normal?
Increased risk of type 2 diabetes mellitus	FH of type 2 diabetes mellitus	Test urine for sugar. Fasting glucose.
No domestic support	**Alone in flat at present.**	**Consider admission for initial care.**

Interpreting the physical examination

The physical examination tends to be focused. The 'open mind' approach, where findings are discovered and their meaning looked up later, is described at the end of this section. If this book is referred to before the examination, the reader could focus on the appearance of the throat and palpation of the neck to look for findings that may differentiate between the four differential diagnoses suggested by the history. The reader should also focus on the BP to see if there is a postural fall, and tremor and lid lag for inadequately treated thyrotoxicosis.

General

Looks unwell, flushed
No tremor or lid lag
Temperature 38.5°C
Bilaterally swollen tonsils, red with linear creamy patches
Bilateral, tender, multiple lymph node enlargement in neck. No lymph node swelling in axillae or groins
CVS
Pulse 110/min, regular, low volume
BP 110/70 reclining, 90/50 standing
Heart sounds normal
No murmurs
RS
Chest shape and movement normal
Breath sounds normal
AS
Not jaundiced
Liver—1 finger breadth below costal margin
Spleen not palpable
CNS
Conscious and alert
No neck stiffness
Hand and leg coordination normal

Reflexes all normal and symmetrical

The presence of linear patches of creamy pus in fissures on the surface of enlarged tonsils occurs commonly in patients with bacterial tonsillitis, but less commonly in agranulocytosis, viral pharyngitis, and glandular fever (where there is usually a grey mucoid film). This finding changes the order of the differential diagnoses, but they all remain possible. A high temperature and lymph node enlargement around the jaw occur in all the differential diagnoses of a sore throat and is a poor differentiator. There was no tremor and lid lag to suggest inadequately treated thyrotoxicosis.

The fall in BP when the patient stands up always occurs at some point in postural hypotension and uncommonly in its other differential diagnoses.

Therefore, the order of the possible diagnoses has changed; this is shown in the problem-structuring note opposite. The format has also changed again from a three-column chart to heading and subheadings.

Problem-structuring note (version 4)

Outline findings: female. Aged 29. Severe sore throat for 2 days, getting worse. Taking carbimazole. Sudden loss of consciousness after getting up from chair, recovery within a minute. PMH of thyrotoxicosis. FH of type 2 diabetes mellitus. No tremor, no lid lag, reflexes normal. Large red tonsils, **linear creamy patches**. Fall in BP on standing.

Acute bacterial (or follicular) tonsillitis? (mainly streptococcal)

Outline evidence: severe sore throat for 2 days, getting worse (18/10/08). **Large red tonsils with linear creamy patches.**

Management: paracetamol 500mg 6 hourly PRN. Examine throat. Request WCC: ↑neutrophils?

Glandular fever (infectious mononucleosis due to Epstein–Barr virus)??

Outline evidence: severe sore throat for 2 days, getting worse (18/10/08). **Large red tonsils with linear creamy patches.**

Management: paracetamol 500mg 6 hourly PRN. Examine throat. Request WCC: lymphocytes atypical? Paul–Bunnell or Monospot® +ve?

Viral pharyngitis?? (less probable)

Outline evidence: severe sore throat for 2 days, getting worse (18/10/08). **Large red tonsils with linear creamy patches.**

Management: paracetamol 500mg 6 hourly PRN. Examine throat. Request WCC: ↓neutrophils, ↑lymphocytes?

Drug induced agranulocytosis? (less probable)

Outline evidence: severe sore throat for 2 days, getting worse (18/10/08). On carbimazole. **Large red tonsils with linear creamy patches.**

Management: paracetamol 500mg 6 hourly PRN. Request WCC: ↓granulocytes (neutrophils, eosinophils, basophils)?

Postural hypotension syncope? Due to dehydration from infection?

Outline evidence: sudden loss of consciousness after getting up from chair, recovery within a minute (18/10/08). **Fall in BP on standing.** Evidence of acute infection.

Management: request U&E. Consider fluids IV to rehydrate.

Thyrotoxicosis now controlled?

Outline evidence: anxiety, weight loss, abnormal thyroid tests in April 2008. No heat or cold intolerance. No tremor, no lid lag, reflexes normal.

Management: carbimazole 5mg od. FT4 and TSH normal?

Increased risk of type 2 diabetes mellitus

Outline evidence: FH of type 2 diabetes mellitus

Management: test urine for sugar. Fasting glucose.

No domestic support

Outline evidence: alone in a flat at present. Parents 200 miles away.

Management: consider admission for initial care.

Interpreting the investigations

Investigations tend to be performed in a focused way like the physical examination. This means that they are done in order to differentiate between diagnostic possibilities created by the history and examination. However, urine testing, full blood count, urea and electrolytes (U&E), and chest X-ray (CXR) are often done routinely in the same way as aspects of the physical examination such as the pulse, temperature, and BP. These are done in case that they will reveal a result which is a good diagnostic lead. This is a form of screening, but if the result is abnormal, then it is investigated in the same way as a presenting complaint. In this case, all the tests, except the CXR were done in order to differentiate between the diagnostic possibilities, and most of the results were helpful.

> *Investigations*
>
> Urine testing: + glucose, no protein, no blood, no ketones
>
> FBC: Hb 12.4g/dL
> WCC 18.3×10^9/L, neutrophils 90%
> No atypical lymphocytes present
>
> Lab blood glucose 8.4mmol/L
> Na 141mmol/L, K 4.3mmol/L, urea 10.1mmol/L, creatinine 112µmol/L
> TSH, T4—results awaited
>
> Monospot® test—result awaited
> Throat swab—result awaited
>
> CXR normal

The presence of glucose in the urine and the random glucose of 8.4mmol/L is suspicious of diabetes mellitus. The WCC of 18.3x10^9/L with 90% neutrophils occurs commonly in bacterial tonsillitis, but never (by definition) in agranulocytosis. This is also very rare in viral pharyngitis and glandular fever so that all these diagnoses drop out of contention. The raised creatinine and urea are common in dehydration and less common in other causes of postural hypotension.

The problem-structuring note opposite shows how the diagnostic opinions and management have changed in the light of these test results.

Medical and surgical sieves

At this point, you can pause and use the medical and surgical sieves from p.14. You can consider whether you have omitted a diagnosis in the social background or environment, the locomotor, nervous, cardiovascular, respiratory, and alimentary systems, the renal system and urinary tract, and the reproductive, endocrine, autonomic, haematological, and immune systems. Within each of these systems, you can consider whether you have forgotten a congenital, infective, traumatic, neoplastic, or degenerative process. If not, you can move on.

Problem-structuring note (version 5)

Outline findings: female. Aged 29. Severe sore throat for 2 days, getting worse. Taking carbamazole. Sudden loss of consciousness after getting up from chair, recovery within a minute. PMH of thyrotoxicosis. FH of type 2 diabetes mellitus. No tremor, no lid lag. Large red tonsils with linear creamy patches. Fall in BP on standing. Urine testing: +ve glucose. Hb 12.4g/dL, WCC 18.3×10⁹/L, neutrophils 90%, no atypical lymphocytes present. Lab blood glucose 8.4mmol/L. Urea 10.1mmol/L. Creatinine 112µmol/L.

Acute bacterial (or follicular) tonsillitis (causing systemic effects, e.g. dehydration)	Severe sore throat for 2 days, getting worse (18/10/08). Large red tonsils with linear creamy patches. **WCC of 18.3×10⁹/L with 90% neutrophils**	Paracetamol 500mg 6 hourly PRN. Begin penicillin V 500mg qds
Probably not glandular fever (infectious mononucleosis due to Epstein–Barr virus)?	Severe sore throat for 2 days, getting worse (18/10/08). Large red tonsils with linear creamy patches. **WCC of 18.3×10⁹/L with 90% neutrophils**	Paracetamol 500mg 6 hourly PRN. Examine throat. Await Monospot® result.
Postural hypotension syncope? Due to dehydration from infection?	Sudden loss of consciousness after getting up from chair, recovery within a minute (18/10/08). Fall in BP on standing. Evidence of acute infection	Fall in BP when standing. Request U&E. Consider fluids IV to rehydrate
Dehydration from infection?	Fall in BP on standing. Evidence of acute infection. Urea 10.1 mmol/L. Creatinine 112 micromol/L	Admit. Encourage oral fluids. For fluids IV if unable to drink 2L in 12h
Thyrotoxicosis now controlled?	Anxiety, weight loss, abnormal thyroid function tests in April 2008. No heat or cold intolerance. No tremor or lid lag. Reflexes normal	Carbimazole 5mg od. Await result of FT4 and TSH
Probable type 2 diabetes mellitus	FH of type 2 diabetes mellitus. Urine glucose +ve. No ketones. Random glucose 8.4 mmol/L	Monitor blood sugar before and 2h after meals. Plan glucose tolerance test
No domestic support	Alone in a flat at present. Parents 200 miles away	Admit for initial care

Writing the diagnosis and management

The positive finding summary could be written out as follows:

> Female. Aged 29. Severe sore throat for 2 days, getting worse. Taking carbima-
> zole for 6 months. Sudden loss of consciousness after getting up from chair,
> recovery within a minute. PMH of thyrotoxicosis (anxiety, weight loss, abnormal
> thyroid function tests). FH of type 2 diabetes mellitus. Large red tonsils with
> linear creamy patches. Fall in BP on standing. Urine testing: +ve glucose. Hb
> 12.4g/dL, WCC 18.3×10⁹/L, neutrophils 90%, no atypical lymphocytes present.
> Lab blood glucose 8.4mmol/L, urea 10.1mmol/L, creatinine 112 μmol/L.

The primary diagnosis (that explains the symptoms that led the patient to
seek help) can be written as:

> Primary diagnosis:
> • Probable acute bacterial (or follicular) tonsillitis (causing systemic effects)

The other diagnoses can be written as:

> Other diagnoses:
> • Postural hypotension syncope due to dehydration from infection
> • Thyrotoxicosis probably now controlled
> • Probable type 2 diabetes mellitus
> • No domestic support currently

The initial plan can be written as:

> Plan:
> • Reassure patient that there is no agranulocytosis and explain other
>   diagnoses
> • Start penicillin V 500mg qds (because of systemic effects)
> • Continue paracetamol 1g qds
> • Continue carbimazole 5mg od
> • Encourage oral fluids (e.g. 2L in 16h)
> • Monitor blood glucose before and 2h after meals
> • Help patient to contact family

It should be noted that this traditional way of writing out the findings does
not give the reader an indication of the writer's thought process. It does
not provide the particular evidence for each diagnosis or specify at which
diagnosis each aspect of the management is directed. This is the approach
mostly used in discharge summaries when patients are discharged from
hospital. In contrast to this, the problem-structuring notes used here do
provide this information (there is a hospital-wide software available to allow
this to be done also for discharge summaries—see the acknowledgement
section of this book).

Case presentations

If you are asked to give a case presentation, then in addition to the positive findings, you should mention negative features. These will imply that you have considered other diagnoses, but were unable to find the supportive features (i.e. that you considered those negative findings to differentiate between your probable diagnosis and those you consider improbable). The information that you require for your case presentation will be found in the 'evidence' column of the latest version of your problem-structuring notes. It is customary to give the history of presenting complaint in some detail, as follows.

Case presentation of Ms AM

Ms AM is a 29-year old secretary who came to the A&E department with a severe sore throat, sweats and malaise for 2 days. She also lost consciousness briefly in A&E 30 minutes after arriving.

She was well until last Friday afternoon 17 October when she developed a **sore throat** at work. It was relieved that day by warm drinks and paracetamol, but when she woke this morning, it was very severe. She remembered that she had been told to report sore throats because she was taking carbimazole and to get a white cell count. She was worried that she might have developed a low white cell count because of this drug. She came to A&E because it was a Saturday morning. When she got up from her seat in the waiting room after being called, she felt dizzy, 'blacked out', and fell to the floor, striking her head. She recovered consciousness within a minute.

There is a past medical history of thyrotoxicosis (as evidenced last April by anxiety, weight loss, abnormal thyroid function tests). There is a family history of type 2 diabetes mellitus. She shares a flat with a friend who is away at present.

On examination, she looked tired and unwell. Her temperature was 38.5. Her pharynx was red with enlarged tonsils, which showed linear creamy patches. There was lymph node enlargement in the angles of the jaw but not elsewhere. Her pulse was 110/min and regular. The BP was 110/70 reclining and 90/50 standing. The heart sounds were normal and there were no murmurs. The chest was clear. The abdomen was soft and there was no splenic enlargement.

Urine testing showed one plus of glucose but no ketones. The white cell count was 18.3×10^9/L, the neutrophils being 90%. There were no atypical lymphocytes present. The laboratory random blood glucose was 8.4mmol/L, The urea was 10.1mmol/L and the creatinine 112 µmol/L.

Clinical opinions

After giving a case presentation, you will be asked to give a clinical opinion and expected to provide the (particular) evidence for your diagnoses. You may be asked if you do not volunteer this information first. The opinion could be based on the latest problem-structuring note.

Clinical opinion on Ms AM

The probable diagnosis is acute follicular tonsillitis (causing systemic effects, e.g. dehydration). This is because she has had a severe sore throat for 2 days, there were large red tonsils with linear creamy patches and a white cell count of 18.3×10^9/L with 90% neutrophils. This should be treated with penicillin because of the systemic effects and the symptoms treated with paracetamol.

There is probably no infectious mononucleosis or agranulocytosis because of the raised neutrophils and absence of atypical lymphocytes. She should be reassured about this.

She has suffered postural hypotension syncope because of the sudden loss of consciousness after getting up from chair with recovery within a minute and the fall in BP on standing. She should not be discharged home until this problem has resolved with rehydration.

She is probably dehydrated from infection because of the pulse of 110/min, fall in BP on standing, urea of 10.1mmol/L and creatinine of 110micromol/L. Fluids need to be encouraged.

The thyrotoxicosis appears to be controlled. The original anxiety and weight loss have resolved and there was no heat or cold intolerance. There was no tremor or lid lag. She should continue on carbimazole 5mg od, pending the result of T4 and TSH measurements.

She probably has type 2 diabetes mellitus because of the FH of this and the random blood sugar of 8.4mmol/L with no urine ketones. She is to have two fasting blood sugars, and her blood sugars monitored before and 2 hours after meals during the admission. A glucose tolerance test will be done if the fasting sugar is not less than 5.6 mmol/L or not more than 7.0 mmol/L on two occasions.

She has little domestic support because she lives alone in her flat this weekend and her parents live 200 miles away. She will be admitted and kept in hospital until she is well enough to self-care.

The 'open mind' approach

The preceding paragraphs described how diagnostic hypotheses were generated as soon as the presenting complaints had been heard. These were displayed in the problem-structuring notes. This approach requires the history taker to have the knowledge to identify the best leads and to know which items of information will differentiate between the possible diagnoses. Alternatively, it depends on the history taker looking up the information in the OHCD at different stages in the history and examination and when the test results become available.

The other option is to take the history and to examine the patient in a mechanical way, without interpreting the findings as they are discovered. The abnormal findings can then be listed at the end and then looked up in the OHCD. The thought process would then follow the same pattern as that described in the problem-structuring notes.

As the history and examination is being performed and the results become known, differential diagnoses may also occur to the assessor consciously or subconsciously in a passive way. This will depend on the assessor's knowledge, which can be helped by reading this book during private study. This can be done by covering the list of diagnoses on the left-hand side of the page, looking at the diagnostic lead on top of the page, and then reading the suggestive and confirmatory findings. The reader should then try to guess the hidden diagnosis and then see if he or she was correct.

The plan of the remainder of this book

An example of a systems enquiry has been given already on pp.32 to 35. The following shows a typical example of the routine physical examination on which the remainder of this book is based.

The 'routine' physical examination

Note the patient's attire, presence of nebulizer masks, sputum pots, medication packets, etc. The general examination is directed mainly at assessing the skin and reticulo-endothelial system (lymph nodes), and the related matters of temperature control and metabolic rate. During the history, the order of questioning could be decided entirely by thought processes (e.g. probing indirectly for a symptom to chase up a diagnostic possibility that comes to mind), but the physical examination is different. It is more efficient to adopt a routine that is smooth and quick, and not to jump about looking for physical signs that might support the diagnostic idea of that moment.

You have already been looking at the patient's face, general appearance, and immediate vicinity (e.g. walking stick, medication packets, etc.) when taking the history. So for the general examination, begin with the hands and work your way up by inspecting (and, when appropriate, palpating) the arms to the shoulders, examine the scalp, ears, eyes, cheeks, nose, lips, take the temperature, examine inside the mouth, then the neck, breasts, axillae, and then the skin of the abdomen, legs, and feet.

Plan of the general examination

Hands, arms, and shoulders
- *Fingernails*
- *Clubbing*
- *Finger nodules*
- *Finger joint deformity*
- *Rashes*
- *Pain and stiffness in the elbow, shoulder, neck*

Head and neck
- *Neck stiffness*
- *Patchy hair loss*
- *Eardrum redness*
- *Perforated eardrum*

Eyes, face, and neck
- *Facial redness, general appearance*
- *Red eye*
- *Iritis*
- *Conjunctival pallor*
- *Temperature—high or low*
- *Mouth lesions*
- *Lumps in the:*
  - *Face*
  - *Submandibular region*
  - *Anterior neck*
  - *Anterior triangle of neck*
  - *Posterior triangle*
  - *Supraclavicular region*

Trunk
- *Breast discharge*
- *Nipple eczema*
- *Breast lumps*
- *Gynaecomastia in male*
- *Axillary lymphadenopathy*
- *Sparse body hair*
- *Hirsutism*
- *Scar pigmentation*
- *Abdominal striae*

Legs
- *Inguinal and generalized lymphadenopathy*
- *Sacral, leg, and heel sores*

Cardiovascular system

Think first of cardiac output, and inspect and feel the hands for warmth or coldness. Feel the radial pulse, take the BP, and check the other pulses in the arms and neck. Next think of venous return and look at the jugular venous pressure (JVP). Then examine the heart itself (palpate, percuss, and then listen to it). Finally, examine output and venous return in the legs by feeling skin temperature, pulses, and looking for oedema of the legs, liver, and lungs.

Cardiac output
- *Peripheral cyanosis*
- *Radial pulse*
  - *Rate*
  - *Rhythm (compare cardiac apex rate, if irregular)*
  - *Amplitude*
  - *Vessel wall*
- *Compare pulses for volume and synchrony*
  - *Radial, brachial, carotid, (femoral, popliteal, posterior, and anterior tibials after the examining the heart)*
- *BP standing and lying in right arm, repeat on left*

Venous return
- *JVP*

The heart
- *Trachea displaced?*
- *Apex beat displaced?*
- *Parasternal heave*
- *Palpable thrill*
- *Auscultation*
  - *Extra heart sounds*
    —Systolic murmurs
    —Diastolic murmurs

Cardiac output and venous return in the legs
- *Skin temperature*
- *Posterior and anterior tibials, popliteal, femoral*
- *Venous skin changes*
- *Vein abnormalities*
- *Calf swelling*
- *Leg oedema*
- *Sacral oedema*
- *Liver enlargement*
- *Basal lung crackles*

Respiratory system

Think of general respiratory structure and function. *Inspect* and think of oxygen and carbon dioxide levels, then the ventilation process which depends on the chest wall and its movement. *Palpate* by feeling for tactile vocal fremitus. *Percuss* and then *auscultate*. Finally, listen for wheezes, thus assessing airways, from small (high-pitched) to large (low-pitched).

General inspection
- *Tremor and muscle twitching*
- *Cyanosis of the tongue and lips*
- *Clubbing*

Chest inspection
- *Respiratory rate*
- *Distorted chest wall*
- *Poor expansion*
- *Paradoxical movement*

Palpation
- *Mediastinum*
  - *Position of trachea*
  - *Position of apex beat*

Tactile vocal fremitus
- *Present or absent (or increased)*

Percussion
- *Hyper-resonant, resonant, normal, dull, or stony dull*

Auscultation
- *Diminished breath sounds*
- *Bronchial breathing*
- *Crackles*
- *Rubs*
- *Wheezes, high- or low-pitched, or polyphonic during inspiration and expiration*

Alimentary and genitourinary systems

Think first of metabolic issues related to general nutrition (obese, normal, thin, cachexia) and ensure that the patient is weighed. Check the mucous membranes, e.g. for signs of vitamin deficiency. Look for skin and eye signs of low fluid volume, and then liver disease. Next, turn your mind to anatomical aspects of the gastrointestinal and genitourinary systems together by inspecting, palpating, and auscultating. Finally, perform examinations (when indicated) that need special equipment, and do the urine tests.

Inspection
- Obesity
- Cachexia
- Oral lesions
- Jaundice
- Hepatic skin stigmata
- Loss of skin turgor
- Low eye tension

Palpation
- Supraclavicular nodes

Inspection of the abdomen
- Abdominal scars
- Veins
- General distension
- Visible peristalsis
- Poor movement

Palpation
- General tenderness
- Localized tenderness
- Hepatic enlargement
- Splenic enlargement
- Renal enlargement
- Abdominal masses

Percussion
- Dull or resonant
- Shifting dullness

Auscultation
- Silent abdomen
- Tinkling bowel sounds
- Bruits

Inspection and palpation again

- *Groin lumps (lymph nodes?)*
- *Scrotal masses*
- *Rectal abnormalities*
- *Melaena, fresh blood*
- *Vaginal and pelvic abnormalities*
- *Urine abnormalities*

Nervous system

If there are no neurological symptoms or signs detected up to this point, then it is customary to perform an abbreviated examination. This is done by commenting on the fact that the patient was conscious and alert, speech was normal, and that there were no cranial nerve abnormalities noted when looking at the face during the history and general examination. Also, you will have been able to note the patient's gait and movements around the hospital bed or consultation room. According to the GALS system, note and record the **G**ait, appearance, and movement of the **A**rms, **L**egs, and **S**pine.

If the patient was not conscious and alert, then the level of consciousness has to be addressed with the Glasgow Coma Scale.

The brief neurological examination consists of checking coordination and reflexes (because this tests the sensory and motor function of the nerves and central connections involved). The findings may be recorded as follows:

Short CNS examination

- Conscious and alert
- Speech normal
- Facial appearance and movement normal
- Finger–nose pointing normal
- Hand tapping and rotating normal
- Heel–toe test normal (ran heel from opposite knee to toe and back)
- Foot tapping (examiner's hand) normal

Reflexes	Right	Left
Biceps normal	+	+
Supinators normal	+	+
Triceps normal	+	+
Knees normal	+	+
Ankles normal	+	+
Plantars normally flexor	↓	↓

The full neurological assessment

The system of examination described here is typical. The general approach is to assess the conscious level (if the patient is not conscious and alert, then it will not be possible to conduct a full neurological examination which needs the patient's cooperation).

The cranial nerve sequence follows in their numbered sequence. Motor function can be assessed next, beginning with inspection for wasting and involuntary movements, and then 'palpation' by testing tone and power. The upper limbs are examined first and then the lower limbs. Sensation is then tested in the upper, then lower limbs, and finally coordination, reflexes, and gait. The order can be changed by addressing the area of abnormality suggested by the history. For example, if the patient complains of difficulty in walking, then it would be sensible to examine gait, then motor and sensory function, and cranial nerves last.

Nervous system
- *Conscious level*
- *Glascow Coma Score*
- *Speech*

Cranial nerves
- *Absent sense of smell*
- *Visual field defects*
- *Decreased acuity*

Ophthalmoscopy
- *Corneal opacity*
- *Lens opacity*
- *Papilloedema*
- *Pale optic disc*
- *Cupped disc*
- *Hypertensive retinopathy*
- *Dot and blot haemorrhages*
- *New vessel formation*
- *Pale/black retinal patches*
- *Ptosis*
- *Pupil*
  - *Constriction*
  - *Irregularities*
  - *Dilatation*
- *Diplopia*
- *Nystagmus*
- *Absent corneal reflex*
- *Loss of facial sensation*
- *Deviation of jaw*
- *Jaw jerk*
- *Facial weakness*
- *Deafness*
- *Loss of taste*
- *Palatal weakness*
- *Neck or shoulder weakness*
- *Paresis of tongue*

Motor function
Upper limbs
- *Arm posture*

- *Hand tremor*
- *Wasting of hand*
- *Wasting of arm*
- *Tone abnormalities*

Weakness of
- *Shoulder abduction and addiction*
- *Elbow flexion*
- *Elbow extension*
- *Wrist extension and flexion*
- *Handgrip*
- *Finger adduction and abduction*
- *Thumb abduction and opposition*
- *Arm incoordination*

Lower limbs
- *Limitation of movement*
- *Wasting*
- *Fasciculation*
- *Tone abnormalities*

Weakness of
- *Hip flexion*
- *Knee extension and flexion*
- *Foot*
  - *Plantar flexion*
  - *Dorsiflexion*
  - *Eversion and inversion*
- *Bilateral spastic paraparesis*
- *Spastic hemiparesis*

Sensation

Upper limb sensation
- *Hypoaesthesia of*
  - *Palm*
  - *Dorsum of hand*
  - *Lateral arm*
  - *Ulnar border of arm*
- *Dissociated sensory loss*
- *Progressive sensory loss*
- *Cortical sensory loss*

Lower limb
- *Hypoaesthesia of*
  - *Inguinal area*
  - *Anterior thigh*
  - *Shin*
  - *Lateral foot*
- *Progressive downward loss*
- *Dissociated sensory loss*
- *Multiple areas of loss*

Reflexes
- *Brisk or*
- *Diminished, in biceps, supinator, triceps, knee, ankle, and plantars*
- *Gait abnormalities*

Mental state examination

Think of the sequence of perception, 'affect', drive and arousal, cognitive processes (check memory of different duration, ability to reason with that memory, and then the nature of beliefs arrived at with such reasoning), and then actions in response to these:

- *Perception*: attentiveness and any hallucination, visual or auditory
- *Mood*: depression or elation
- *Mental*: *drive* rate of speech, anxiety
- *Cognition*: (6/10 or less correct implies impairment)
- *Orientation*: time to nearest hour, year, address of hospital
- *Short-term memory*: repeat a given name and address, name 2 staff
- *Long-term memory*: own age, date of birth, current monarch, dates of wars
- *Concentration*: count backwards from 20 to 1
- *Beliefs*: patient's perception and insight of health, self-confidence, any extreme convictions
- *Activity*: physical and social activity, employment, physical signs of drug use

Basic blood and urine test results

First check the patient's name, gender, age, and address to make sure whose sample you are handling and whose results you are interpreting. The following are interpreted in Chapter 11.

Urine testing
- *Microscopic haematuria*
- *Asymptomatic proteinuria*
- *Glycosuria*
- *Raised urine or plasma bilirubin*
  - *Hepatocellular jaundice*
  - *Obstructive jaundice*

Biochemistry
- *Hypernatraemia*
- *Hyponatraemia*
- *Hyperkalaemia*
- *Hypokalaemia*
- *Hypercalcaemia*
- *Hypocalcaemia*
- *Raised alkaline phosphatase*

Haematology
- *Low haemoglobin*
- *Microcytic anaemia*
- *Macrocytic anaemia*
- *Normocytic anaemia*
- *Very high ESR or CRP*

Abnormal chest X-ray appearances

Many CXR appearances may be recognizable immediately as indicating a specific diagnosis, but if not, the appearances below are considered in Chapter 12.

- Area of uniform opacification with a well-defined border
- Rounded opacity (or opacities)
- Multiple 'nodular' shadows and 'miliary mottling'
- Diffuse, poorly defined hazy opacification
- Increased linear markings
- Dark lung/lungs
- Abnormal hilar shadowing
- Upper mediastinal widening
- Abnormal cardiac shadow

References

1. Llewelyn DEH, Ewins DL, Horn J, Evans TGR, McGregor AM (1988). Computerised updating of clinical summaries: new opportunities for clinical practice and research. *BMJ* 297, 1504–6.

General and endocrine symptoms and physical signs

General principles

The findings are discussed in a sequence of the general examination. You will have been looking at the patient's face during the history. Begin with fingernail and joints, backs and fronts of hands, arms, elbows, moving up to the neck and scalp, then down to the face, mouth, the throat, the breasts, axillae, trunk, and groin. Note any skin abnormalities.

Fingernail abnormality

Classify fingernail changes by 'naming' them first. Some have very few causes and are good diagnostic leads.

Classification	
Clubbing due to many causes (see 📖pp.72–73)	*Confirmed by*: angle lost between nail and finger (no gap when nails of same finger on both hands apposed, bogginess of nail bed, increased nail curvature, both longitudinally and transversely, and drumstick finger appearance).
Terry's lines due to many causes (see 📖p.74)	*Confirmed by*: nail tips having dark pink or brown bands.
Nail fold infarcts due to vasculitis due to many causes (see 📖p.76)	*Confirmed by*: dark blue-black areas in nail fold.
Koilonychia due to iron deficiency anaemia (occasionally ischaemic heart disease or syphilis)	*Suggested by*: spoon-shaped nails. *Confirmed by*: ↓Hb, ↓ferritin from iron deficiency (basal or exercise **ECG** for ischaemic heart disease; **serology** for syphilis).
Onycholysis due to psoriasis, hyperthyroidism	*Suggested by*: nail thickened, dystrophic, and separated from the nail bed. *Confirmed by*: clinical appearance and evidence of cause, e.g. skin changes of psoriasis or ↑**FT4** ± ↑**FT3** and ↓**TSH**.
Beau's lines due to any period of severe illness	*Suggested by*: transverse furrows. *Confirmed by*: history of associated condition.
Longitudinal lines due to lichen planus, alopecia areata, Darier's disease	*Suggested by*: transverse furrows (ending in triangular nicks and nail dystrophy in Darier's disease).
Onychomedesis due to any period of severe illness	*Suggested by*: shedding of nail. *Confirmed by*: history of associated condition.
Muehrcke's lines due to hypoalbuminaemia	*Suggested by*: paired, white, parallel, transverse bands. *Confirmed by*: serum albumin <20g/L.

Nail pitting due to psoriasis or alopecia areata	*Suggested by:* small holes in nail. *Confirmed by:* rash on extensor surfaces with silvery scales (psoriasis) or circumscribed areas of hair loss (alopecia areata).
Splinter haemorrhages due to infective endocarditis (sometimes due to manual labour)	*Suggested by:* fine, longitudinal, haemorrhagic streaks under the nail. *Confirmed by:* history of manual labour (or fever, changing heart murmurs, and bacterial growth on several **blood cultures**).
Chronic paronychia due to chronic infection of nail bed	*Suggested by:* red, swollen, and thickened skin in nail fold. *Confirmed by:* response to antibiotics (erythromycin for bacterial infection or nystatin for fungal infection).
Mee's lines due to arsenic poisoning or renal failure, Hodgkin's disease, heart failure	*Suggested by:* single, white, transverse bands. *Confirmed by:* presence of associated conditions.
'Yellow' nails due to lymphoedema, bronchiectasis, hypo-albuminaemia	*Suggested by:* colour! *Confirmed by:* presence of associated condition.

Clubbing

Present when the angle is lost between nail and finger (no gap when nails of same finger on each hand apposed). Initial investigations (other tests in **bold** below): FBC, ESR/CRP, CXR.

Main differential diagnoses and typical outline evidence, etc.	
Subacute bacterial endocarditis	*Suggested by:* general malaise, weight loss, pallor, low grade fever, changing heart murmurs ± past medical history (PMH) of valve or congenital heart disease. *FBC:* ↓Hb, ↑WBC. ↑↑ESR, ↑↑CRP.
	Confirmed by: growth of organism, e.g. Streptococcus viridians after **serial blood cultures** ± endocardial vegetations on **transoesophageal echocardiography**.
	Initial management: treated on high index of suspicion, admit, avoid antibiotics before blood cultures, consult microbiology, initial benzylpenicillin and gentamicin IV for 4wk with gentamicin levels.
Cyanotic congenital heart disease	*Suggested by:* long past history, central cyanosis.
	Confirmed by: **echocardiogram** appearances.
	Initial management: O₂ therapy, treat heart failure and infection, consider surgical intervention.
Bronchial carcinoma	*Suggested by:* malaise, increased cough, weight loss, haemoptysis. Smoking history. Opacity (suggestive of mass ± pneumonia ± effusion) on **CXR** and **CT** *scan*.
	Confirmed by: **bronchoscopy** appearances and histology.
	Initial management: control of pain and infection. Non-small cell tumours: excision, radiotherapy, or combined radiotherapy and chemotherapy depending on staging. Small cell tumours: chemotherapy or palliative radiotherapy.
Bronchiectasis	*Suggested by:* chronic cough, productive of copious purulent, often rusty-coloured sputum.
	Confirmed by: **CXR** and **CT** *scan:* thickened 'tram line' (dilated) bronchi. *Bronchoscopy* appearances.
	Initial management: postural drainage, antibiotics according to sputum culture and sensitivity, bronchodilators (e.g. nebulized salbutamol), steroids, (e.g. prednisolone). Consider surgery.
Lung abscess	*Suggested by:* cough, very ill, spiking fever, PMH of lung disease.
	Confirmed by: **CXR**: mass containing fluid level (air above pus).
	Initial management: antibiotics according to sputum culture and sensitivity for up to 6wk, aspiration, and antibiotic instillation, surgical excision.

Empyema	*Suggested by:* cough, very ill, fever, stony dull over one lung.
	Confirmed by: ↑neutrophil WBC. **CXR:** long opacity on one view. Aspiration of pus, culture and sensitivity.
	Initial management: antibiotics, chest drain.
Fibrosing alveolitis	*Suggested by:* cough, fine crackles, especially bases.
	Confirmed by: **CXR:** bilateral diffuse nodular shadows or honeycombing (late finding).
	Initial management: oral steroids (e.g. prednisolone) for up to 4mo, then reduce, immunosuppressants (e.g. azathioprine), or both.
Hepatic cirrhosis	*Suggested by:* long history of liver disease, e.g. due to high alcohol intake, ascites, prominent abdominal veins. In males: spider naevi, gynaecomastia.
	Confirmed by: **↓serum albumin**, abnormal **liver function tests. (LFT). Liver biopsy** findings.
	Initial management: no alcohol, low salt diet if ascites, vitamin K *if ↑prothrombin time*, anti-flu and pneumococcal vaccination, colestyramine if pruritus
Crohn's disease	*Suggested by:* history of chronic diarrhoea and abdominal pain, low weight.
	Confirmed by: **colonoscopy *and biopsy*, barium enema, *and* barium meal *and follow-through*.**
	Initial management: oral prednisolone if mild. Steroids IV if severe, immunosuppressants (e.g. methotrexate), immunotherapy (e.g. infliximab).
Ulcerative colitis	*Suggested by:* history of intermittent diarrhoea with blood and mucus, low weight.
	Confirmed by: **colonoscopy** and **biopsy**.
	Initial management: prednisolone PO + mesalazine, prednisolone enemas. If severe, hydrocortisone IV followed by prednisolone PO and sulfasalazine ± surgery.

Terry's lines: dark pink or brown bands on nails

Initial investigations (other tests in **bold** below): FBC, LFT, CXR, ESR/CRP.

Main differential diagnoses and typical outline evidence, etc.	
Hepatic cirrhosis	*Suggested by:* long history of liver disease, e.g. due to high alcohol intake, ascites, prominent abdominal veins. In males: spider naevi, gynaecomastia.
	Confirmed by: ↓serum albumin, abnormal **LFT**. **Liver biopsy** findings.
	Initial management: no alcohol, dietary advice, low salt diet if ascites, vitamin K *if ↑prothrombin time*, anti-flu and pneumococcal vaccination, cholestyramine for pruritus.
Congestive cardiac failure	*Suggested by:* dyspnoea, orthopnoea, paroxysmal nocturnal dyspnoea (PND), ↑JVP, gallop rhythm, basal inspiratory crackles, ankle oedema.
	Confirmed by: **CXR** and **echocardiography**.
	Initial management: identify and treat any causes, e.g. valve disease, anaemia or thyroid disease, chest infections, stop smoking, diuretics (e.g. furosemide), ACE inhibitors (e.g. ramipril), β-blockers (e.g. carvedilol), spironolactone, and digoxin.
Diabetes mellitus (DM)	*Suggested by:* thirst, polydipsia, polyuria, fatigue, family history.
	Confirmed by: **fasting blood glucose** ≥7.0mmol/L on two occasions OR fasting, random or 2h **GTT** glucose ≥11.1mmol/L once only with symptoms.
	Initial management: diabetic diet, lifestyle advice, e.g. exercise, no smoking, follow-up plan. Insulin for all type 1 and type 2 diabetics on maximum oral treatment. For type 2 DM, metformin as 1st line.
Cancer somewhere	*Suggested by:* weight loss and anorexia with symptoms developing over months, bone pain.
	Confirmed by: careful history, examination, **CXR, FBC, ESR,** and follow-up.
Old age	*Suggested by:* age >75y.
	Confirmed by: no other illness discovered on follow-up.

Vasculitic nodules on fingers

Nodules and dark lines in nail folds which are focal areas infarction, which suggest local vasculitis. Initial investigations (other tests in **bold** below): FBC, ESR/CRP.

Main differential diagnoses and typical outline evidence, etc.	
Systemic lupus erythematosus (SLE)	*Suggested by:* swelling of distal interphalangeal (IP) joints, any other large joints, malar rash, pleural effusion, especially in Afro-Caribbean female. Multisystem dysfunction.
	Confirmed by: **FBC**: ↓Hb, ↓WBC. ↑**ESR** or ↑**CRP**. **Antinuclear antibody** +ve, especially if directed at **double-stranded DNA**.
	Initial management: NSAIDs for mild disease, topical steroids, sunblocks for rashes. Antimalarials, e.g. hydroxychloroquine for joint pain. For systemic disease and renal disease: oral steroids and immunosuppressants. Plasmapharesis for severe cases.
Subacute bacterial endocarditis ('Osler nodes')	*Suggested by:* general malaise, weight loss, pallor, low grade fever, changing heart murmurs ± PMH of valve or congenital heart disease. **FBC**: ↓Hb, ↑WCC. ↑↑**ESR**, ↑↑**CRP**.
	Confirmed by: growth of organism, e.g. Streptococcus viridians after **serial blood cultures** ± endocardial vegetations on **transoesophageal echocardiography**.
	Initial management: treated on high index of suspicion, admit, avoid antibiotics before blood cultures, consult microbiology, initial benzylpenicillin and gentamicin IV for 4wk with gentamicin levels.

Hand arthropathy

Look at the finger joints (IP joints), the knuckles (the metacarpo-phalangeal or MP joints), and compare. Finally look at the wrist. Initial investigations (other tests in **bold** below): FBC, RF, ANA X-ray hands

Main differential diagnoses and typical outline evidence, etc.	
Primary (post-menopausal) osteoarthrosis	*Suggested by:* Heberden's nodes (paired bony nodes on terminal IP joints).
	Confirmed by: **X-ray** appearances of affected joints.
	Initial management: analgesics and NSAIDs if not contraindicated + gastric acid reduction, e.g. proton pump inhibitor (PPI).
Rheumatoid arthritis (RA)	*Suggested by:* swelling and deformity of phalangeal joints (with ulnar deviation), wrist, and 'rheumatoid nodules'.
	Confirmed by: +ve **rheumatoid factor. X-ray** appearances of affected joints.
	Initial management: physiotherapy and occupational therapies, analgesics, and NSAIDs + gastric acid reduction (e.g. PPI), low dose prednisolone, disease-modifying drugs (DMARDs) (e.g. methotrexate), immunotherapy, e.g. infliximab.
Psoriatic arthropathy	*Suggested by:* swelling and deformity of distal (or all) IP joints. **X-ray** appearances of affected joints.
	Confirmed by: dry rash with silvery scales (especially near elbow extensor surface).
	Initial management: NSAIDs, e.g. diclofenac + gastric acid reduction (e.g. PPI), DMARDS, e.g. methotrexate, leflunomide; immunotherapy e.g. infliximab.
SLE	*Suggested by:* swelling and deformity of all (or distal) IP joints, butterfly facial rash, signs of pleural/pericardial effusion, renal impairment.
	Confirmed by: +ve **anti-nuclear factor, ↑DNA antibodies.**
	Initial management: NSAIDs for mild disease, sunblocks and topical steroids for rashes, antimalarials, e.g. hydroxychloroquine for joint pain, for systemic or renal disease, oral steroids and immunosuppressants. Plasmapharesis for severe cases.

Lumps around the elbow

Inspect and palpate with care as not to hurt. Initial investigations (other tests in **bold** below): FBC, RF, Pl urate, X-ray elbow.

Main differential diagnoses and typical outline evidence, etc.	
Osteoarthritis	*Suggested by:* joint deformity, intermittent pain and swelling, paired Heberden's nodes over distal ip joints in primary osteoarthritis.
	Confirmed by: clinical appearance if gross. If mild, **X-ray** showing loss of joint space (due to atrophy of cartilage) and –ve **rheumatoid factor**.
	Initial management: analgesics and NSAIDs + gastric acid reduction, e.g. PPI.
Rheumatoid nodules	*Suggested by:* mobile subcutaneous nodule.
	Confirmed by: history or joint changes of rheumatoid arthritis and +ve **rheumatoid factor**.
	Initial management: physiotherapy and occupational therapies, analgesics and NSAIDs + gastric acid reduction (e.g. PPI), low dose prednisolone, DMARDs (e.g. methotrexate), immunotherapy, e.g. infliximab.
Xanthomatosis	*Suggested by:* pale subcutaneous plaques attached to underlying tendon.
	Confirmed by: **hyperlipidaemia** on blood testing.
	Initial management: treat hyperlipidaemia, excision or electrocautery if unsightliness remains.
Gouty tophi	*Suggested by:* irregular hard nodules, risk factors or PMH of gout.
	Confirmed by: ↑**plasma urate. Biopsy:** urate crystals present.
	Initial management: allopurinol, local excision of tophi if required.

Neck stiffness

Distinguish between limited range of neck movement and neck stiffness throughout range of movement. Initial investigations (other tests in **bold** below): FBC, X-ray neck.

- Limited neck range of movement.

Main differential diagnoses and typical outline evidence, etc.	
Chronic cervical spondylosis with osteophytes	*Suggested by:* no fever or associated symptoms.
	Confirmed by: limitation in range of neck movement, but no stiffness within free range of movement. **WCC** normal, no fever, no neurological signs, **neck X-ray** appearance.
	Initial management: analgesics, muscle relaxants, and NSAIDs (if no contraindication) + gastric acid reduction (e.g. PPI), intermittent cervical collar, physiotherapy.

- Neck stiffness throughout range of movement.

Bacterial meningitis	*Suggested by:* gradual headache over days, photophobia, vomiting. Fever, ↑neutrophil count. Petechial rash (in meningococcal meningitis).
	Confirmed by: **lumbar puncture:** turbid CSF, ↑CSF neutrophil count with ↓glucose. Bacteria on microscopy. Growth of bacteria on culture of CSF.
	Initial management: benzylpenicillin IV/IM while awaiting transport to hospital (cefotaxime for penicillin allergic patients), gain IV access, ABCs, contact tracing, and treatment.
Viral meningitis	*Suggested by:* gradual headache over days. Fever, ↑lymphocyte count, normal neutrophil count.
	Confirmed by: **lumbar puncture:** clear CSF. ↑CSF lymphocyte count↑ with normal glucose. No bacteria on microscopy. No growth of bacteria on CSF culture.
	Initial management: analgesia, reassure that illness is self-limiting; if features suspicious of encephalitis, aciclovir.
Meningism due to viral infection	*Suggested by:* gradual headache over days. Fever, ↑lymphocyte count, normal neutrophil count.
	Confirmed by: **lumbar puncture:** clear CSF. Normal CSF white cell count. No bacteria on microscopy. No growth of bacteria on CSF culture.
	Initial management: analgesia, reassure that illness is self-limiting.

Subarachnoid haemorrhage	*Suggested by:* sudden onset of headache over seconds. Variable degree of consciousness. No fever. Normal WCC.
	Confirmed by: **CT or MRI *brain scan appearance*. Lumbar puncture**: bloodstained CSF that does not clear in successive bottle collection (may be negative if <2h after the bleed, or presence of xanthochromia in CSF (12h to 2wk after the haemorrhage).
	Initial management: discuss with neurosurgeons, regular monitoring of vital signs and Glasgow coma scale. If no rebleeding, clipping of an aneurysm ± clot evacuation if surgically feasible.
Acute cervical spondylitis	*Suggested by:* gradual neck pain (occasionally a headache) over hours or days. Immobile neck. Usually past history of similar episodes. No fever.
	Confirmed by: above history.
	Initial management: analgesics and NSAIDs if not contraindicated + gastric acid reduction (e.g. PPI), cervical collar, physiotherapy.
Posterior fossa tumour	*Suggested by:* headache, papilloedema.
	Confirmed by: **CT or MRI *scan*** appearances.
	Initial management: analgesia, dexamethasone to reduce brain oedema, treat seizures with anti-epileptics, assessment for resection or palliative surgery, palliative radiotherapy.
Anxiety with semi-voluntary resistance	*Suggested by:* improvement with reassurance or temporary distraction.
	Confirmed by: resolution after rest and observation.
	Initial management: analgesia, reassurance.

Hair loss in a specific area

Examine overall and then gently part hair to examine scalp. Use magnifying glass if hair is abnormal. Initial investigations (other tests in **bold** below): FBC, ferritin, TSH.

Main differential diagnoses and typical outline evidence, etc.	
Alopecia areata	*Suggested and confirmed by:* well circumscribed loss with exclamation mark hairs.
	Initial management: reassurance, advise patient not to scratch, usually no treatment needed, if slow to resolve, local triamcinolone.
Alopecia totalis	*Suggested and confirmed by:* total hair loss on head.
	Initial management: treat underlying problems, e.g. stress, iron deficiency, hypothyroidism, wig, local minoxidil for androgenic alopecia.
Polycystic ovary syndrome	*Suggested by:* bitemporal recession and occipital thinning. Hirsutism on trunk. Onset near puberty. Obesity.
	Confirmed by: ↑**testosterone** and ↓**SHBG**. ↑**LH**, **ovarian US scan**.
	Initial management: metformin to reduce insulin resistance. Combined oestrogen 'pill' to ↑SHBG and ↓free androgen. Co-cyprindiol (contains cyproterone) for hirsutism. Clomifene to induce ovulation.
Testosterone-secreting ovarian tumour	*Suggested by:* bitemporal recession and occipital thinning. Rapid onset over months.
	Confirmed by: ↑↑**testosterone** and ↓**LH**, *ovarian US scan*, and **laparoscopy** appearance.
	Initial management: resection of tumour.

Diffuse hair loss

Examine trunk, pubic and limb hair too (alopecia universalis). Initial investigations (other tests in **bold** below): FBC, ferritin.

Main differential diagnoses and typical outline evidence, etc.	
Cytotoxic drugs	*Suggested by:* mainly head hair loss. History of recent cytotoxic drugs.
	Confirmed by: improvement after stopping cytotoxic drug.
	Initial management: explain, offer temporary wig.
Iron deficiency	*Suggested by:* mainly head hair loss. Koilonychia, pallor of conjunctivae.
	Confirmed by: ↓Hb, ↓MCV, ↓MCHC, **↓ferritin**. Improvement if iron stores restored.
	Initial management: iron replacement, e.g. ferrous sulphate, investigate and treat the underlying cause.
Severe illness	*Suggested by:* mainly head hair loss. History of recent severe illness.
	Confirmed by: improvement with restoration of health.
	Initial management: explain expected outcome.
Hypogonadism	*Suggested by:* loss of hair from axilla, pubic area.
	Confirmed by: **↓testosterone** or **↓oestrogen** with **↑FSH** and **↑LH** in primary gonadal failure; normal or ↓LH, normal or ↓FSH if 2° to pituitary disease.
	Initial management: cyclical oestrogen in female or testosterone replacement therapy in men (IM, gel, patch or implant, provided prostatic-specific antigen normal.
Recent pregnancy	*Suggested by:* mainly head hair loss. Recent pregnancy.
	Confirmed by: improvement after delivery.
	Initial management: explanation and reassurance.

External ear abnormalities

Inspect the pinna for scars and other abnormalities. Examine the auditory meatus by first pulling the pinna up and back to straighten the cartilaginous bend. (In infants, pinna is pulled back and down.) Swab any discharge and remove any wax. Initial investigations (other tests in **bold** below): swab, culture, and sensitivity.

Main differential diagnoses and typical outline evidence, etc.	
Congenital anomalies	*Suggested by:* malformed pinna, accessory tags, auricles and pre-auricular pit, sinus, or fistula and microtia (no pinna ± atresia of ear canal).
	Confirmed by: above clinical appearances. **CT and MRI scans** to exclude other associated abnormalities.
	Initial management: rule out associated middle and inner ear abnormalities, hearing assessment, no treatment if minor ± hearing aids, surgical intervention if major.
Infected pre-auricular sinus	*Suggested by:* looking like a small dimple anterior to tragus with a discharge.
	Confirmed by: deep tract that lies close to the facial nerve. Swab, culture, and sensitivity.
	Initial management: antibiotics according to culture and sensitivity, excision if recurrent infection.
Chondrodermatitis nodularis chronica helicis	*Suggested by:* painful nodular lesions on the upper margin of the pinna in men (helical rim) or antihelix (in women), pain wakes up patient at night.
	Confirmed by: clinical appearance.
	Initial management: avoid pressure (lying on other side), local triamcinolone or excision.
Pinna haematoma resulting in a 'cauliflower' ear	*Suggested by:* history of blunt trauma.
	Confirmed by: appearance of bleeding in the subperi-chondrial plane that elevates the perichondrium to form a haematoma.
	Initial management: aspiration with a wide bore needle followed by firm pressure dressing; failing this, incision and drainage.
Exostosis (localized bony hypertrophy) may cause buildup of wax or debris or conductive deafness	*Suggested by:* palpable bony projections in the ear canals, accumulated wax difficult to clear ± history of much swimming in cold water.
	Confirmed by: sessile, smooth, often multiple, bilateral bony overgrowths of the ear canals.
	Initial management: no treatment, if wax clearing is a problem, then surgical removal of exostoses.

Wax (cerumen)—may cause conductive deafness if it impacts	*Suggested by:* hearing difficulty, irritation feeling in the ear, dark brown, shiny, soft mass.
	Confirmed by: improvement in hearing after removal.
	Initial management: slightly warm olive oil drops, ear syringing, or suctioning.
Foreign bodies in the ear	*Suggested by:* visible foreign body and inflammation (in child or learning-disabled patient).
	Confirmed by: retrieval of foreign body.
	Initial management: removal by gentle syringing or forceps. (A button battery needs to be removed immediately.) If an insect, some olive oil first.

Painful ear

Consider referred pain from neck, (C3, C4 and C5), throat, and teeth, and examine these too. Insert the largest comfortable aural speculum gently. Initial investigations (other tests in **bold** below): swab, culture, and sensitivity.

Main differential diagnoses and typical outline evidence, etc.	
Otitis externa (swimmer's ear) due to eczema, psoriasis, trauma, *Pseudomonas*, fungal infection	*Suggested by:* itching, irritation, pain, discharge, and tragal tenderness, recent ear syringing. *Confirmed by:* acute inflammation of the skin of the meatus, **culture of swab**, intact tympanic membrane. *Initial management:* analgesics, if mild—antibiotics and steroid drops. If severe, clear debris and keep ear dry, ear canal dressing with ribbon gauze impregnated with antiseptic and changed daily. No swimming.
Malignant necrotizing otitis externa	*Suggested by:* pain, discharge, and tragal tenderness in a diabetic, elderly, or immunosuppressed person, facial palsy. *Confirmed by:* **X-ray** showing local bone erosion, isotope bone scan, and **white cell scan**. *Initial management:* aural toilet, local and systemic antibiotics. If severe, check cranial nerves, surgical debridement.
Furunculosis (staphylococcal abscess in hair follicle) often diabetic	*Suggested by:* acutely painful throbbing ear, pain is worse on moving the pinna or pressing on tragus. *Confirmed by:* appearance of a boil in the meatus. *Initial management:* insertion of wick soaked in icthammol to ease pain, analgesics, and oral antibiotics.
Bullous myringitis (associated with influenza infection or *Mycoplasma pneumoniae*)	*Suggested and confirmed by:* extremely painful haemorrhagic blisters on the drum and deep meatal skin, and fluid behind the drum. *Initial management:* analgesia.
Barotrauma (aerotitis)	*Suggested by:* history of ear pain during descent in an aircraft or diving. *Confirmed by:* relief by decompression (e.g. holding nose and swallowing). *Initial management:* repeated Valsalva manoeuvre to open up the Eustachian tube, with use of topical nasal decongestants. Consider myringotomy if intractible.
Temporo-mandibular joint dysfunction	*Suggested by:* earache, facial pain, and joint clicking or popping related to malocclusion, teeth-grinding or joint derangement. *Confirmed by:* tenderness exacerbated by lateral movement of the open jaw, or trigger points in the pterygoids. *Initial management:* simple analgesics, e.g. paracetamol, NSAIDs, muscle relaxants, correction of malocclusive bite.

Discharging ear

Examine the eardrum quadrants in turn. Note colour, translucency, and any bulging or retraction of the membrane. Note size, position, and site (marginal or central) of any perforations. Drum movement during a Valsalva manoeuvre also depends on a patient's eustachian tube. Initial investigations (other tests in **bold** below): swab, culture, and sensitivity.

Main differential diagnoses and typical outline evidence, etc.	
Acute otitis media (due to *Pneumococcus*, *Haemophilus*, *Streptococcus*, and *Staphylo-coccus*, occasionally complicated by mastoiditis)	*Suggested by:* rapid onset over hours of throbbing and severe pain and fever, irritability, anorexia, or vomiting after an upper respiratory tract infection.
	Confirmed by: bulging red drum or profuse purulent discharge for 48h after drum perforates. Swab, culture and sensitivity.
	Initial management: analgesics, antibiotics if symptoms persist after 24h, myringotomy if bulging persists.
Otitis media with effusion (serous, secretory, or glue ear) usually in young children	*Suggested by:* gradual onset over weeks or months of deafness and intermittent ear pain.
	Confirmed by: loss of drum's light reflex or retraction relieved by grommets.
	Initial management: advise that it may improve spontaneously; treat predisposing conditions, e.g. allergic rhinitis, cleft palate. If persists, insertion of grommets ± adenoidectomy.
Chronic suppurative otitis media (may lead to cholesteatoma, petrositis, labyrinthitis, facial palsy, meningitis, intracranial abscess)	*Suggested by:* offensive purulent discharge, hearing loss, but no pain.
	Confirmed by: central drum perforation, swab, culture and sensitivity.
	Initial management: local and systemic antibiotics based on culture and sensitivity; regular aural toilet. If severe, myringoplasty and cortical mastoidectomy.
Cholesteatoma (locally destructive stratified squamous epithelium)	*Suggested by:* foul discharge, deafness, headache, ear pain, facial paralysis, and vertigo.
	Confirmed by: continuing mucopurulent discharge, swab, culture and sensitivity, pearly white soft matter (keratin) in attic or posterior marginal perforation.
	Initial management: if early retraction pocket, clean and remove keratin. If advanced, mastoid surgery.

Chronic otitis externa	*Suggested by:* watery discharge, itching, bilateral symptoms, painless and relapsing.
	Confirmed by: erythema and weeping of meatus.
	Initial management: keep ears dry, regular aural toilets, avoid local antibiotic drops, oral antibiotics when indicated according to culture and sensitivity.
Auditory canal trauma	*Suggested by:* bloody discharge.
	Confirmed by: history of trauma, laceration, and erythema.
	Initial management: analgesics, stop bleeding with pressure + dressing, suturing if needed.
CSF otorrhoea	*Suggested by:* history of head or facial trauma or surgery.
	Confirmed by: halo sign on filter paper.
	Initial management: observation, prophylactic antibiotics.

Striking facial appearance

Best recognized when meeting patient for the first time, but there is a wide normal variation. Initial investigations (other tests in **bold** below): TSH, ±FT4

Main differential diagnoses and typical outline evidence, etc.	
Parkinson's disease	*Suggested by:* rigidity, lack or slowness of movements, no arm swing on walking, mask-like (akinetic) face ± hand or head tremor.
	Confirmed by: response to dopaminergic drugs. **CT and MRI scans** to eliminate other diagnoses. (Failure to respond to levodopa indicates no idiopathic Parkinson's disease.)
	Initial management: in early disease avoid dopa preparations; use dopamine releasing agents (e.g. amantadine), monoamine oxidase inhibitors (e.g. selegiline) or anticholinergics (e.g. trihexyphenidyl). In more severe disease, use levodopa or dopamine agonists.
Huntington's chorea (or drug effect)	*Suggested by:* choreiform—jerky, purposeless facial movement or athetosis (writhing facial movement), tongue protrusion, and a bizarre gait.
	Confirmed by: family history or response to withdrawal of drug or dose reduction (if due to drug effect); also **genetic studies**.
	Initial management: symptomatic, e.g. tetrabenazine and haloperidol to reduce involuntary movements.
Bilateral upper or lower motor neurone lesion (due to motor neurone disease, cerebrovascular disease, myasthenia gravis)	*Suggested by:* paucity of movement of face, muscle weakness, and fasciculation.
	Confirmed by: other features of cause and **MRI** or **CT scan**.
	Initial management: supportive including physiotherapy, occupational, and speech therapies. Psychological support.
Thyrotoxicosis due to Graves's disease, single or multiple toxic nodules	*Suggested by:* anxious-looking, thin, with lid retraction and lag, tremor, hyperreflexic, diffuse goitre in Graves's, visible or palpable nodules(s) if toxic nodules.
	Confirmed by: ↓TSH and ↑T3 or ↑T4 or both. **Thyroid antibodies** +ve if Graves's. **US scan or isotope scan** appearance.
	Initial management: propranolol 40-80mg 8 hourly to control symptoms. Carbimazole 40mg od reduced to 5–15mg od over 1–3mo period depending on TFT results; continue for 6–18mo. Radioiodine therapy if hot nodule(s) or relapse of Graves's disease after full course.

Hypothyroidism	*Suggested by:* puffy face, obesity, cold intolerance, tiredness, constipation, bradycardia. *Confirmed by:* ↑**TSH**, ↓**FT4**. *Initial management:* levothyroxine 50mcg od; if elderly or if angina, 25mcg od. Check TFT after 4–8wk and adjust dose accordingly.
Acromegaly	*Suggested by:* large wide face, embossed forehead, jutting jaw (prognathism) widely spaced teeth, and large tongue. *Confirmed by:* ↑**IGF**, failure to suppress GH to <2mU/L with **oral GTT**. **Skull X-ray** showing bony abnormalities. **Hand X-ray** showing typical tufts on terminal phalanges. **MRI or CT** *head scan* showing enlarged pituitary fossa. *Initial management:* treat diabetes and hypertension. Somatostatin or trans-sphenoidal hypophysectomy with or without radiotherapy.
Cushing's syndrome pituitary-driven Cushing's disease or autonomous adrenal Cushing's or glucocorticoid therapy	*Suggested by:* round, florid face (and trunk with purple striae) with thinner arms and legs, hirsutism in females. Inability to rise from squatting position (due to proximal myopathy). *Confirmed by:* ↑**midnight cortisol** and/or failure to suppress on **dexamethasone suppression test** 0.5mg 6 hourly for 48h or drug history of glucocorticoids. *Initial management:* treat any infection, DM, hypertension and hypokalaemia. Consider metopirone® for temporary control. Plan pituitary adenectomy if Cushing's disease or adrenalectomy for adrenal adenoma + radiotherapy for carcinoma.

Proptosis of eye(s) or exophthalmos

Prominent eye suggested by sclera showing between the cornea and upper lid margin (may also be due to lid retraction due to sympathetic overactivity or lung disease). If in doubt, look down on eyes from above. (In myopia there is a large eyeball but the sclera is not visible.) Initial investigations (other tests in **bold** below): TSH±FT₄, CT orbit.

Main differential diagnoses and typical outline evidence, etc.	
Ophthalmic Graves's disease (± thyrotoxicosis)	*Suggested by:* bilateral (usually) exophthalmos, goitre, pretibial myxoedema, and lid retraction. Eyes not closing during sleep if severe.
	Confirmed by: ↑titre of thyroid antibodies (with ↓**TSH**, and ↑**T4** or ↑**T3**). **CT scan** appearance.
	Initial management: if mild, dark glasses, eye lubricants before bed or artificial tears during day. In severe cases, steroids PO or IV, external radiation or orbital decompression. Treat thyrotoxicosis.
Orbital cellulitis (medical emergency)	*Suggested by:* pain, fever, unilateral lid swelling, decreased vision, and double vision. Neurological signs in advanced disease.
	Confirmed by: **CT or MRI** *scan* appearance, and response to antibiotics.
	Initial management: antibiotics IV in hospital.
Cortico-cavernous fistula	*Suggested by:* unilateral engorgement of eye surface vessels, lid and conjunctiva, pulsatile with bruit over eye.
	Confirmed by: **CT or MRI** *scan* appearance.
	Initial management: pain control only.
Orbital tumours—rarely 1°, often 2°, especially reticulosis	*Suggested by:* unilateral proptosis and displacement of the eyeball. Lymph node, liver or spleen enlargement.
	Confirmed by: **CT or MRI** *scan* appearance.
	Initial management: pain control and treat eye infection, surgical decompression.

Red eye

Gritty pain suggests external cause. Aching pain suggests internal cause. Light sensitivity always accompanies inflammation in the eye. Fluorescein (Fl) yellow dye glows green with a blue examination light and stains all epithelial breaks. Initial investigations (other tests in **bold** below): Fl stain, swab culture and sensitivity.

Main differential diagnoses and typical outline evidence, etc.	
Spontaneous subconjunctival haemorrhage	*Suggested by:* painless bright red area on conjunctiva (oxygenated blood) and no light sensitivity.
	Confirmed by: clinical appearance and resolution over days. No Fl staining of cornea (not done often).
	Initial management: no treatment, resolves spontaneously; if sustained hypertension, treat.
Conjunctivitis due to bacterial infection	*Suggested by:* red sticky eyes, dilated blood vessels on the eyeball and the tarsal (lid) conjunctiva with a purulent discharge ± bilateral ± gritty pain.
	Confirmed by: above clinical appearance. Not light-sensitive and no Fl stain of cornea.
	Initial management: antibacterial eye drops, treat any underlying cause, e.g. dry eyes, blepharitis.
Conjunctivitis due to viral infection	*Suggested by:* red eyes with dilated vessels on the eyeball only, sometimes in one quadrant around the cornea with a watery 'tap running' discharge. Gritty pain ± impaired vision.
	Confirmed by: Fl stain showing dendritic (branching) pattern and resolution with topical antiviral.
	Initial management: aciclovir if herpetic infection.
Conjunctivitis due to allergy	*Suggested by:* red eyes with pink swollen conjunctiva and white stringy mucoid discharge, usually bilateral, episodic, and seasonal.
	Confirmed by: no Fl stain, and no visual loss and resolution with cromoglicate (over 6wk) or steroid eye drops.
	Initial management: advise to avoid allergens, topical sodium cromoglicate with oral antihistamine.
Giant papillary conjunctivitis	*Suggested by:* patient wearing soft contact lens, history of eye surgery. Eye red, itchy, and watery.
	Confirmed by: conjunctiva: cobblestone appearance.
	Initial management: remove irritating sutures, suspend contact lens until recovery. Advise about lens hygiene and minimize wearing time.

Corneal ulcer (ulcerative keratitis) due to abrasion or Herpes simplex, Pseudomonas, Candida, Aspergillus, protozoa	*Suggested by:* painful, watering, light-sensitive, deeply red eye with yellowish abscess in the cornea, purulent discharge, and blurring of vision. *Confirmed by:* slit lamp examination after **Fl *instillation showing*** hypopyon (pus in the eye). Dendritic staining pattern in herpes. *Initial management:* analgesics, cycloplegic eye drops (e.g. cyclopentolate) to ease pain, aciclovir in herpetic infections, eye patching for at least 24h. No steroid eye drops until a herpes infection is excluded.
Episcleritis	*Suggested by:* localized red eye with superficial vessel dilatation, mild pain, no visual loss or light sensitivity, history of recurrent episodes. *Confirmed by:* one drop of phenylephrine 2.5% causing a blanching of the lesion. *Initial management:* if mild, settles spontaneously; if not steroid eye drops and NSAIDs.
Scleritis associated with RA, SLE	*Suggested by:* localized area of dark red, dilated superficial and deep vessel on the sclera with aching pain and tenderness. Features of associated illness. *Confirmed by:* failure to blanch with one drop of 2.5% phenylephrine. *Initial management:* urgent referral for monitoring of progress ± systemic steroids.
Acute closed-angle glaucoma	*Suggested by:* severely painful red eye with marked visual loss, accompanied by nausea and vomiting ± history of haloes around lights and severe headache with blurred vision. *Confirmed by:* dull grey cornea, non-reacting and irregular pupil with **raised ocular pressures**. *Initial management:* analgesics and antiemetics, β-blocker drops, e.g. timolol; oral acetazolamide. Prevent recurrence by laser iridotomy.
Iritis or anterior uveitis	*Suggested by:* redness around cornea, haze in front of iris, and severe photophobia. *Confirmed by:* small, non-reacting and irregular pupil, **slit lamp examination** showing flare, cells and, hypopyon (pus in eye). *Initial management:* topical steroids, e.g. prednisolone. Systemic steroids and immunosuppressants if severe.

Iritis (anterior uveitis)

Redness in cornea next to iris (circumcorneal injection) with muddy appearance of fluid in front of iris. The eye is painful, red, and watering with photophobia and blurred vision. All cases are referred for specialist ophthalmic management and follow-up to prevent long-term damage with adhesions and glaucoma. Initial investigations (other tests in **bold** below): slit lamp examination, swab, culture and sensitivity, RF, CXR.

Main differential diagnoses and typical outline evidence, etc.	
Trauma (usually surgical)	*Suggested by:* impact accident, recent surgery. *Confirmed by:* **slit lamp examination** showing blood in the front of the eye and 'D' shaped distortion of the pupil if torn from its base or perforation if the pupil is pointing. *Initial management:* symptomatic: analgesia, dark glasses, specialist management.
Infection: Herpes simplex, zoster, TB, syphilis, leprosy, protozoa, fungi	*Suggested by:* general malaise, fever, leucocytosis. *Confirmed by:* **bacteriological culture** of eye swab or **viral immunology**. *Initial management:* symptomatic: analgesia, dark glasses, treatment according to virology or culture and sensitivity, specialist management.
Autoimmune diseases: ankylosing spondylitis, Reiter's disease, juvenile chronic arthritis, immune ocular disease	*Suggested by:* arthritis, anaemia, no obvious fever, raised ESR. *Confirmed by:* **immunology** (seronegative for Rheumatoid factor). **Protein electrophoresis**. *Initial management:* symptomatic: analgesia, dark glasses, specialist management with oral steroids and immunosuppressive agents.
Sarcoidosis	*Suggested by:* history of dry cough, breathlessness, malaise, fatigue, weight loss, enlarged lacrimal glands, erythema nodosum. Raised serum ACE. *Confirmed by:* **CXR** appearances (e.g. bilateral lymphadenopathy), **tissue biopsy** showing non-caseating granuloma. **Slit lamp examination** showing large keratic precipitates. *Initial management:* analgesia, NSAIDs for pain and erythema nodosum. If severe, oral steroids and immunosuppressive agents.
Ulcerative colitis	*Suggested by:* history of diarrhoea with mucus and blood. *Confirmed by:* **colonoscopy** appearance and **biopsy** histology. *Initial management:* prednisolone PO + mesalazine, prednisolone retention enemas; if severe, hydrocortisone IV followed by prednisolone PO and sulfasalazine; surgery.

Crohn's disease   *Suggested by:* history of abdominal pain, diarrhoea, weight loss.

Confirmed by: **colonoscopy, barium enema** and **meal** and follow-through.

Initial management: prednisolone for 2wk for mild attacks. Steroids IV in severe cases. Immuno-suppressants (e.g. methotrexate), immunotherapy (e.g. infliximab).

Clinical anaemia

Subconjunctival pallor (± face, nail and hand pallor). Initial investigations (other tests in **bold** below): FBC.

Main differential diagnoses and typical outline evidence, etc.	
Microcytic due to iron deficiency, thalassaemia, etc (see 📖p.716)	*Suggested by:* history of blood loss or family history of haemoglobinopathy (especially in Mediterranean origin) and sideroblastic anaemia.
	Confirmed by: **FBC:** ↓Hb and ↓MCV.
Macrocytic (see 📖p.718)	*Suggested by:* family history of pernicious anaemia, antifolate, and cytotoxic drugs or alcohol.
	Confirmed by: **FBC:** ↓Hb and ↑MCV. **Film:** hypersegmented polymorphs in B12 deficiency.
Normocytic (see 📖p.720)	*Suggested by:* history of chronic intercurrent illness, e.g. chronic renal failure, anemia of chronic disease, etc.
	Confirmed by: **FBC:** ↓Hb and normal MCV.
Hypoplastic or aplastic	*Suggested by:* gradual onset without blood loss and potentially causal medication.
	Confirmed by: **FBC:** ↓Hb and normal MCV and **bone marrow biopsy:** atrophic.
	Initial management: stop potential causative drugs. If persistent and severe, consider blood and platelet transfusion, combination immunosuppressants and bone marrow transplantation.
Leukaemia	*Suggested by:* gradual onset and large spleen or LN (rapid deterioration in acute leukaemia).
	Confirmed by: **FBC:** ↓Hb and normal MCV, ↑↑WCC. **Bone marrow biopsy:** replacement by leukaemic cells.
	Initial management: blood and platelet transfusions, chemotherapy, and bone marrow transplantation.

Fever

Temperature >37°. Fever is not a 'good lead'. The causes suggested here are broad. The approach is to listen carefully and examine for better diagnostic leads. Initial tests: FBC, MSU, blood cultures, viral and autoimmune serology (other tests in **bold** below):

Main differential diagnoses and typical outline evidence, etc.	
Infection	*Suggested by:* low grade or high fever with ↑WCC and usually symptoms and signs pointing to a focus.
	Confirmed by: **serology** ± **cultures** of blood and other body fluids.
Thrombus, tissue necrosis, neoplasm, autoimmune diseases, drugs	*Suggested by:* low grade fever, history of severe illness or trauma WCC normal.
	Confirmed by: specific tests, e.g. **CXR, Doppler US scan of leg veins.**

Possible hypothermia

Temperature <35°C—but confirm with low reading thermometer—it could be lower. Also confirm with rectal temperature. Initial investigations (other tests in **bold** below): FBC, TSH, FT4

Main differential diagnoses and typical outline evidence, etc.	
True hypothermia due to prolonged exposure to cold or hypothyroidism	*Suggested by:* history of immersion or cold weather exposure. Temperature <35° with low reading rectal thermometer.
	Confirmed by: temperature chart using low reading rectal thermometer.
	Initial management: rewarm patient slowly, e.g. 0.5°C/h (faster may be fatal). Ventilation, IV access, antibiotics, and bladder catheterization. Liaise with GP and social services before discharge to prevent recurrence.

Mouth lesions

Examine lips, buccal mucosa, teeth, tongue, tonsils, and pharynx. Initial investigations (other tests in **bold** below): FBC

Main differential diagnoses and typical outline evidence, etc.	
Local aphthous ulcers	*Suggested by:* red, painful ulcer with associated lymph node enlargement.
	Confirmed by: spontaneous resolution within days.
	Initial management: topical oral ointment.
Local infection and gingivitis	*Suggested by:* vesicles in *Herpes simplex*, creamy white plaques in oral candidiasis.
	Confirmed by: spontaneous resolution or after oral antiseptic or antifungal treatment within days.
	Initial management: oral antiseptic or antifungal.
Carious teeth	*Suggested by:* intermittent toothache, broken and/or severely discoloured teeth.
	Confirmed by: formal dental examination.
	Initial management: oral antiseptic, referral for course of dental treatment.
Traumatic ulceration	*Suggested by:* jagged ulcers or lacerations.
	Confirmed by: history of trauma, injury, ill-fitting dentures, shallow, painful ulcers.
	Initial management: referral for dental assessment.
Vitamin deficiency e.g. B_{12}, riboflavine, nicotinic acid	*Suggested by:* atrophic glossitis, fissured tongue; 'raw beef' in B_{12} deficiency, magenta in riboflavin deficiency.
	Confirmed by: response to vitamin supplements.
	Initial management: treat underlying conditions, e.g. malabsorption, refer to dietitian, advise well balanced diet and vitamin supplements.
Hereditary haemorrhagic telangiectasia	*Suggested by:* telangiectasia on the face, around the mouth, on the lips and tongue, epistaxis, anaemia.
	Confirmed by: family history and examination of relatives.
Peutz–Jegher's syndrome (associated with intestinal polyps)	*Suggested by:* peri-oral pigmentation (not the tongue).
	Confirmed by: finding polyps on **colonoscopy**.
	Initial management: referral for long-term follow-up with colonoscopy and removal of suspect lesions.

Red pharynx and tonsils

Initial investigations (other tests in **bold** below): FBC

Main differential diagnoses and typical outline evidence. etc.	
Viral pharyngitis	*Suggested by:* sore throat, pain on swallowing, fever, cervical lymphadenopathy and injected fauces. ↑lymphocytes, normal or ↓leucocytes.
	Confirmed by: –ve **throat swab** for bacterial culture, dehydration: resolution within days.
	Initial management: gargles/lozenges, paracetamol, etc.
Acute follicular tonsillitis (streptococcal)	*Suggested by:* severe sore throat, pain on swallowing, fever, enlarged tonsils with white patches (like strawberries and cream). Cervical lymphadenopathy, especially in angle of jaw. Fever, ↑leucocytes in WCC.
	Confirmed by: **throat swab** for culture and sensitivities of organisms.
	Initial management: analgesic, antibiotics, e.g. penicillin V or cephalosporin or clavulanic acid + amoxicillin.
Infectious mononucleosis (glandular fever) due to Epstein–Barr virus	*Suggested by:* very severe throat pain with enlarged tonsils covered with grey mucoid film. Petechiae on palate. Profound malaise. Generalized lymphadenopathy, splenomegaly.
	Confirmed by: ↑atypical lymphocytes in WBC. **Paul–Bunnell** or **Monospot®** test +ve. **Viral titres**.
	Initial management: gargles/lozenges, analgesics, e.g. paracetamol (amoxicillin causes rash, aspirin may cause Reye syndrome).
Candidiasis of buccal or oesophageal mucosa	*Suggested by:* painful dysphagia, white plaque, history of immunosuppression/diabetes/recent antibiotics.
	Confirmed by: **oesophagoscopy** showing erythema and plaques, **brush cytology ± biopsy** showing spores and hyphae.
	Initial management: analgesics, antifungal lozenges or solutions, e.g. nystatin suspension or oral fluconazole.
Agranulocytosis e.g. antithyroid drugs	*Suggested by:* sore throat, history of taking a drug (e.g carbimazole) or contact with noxious substance.
	Confirmed by: low or absent neutrophil count.
	Initial management: stop offending drug, broad-spectrum antibiotics IV or PO, if febrile.
Also with oropharyngeal ulceration;	Herpes zoster infection, Herpes simplex infection, local herpangina, aphthous ulceration, etc.
without oropharyngeal ulceration	Reflux oesophagitis, epiglottitis, blood dyscrasia, etc.

'Parotid' swelling

Swelling from anterior border of masseter muscle (teeth clenched) to lower half of ear and from zygoma to angle of jaw. Initial investigations (other tests in **bold** below): FBC

Main differential diagnoses and typical outline evidence, etc.	
Parotid duct obstruction (usually due to stone)	*Suggested by:* intermittent infection or no discharge from duct.
	Confirmed by: **plain X-ray** showing radio-opaque stone or **sialography** to show filling defect.
	Initial management: analgesia, referral for surgery.
Parotid tumour	*Suggested by:* no obvious features of alterative non-malignant or infective condition.
	Confirmed by: urgent surgical referral for **biopsy** or exploration.
	Initial management: referral for surgery.
Mumps parotitis	*Suggested by:* acute painful swelling of whole gland(s), contact with other cases.
	Confirmed by: bilateral swelling or associated pancreatitis or orchitis (rising mumps **viral titre**).
	Initial management: analgesia, fluids, etc.
Suppurative parotid infection	*Suggested by:* hot, tender, fluctuant swelling with high fever. No discharge from duct orifice.
	Confirmed by: WBC: ↑neutrophils response to antibiotics, drainage.
	Initial management: referral for surgery.
Non-suppurative parotitis from ascending infection along parotid duct	*Suggested by:* unilateral swelling, oral sepsis or poor general condition, fever.
	Confirmed by: WCC: ↑neutrophils, resolution with antibiotics.
	Initial management: analgesia, broad-spectrum antibiotics.
Parotid Sjögren's syndrome	*Suggested by:* dry mouth and eyes with no tears.
	Confirmed by: **rheumatoid factor** +ve, **anti Ro (SSA)** and **anti-La (SSB)** +ve.
	Initial management: oral lubricants (e.g. gelatin lozenge) and eye lubricant (e.g. methylcellulose).
Parotid sarcoidosis	*Suggested by:* history of dry cough, enlarged lacrimal glands, erythema nodosum, ↑serum ACE.
	Confirmed by: **CXR** appearances (e.g. bilateral lymphadenopathy) and **tissue biopsy** showing non-caseating granuloma.
	Initial management: oral lubricants, e.g. gelatin lozenge, NSAID if associated polyarthalgia; oral steroids if associated hypercalcaemia, or lung, heart, neurological involvement.

Lump in the face (non-parotid lesion)

Main differential diagnoses and typical outline evidence, etc.

Pre-auricular lymph node inflammation	*Suggested by:* tender, nodular swelling in front of ear.
	Confirmed by: above clinical features, spontaneous resolution, histology.
	Initial management: review in days. If no spontaneous resolution, refer for excision biopsy.
Pre-auricular lymphoma	*Suggested by:* non-tender, nodular swelling in front of ear.
	Confirmed by: **biopsy** with or without or excision.
	Initial management: surgical referral.
Basal cell carcinoma	*Suggested by:* painless ulcer with rolled edge.
	Confirmed by: **biopsy** appearance.
	Initial management: surgical referral.
Sebaceous cyst	*Suggested by:* fluctuant swelling with central punctum.
	Confirmed by: **incision** and content evacuation.
	Initial management: no treatment, antibiotics if infected, surgical referral if persistent.
Subcutaneous abscess	*Suggested by:* tender fluctuant swelling.
	Confirmed by: **incision** when pointing.
	Initial management: incision ± antibiotic.
Dental abscess	*Suggested by:* tenderness of underlying tooth (tap gently).
	Confirmed by: **dental exploration**.
	Initial management: dental referral.
Skin melanoma	*Suggested by:* painless swelling with pigment and red edge.
	Confirmed by: **wide excision biopsy** and histology.
	Initial management: surgical excision

Submandibular lump—not moving with tongue nor on swallowing

Below the mandible and above the digastric muscle. Initial investigations (other tests in **bold** below): FBC.

Main differential diagnoses and typical outline evidence, etc.	
Mumps sialitis	*Suggested by:* acute painful swelling of whole gland(s), contact with others cases.
	Confirmed by: bilateral swelling or associated pancreatitis or orchitis. (↑*mumps titre* if in doubt.)
	Initial management: analgesia, maintain hydration.
Non-suppura-tive sialitis from ascending infection along duct	*Suggested by:* unilateral swelling, oral sepsis, or poor general condition.
	Confirmed by: discharge from duct orifice. Resolution with antibiotics.
	Initial management: rehydration, antibiotics, oral hygiene, lemon drops to stimulate saliva production. Surgical drainage if intractable.
Suppurative salivary infection	*Suggested by:* hot, tender, fluctuant swelling with high fever. No discharge from duct orifice.
	Confirmed by: **US scan**, appearance.
	Initial management: **incision and** drainage ± antibiotics.
Salivary duct obstruction (usually due to stone)	*Suggested by:* intermittent infection or no discharge from duct.
	Confirmed by: **US scan** response to stomaplasty.
	Initial management: rehydration, analgesia, and antibiotics if fever and ↑WCC. Await spontaneous passage of small stone. Surgical removal if large.
Salivary Sjögren's syndrome	*Suggested by:* dry mouth and eyes with no tears.
	Confirmed by: **rheumatoid factor** +ve, **anti-Ro (SSA)** and **anti-La (SSB)** +ve.
	Initial management: oral lubricants (e.g. gelatin lozenge) and eye lubricant (e.g. methylcellulose).
Salivary sarcoidosis	*Suggested by:* dry cough, enlarged lacrimal glands, and erythema nodosum.
	Confirmed by: **CXR** appearances (e.g. bilateral lymphadenopathy) and tissue biopsy showing non-caseating granuloma.
	Initial management: oral lubricants, e.g. gelatin lozenge, NSAID if associated polyarthalgia; oral steroids if associated hypercalcaemia, or lung, heart, neurological involvement.
Salivary tumour due to ad-enocarcinoma, squamous cell tumour, etc.	*Suggested by:* no obvious features of alternative non-malignant or infective condition.
	Confirmed by: **biopsy or surgical exploration**.
	Initial management: surgical excision

Submandibular lymph node inflammation	*Suggested by:* tender, solid, nodular swelling between rami of mandible, especially <20y of age.
	Confirmed by: above clinical features or **US scan**.
	Initial management: await spontaneous resolution.
Submandibular lymph node malignancy	*Suggested by:* non-tender, solid nodular swelling between rami of mandible, especially age >20y.
	Confirmed by: **US scan, biopsy** appearance.
	Initial management: surgical excision.
Ranula	*Suggested by:* transilluminable cyst lateral to midline, with domed, bluish discoloration in floor of mouth lateral to frenulum.
	Confirmed by: clinical appearance, **US scan**, and *histology* after excision.
	Initial management: surgical excision
Submental dermoid	*Suggested by:* midline cyst and age <20 years.
	Confirmed by: **histology** after excison.
	Initial management: surgical excision

Anterior neck lump—moving with tongue and swallowing

Suggests extrathyroid tissue. Initial investigations (other tests in **bold** below): Ultrasound (US) scan

Main differential diagnoses and typical outline evidence, etc.	
Thyroglossal cyst	*Suggested by:* fluctuant, cystic lump in midline or just to the left.
	Confirmed by: **US scan** shows cystic lesion, **radioisotope scan** (cyst is cold), **CT scan**, **histology** of excised tissue.
	Initial management: surgical excision shows cyst.
Ectopic thyroid tissue	*Suggested by:* solid lump in midline or just laterally.
	Confirmed by: **US scan** shows non-cystic lesion, **radioisotope scan:** nodule taking up iodine, **CT scan**, **histology** of excised tissue.
	Initial management: surgical excision

Neck lump—moving with swallowing but not with tongue

Suggests a goitre (or something attached to thyroid gland).
The following are preliminary diagnoses (see also 🕮pp.154 and 156).
Initial investigations (other tests in **bold** below): TSH, FT4

Main differential diagnoses and typical outline evidence, etc.	
Thyrotoxic goitre	*Suggested by:* sweating, fine tremor, tachycardia, weight loss, lid lag.
	Confirmed by: ↑FT4 ± ↑FT3 and ↓↓TSH. **US scan** appearance, **isotope scan** appearance.
	Initial management: propranolol to control symptoms. Carbimazole 40mg od reduced to 5–15mg over 1–3mo period. FBC before starting treatment, warn about agranulocytosis, sore throat.
Hypothyroid goitre	*Suggested by:* cold intolerance, tiredness, constipation, bradycardia.
	Confirmed by: ↑TSH, ↓FT4. **US scan ± thyroid antibodies** +ve.
	Initial management: levothyroxine 25–50mcg od. Regular checks on TFT.
Euthyroid goitre	*Suggested by:* no sweating, no fine tremor, no weight change, no cold intolerance, no tiredness, no lid lag, normal bowel habit, normal pulse rate.
	Confirmed by: normal *FT4*, and normal *TSH*.
	Initial management: no treatment. Surgery if causing symptoms of compression in neck or thoracic inlet.

Bilateral neck mass—moving with swallowing but not with tongue

(Central mass crossing the midline). Initial investigations (other tests in **bold** below): TSH, FT4, ultrasound scan of goitre.

Main differential diagnoses and typical outline evidence, etc.	
Graves's disease	*Suggested by:* clinical thyrotoxicosis, exophthalmos, pretibial myxoedema. No nodules.
	Confirmed by: ↑**FT4** or ↑**FT3** and ↓**TSH** and **TSH receptor antibody** +ve. Diffusely increased uptake on **thyroid isotope scan**.
	Initial management: propranolol 40 to 80mg 8 hourly to control symptoms. Carbimazole 40mg od reduced to 5–10mg over 1–3mo with monthly TFT. FBC before starting. Written warning for agranulocytosis causing sore throat. Radioiodine or thyroidectomy offered if relapse after 6–18mo carbimazole.
Hashimoto's thyroiditis	*Suggested by:* clinically euthyroid or hypothyroid (or rarely transient thyrotoxicosis). Multiple nodules in large gland.
	Confirmed by: ↑**FT4** transiently then ↓**FT4** and ↑**TSH**, ↑↑**thyroid antibody titre**. Diffuse poor uptake on **thyroid isotope scan**.
	Initial management: analgesic, oral steroid if persistent pain. Thyroxine if TSH persistently ↑.
'Simple' goitre	*Suggested by:* clinically euthyroid. Not nodular.
	Confirmed by: **FT4** and **FT3** normal, **TSH** normal and **thyroid antibodies** –ve.
	Initial management: reassurance, no treatment.
Toxic multinodular goitre	*Suggested by:* multiple nodules and clinically thyrotoxic.
	Confirmed by: ↑**FT4** or ↑**FT3**, and ↓**TSH** and nodules on **US scan or thyroid isotope scan**.
	Initial management: carbimazole (± β-blocker for symptoms). Radioiodine very effective (not used if compression of adjacent structures in the neck and thoracic inlet—surgery offered instead).
Non-toxic multinodular goitre	*Suggested by:* multiple nodules, clinically euthyroid.
	Confirmed by: **FT4** or **FT3** normal **TSH** normal. Nodules on **US scan or thyroid isotope scan**.
	Initial management: surgery only if symptomatic.
Thyroid enzyme deficiency (rare)	*Suggested by:* presentation in childhood, clinically hypothyroid or euthyroid. Smooth goiter, not nodular.
	Confirmed by: ↓**FT4** and ↓**TSH** but with abnormal (high or low) *radioiodine uptake*. Thyroid antibodies –ve.
	Initial management: thyroxine replacement.

Solitary thyroid nodule

Initial investigations (other tests in **bold** below): TSH, FT4, ultrasound scan of thyroid.

Main differential diagnoses and typical outline evidence, etc.	
Autonomous toxic thyroid nodule	*Suggested by:* single nodule and 'clinically thyrotoxic': weight loss, frequent bowel movement, ↑pulse rate, sweats, tremor.
	Confirmed by: ↑*FT4* or ↑*FT3*, ↓*TSH,* and single hot nodule thyroid isotope (iodine or technetium) scan.
	Initial management: plan radioactive iodine therapy (treatment of choice) control symptoms with β-blocker ± carbimazole until euthyroid.
Thyroid carcinoma: papillary 60%, follicular 25%, medullary 5%, lymphoma 5%, anaplastic <1%	*Suggested by:* single nodule and clinically euthyroid.
	Confirmed by: normal *FT4* or *FT3*, normal *TSH* and single cold nodule **thyroid isotope scan**. Solid on **US scan**. Malignant cells on **needle aspiration** or **excision**.
	Initial management: total thyroidectomy, radioactive iodine for residual tissue and any tumour. Plan follow-up scans and eradication of any recurrence.
Thyroid adenoma	*Suggested by:* single nodule and clinically euthyroid.
	Confirmed by: normal *FT4* or *FT3*, normal *TSH* and single cold nodule **thyroid isotope scan**. Solid on **US thyroid scan**. No malignant cells on **needle aspiration** or **excision**.
	Initial management: partial thyroidectomy.
Thyroid cyst	*Suggested by:* single nodule and clinically euthyroid.
	Confirmed by: normal *FT4* or *FT3*, normal *TSH* and single cold nodule **thyroid isotope scan**. Cyst on **US scan**. Disappears on **needle aspiration** and no malignant cells then or if removed.
	Initial management: needle aspiration; surgery if persistent recurrence.

Lump in anterior triangle

Below digastric and in front of sternomastoid muscles. Initial investigations (other tests in **bold** below): FBC, ultrasound scan.

Main differential diagnoses and typical outline evidence, etc.	
Lymph node inflammation	*Suggested by:* tender, solid nodular swelling.
	Confirmed by: above clinical features, **CT scan**.
	Initial management: reassurance, follow-up until resolved.
Acute abscess	*Suggested by:* hot, tender, fluctuant swelling with high fever, WCC: ↑neutrophils.
	Confirmed by: clinical features and discharge of pus after incision.
	Initial management: incision.
Tuberculosis ('cold') abscess	*Suggested by:* fluctuant swelling with low grade or no fever.
	Confirmed by: acid-fast bacilli (AFB), on microscopy or culture and sensitivity of **aspirate**.
	Initial management: refer to TB specialist for provisional treatment pending result of culture and sensitivity with isoniazid, pyrazinamide, rifampicin for 2mo. If malnourished, add pyridoxine. Refer for contact tracing.
Branchial cyst	*Suggested by:* fluctuant swelling at anterior border of sternomastoid muscle, <20y of age.
	Confirmed by: **US scan, CT scan**, surgical anatomy, appearance and *histology* on excision.
	Initial management: surgical referral for excision.
Cystic hygroma	*Suggested by:* fluctuant swelling that transilluminates well, <20y of age.
	Confirmed by: **US scan, CT scan**, surgical anatomy, appearance and histology on **excision**, or regression with sclerosant.
	Initial management: surgical referral for excision.
Pharyngeal pouch	*Suggested by:* intermittent, fluctuant swelling (usually on left) and dysphagia.
	Confirmed by: **barium swallow** fills pouch.
	Initial management: surgical referral for excision.
Carotid body tumour (chemo-dectoma)	*Suggested by:* mobile, arising from carotid bifurcation (upper third of sternomastoid), soft, and gently pulsatile.
	Confirmed by: **US scan, CT scan**, surgical anatomy, appearance and histology on excision.
	Initial management: surgical referral for excision.
Hodgkin's or non-Hodgkin's lymphoma	*Suggested by:* non-tender, solid nodular swelling between rami of mandible, especially >20y of age ± fever, weight loss. Chest pain with alcohol in Hodgkin's.
	Confirmed by: **US scan, CT scan**, *biopsy* with or without or excision.
	Initial management: plan radiotherapy or chemotherapies depending on the stage of disease.

Lump in posterior triangle of neck

Behind sternomastoid and in front of trapezius. Initial investigations (other tests in **bold** below): FBC, ultrasound scan.

Main differential diagnoses and typical outline evidence, etc.	
Acute abscess	*Suggested by:* hot, tender fluctuant swelling with high fever, WCC: ↑neutrophils.
	Confirmed by: clinical features and discharge of pus after incision.
	Initial management: incision.
Cystic hygroma	*Suggested by:* fluctuant swelling that transilluminates well, <20y of age.
	Confirmed by: **US scan, CT scan**, surgical anatomy, appearance and histology on excision, or regression with sclerosant.
	Initial management: surgical referral for excision.
Lymph node inflammation	*Suggested by:* tender, solid nodular swelling.
	Confirmed by: above clinical features, **US scan**.
	Initial management: reassurance, follow-up until resolved.
Hodgkin's or non-Hodgkin's lymphoma	*Suggested by:* non-tender, solid nodular swelling. Chest pain with alcohol in Hodgkin's.
	Confirmed by: **US scan, CT scan, *biopsy*** with or without or excision.
	Initial management: plan radiotherapy or chemotherapy depending on stage of disease.
Metastasis in lymph node	*Suggested by:* non-tender, solid nodular swelling.
	Confirmed by: **US scan, CT scan, *biopsy*** ± excision.
	Initial management: plan radiotherapy or chemotherapy depending on 1° and stage of disease.
Tuberculous ('cold') abscess	*Suggested by:* non-tender, cystic swelling >50y of age.
	Confirmed by: US scan, **CT scan, *aspiration*** biopsy or excision, culture of *AFB*.
	Initial management: refer to TB specialist for provisional treatment pending result of culture and sensitivity with isoniazid, pyrazinamide, rifampicin ±ethambutol for 2mo. If malnourished, add pyridoxine. Refer for contact tracing.

Supraclavicular lump(s)

Initial investigations (other tests in **bold** below): ultrasound scan.

Main differential diagnoses and typical outline evidence, etc.	
Lymph node inflammation	*Suggested by:* tender, solid nodular swelling, especially <20y of age.
	Confirmed by: clinical features. **US scan**: solid lesion.
	Initial management: reassurance, follow-up to ensure resolution.
Lymphoma	*Suggested by:* rubbery, matted nodes.
	Confirmed by: lymph node *biopsy*.
	Initial management: radiotherapy or chemotherapy depending on stage
Lymph node↑s to gastric or lung carcinoma	*Suggested by:* rock-hard, fixed nodes, Virchow's node in left supraclavicular fossa (Troisier's sign).
	Confirmed by: lymph node *biopsy, gastroscopy, bronchoscopy.*
	Initial management: radiotherapy or chemotherapy depending on 1° source and stage
Aneurysm of subclavian artery	*Suggested by:* pulsatile cyst.
	Confirmed by: **US** *scan* and *MRI scan* or *angiography.*
	Initial management: surgical referral for assessment of feasibility of excision and repair.

Galactorrhoea

Spontaneous or expressible milky fluid. Initial investigations (other tests in **bold** below): prolactin, TSH, FT4, pregnancy test.

Main differential diagnoses and typical outline evidence, etc.	
1° hyperprolacti-naemia	*Suggested by:* infertility, oligomenorrhoea, or amenorrhoea.
	Confirmed by: ↑**prolactin** and normal **TSH** and T4. **Pituitary CT or MRI scan:** normal.
	Initial management: dopamine agonists, e.g. long-term bromocriptine or cabergoline.
Prolactinoma	*Suggested by:* infertility, oligomenorrhoea, or amenorrhoea. In large tumours, field defects and loss of 2° sexual characteristics.
	Confirmed by: ↑**prolactin** and normal **TSH** and **T4**. Micro- or macro-adenoma on **pituitary CT or MRI scan**.
	Initial management: dopamine agonist, e.g. bromocriptine and cabergoline. Surgical intervention if intolerance to medical treatment or presence of field defect or other pressure effects.
Pregnancy	*Suggested by:* amenorrhoea, frequency of urine, etc. in woman of childbearing age.
	Confirmed by: **pregnancy test** +ve.
	Initial management: explanation.
1° hypothyroidism	*Suggested by:* cold intolerance, tiredness, constipation, bradycardia.
	Confirmed by: ↑**TSH**, ↓**FT4**.
	Initial management: levothyroxine, e.g. 50mcg od. Check TFT after 1–2mo and titrate dose.
Drugs	*Suggested by:* taking chlorpramazine and other major tranquilizers, metoclopramide, domperidone.
	Confirmed by: ↑**prolactin**, resolution and lowering of **prolactin** after stopping suspect drug.
	Initial management: stop causative drug
'Idiopathic galactorrhoea'	*Suggested by:* galactorrhoea, no other findings.
	Confirmed by: normal **prolactin**.
	Initial management: short course (e.g 4wk) of dopamine agonists, e.g. cabergoline.

Nipple abnormality

Initial investigations (other tests in **bold** below): swab of discharged, culture, and sensitivity.

Main differential diagnoses and typical outline evidence, etc.	
Paget's disease of nipple with underlying carcinoma	*Suggested by:* breast nipple 'eczema'.
	Confirmed by: in situ malignant change on **histological examination** of **skin scrapings**.
	Initial management: surgical excision or mastectomy combined with endocrine therapy and chemotherapy.
Duct ectasia and chronic infection	*Suggested by:* green or brown nipple discharge.
	Confirmed by: chronic inflammation on **histology** of excised ducts.
	Initial management: analgesics for breast pain, surgical excision of lumps, antibiotics for infection.
Duct papilloma	*Suggested by:* bleeding from nipple.
	Confirmed by: excision of affected ducts. Benign **histology** of **excised ducts**.
	Initial management: surgical referral for excision of affected ducts.
Mammillary fistula	*Suggested by:* discharge from para-areolar region aged 30–40.
	Confirmed by: excision of affected ducts. Benign **histology** of excised ducts.
	Initial management: surgical referral for excision of affected ducts.

Breast lump(s)

Initial investigations (other tests in **bold** below): mammography.

Main differential diagnoses and typical outline evidence, etc.	
Benign fibrous mammary dysplasia	*Suggested by:* generally painful breast lumpiness, greatest near axilla. Cyclically related to periods.
	Confirmed by: relief on **aspiration** of cysts, diuretics or oestrogen suppression.
	Initial management: surgical referral for aspiration of cysts.
Fibroadenoma	*Suggested by:* smooth and mobile lump ('breast mouse'), usually in ages 15–30y.
	Confirmed by: appearance on **mammogram** confirmed by benign *histology* after excision.
	Initial management: surgical referral for excision of adenoma.
Cyst(s)	*Suggested by:* spherical, fluctuant lump, single or multiple, painful before periods.
	Confirmed by: cysts on **mammography**, benign tissue after excision.
	Initial management: surgical referral for excision of cyst.
Acute or chronic abscess	*Suggested by:* fluctuant lump, hot and tender, acute presentation often in puerperium. Chronic after antibiotics.
	Confirmed by: response to drainage, chronic abscess excision, and **histology** to exclude carcinoma.
	Initial management: surgical referral for drainage.
Fat necrosis or sclerosing adenosis	*Suggested by:* firm, solitary localized lump.
	Confirmed by: appearance on mammogram confirmed by benign **histology** after excision.
	Initial management: surgical referral for excision of affected tissue.
Carcinoma infiltrating ductal cancer or invasive lobar cancers	*Suggested by:* fixed, irregular, hard, painless lump, nipple retraction, fixed to skin (peau d'orange) or muscle, and local, hard or firm, fixed nodes in axilla.
	Confirmed by: **mammography** showing ill-defined, spiculate borders, faint linear or irregular calcification, and abnormal adjacent structures. Malignant *histology on after* **breast aspiration** or **excision**.
	Initial management: surgical referral for excision.

Gynaecomastia

These findings should have been discovered during the general examination. Breast swelling in male with disc of firm tissue. If there is no disc, it is fatty tissue only. Initial investigations (other tests in **bold** below): LH, FSH, plasma Testosterone, oestrogens.

Main differential diagnoses and typical outline evidence, etc.	
Immature testis	*Suggested by:* adolescence and no testicular lump.
	Confirmed by: normal testosterone, oestrogen and LH levels normal, **US scan of testis**.
	Initial management: explanation and reassurance that spontaneous resolution can be expected over months.
Digoxin, spironolactone	*Suggested by:* taking of drug and no testicular lump.
	Confirmed by: improvement when drug stopped.
	Initial management: stop suspect drug.
High alcohol intake	*Suggested by:* high alcohol intake and no testicular lump.
	Confirmed by: improvement when alcohol stopped.
	Initial management: stop alcohol.
Hepatic cirrhosis	*Suggested by:* long history of high alcohol intake (usually), spider naevi, abnormal liver size (large or small) and consistency (fatty or hard).
	Confirmed by: **LFT** abnormal, **↓LH, ↑oestrogens, ↓testosterone**.
	Initial management: dietary and alcohol advice, avoid sedatives and opiates. Vitamin K *if* ↑*prothrombin time*. Colestyramine for pruritus. Spironolactone + furosemide for oedema, ascites. Interferon-alpha to delay development of hepatoma.
Testicular tumours	*Suggested by:* scrotal mass ± pain, tenderness if haemorrhage occurs (sometimes in undescended testis).
	Confirmed by: **testicular US scan**, inguinal exploration, ↑*alpha-fetoprotein*, ↑*β-hCG*.
	Initial management: surgical referral for orchidectomy, radiotherapy or chemotherapy. (Seminomas radiosensitive, teratomas sensitive to combination chemotherapy).
Hypogonadism (1° testicular disease, or 2° to low LH from pituitary defect or tumour)	*Suggested by:* sparse pubic hair, no drug or alcohol history, poor libido.
	Confirmed by: ↓**testosterone**, ↑**LH** (in 1° testicular disease), ↓**LH** or normal (if 2° to pituitary diseases).
	Initial management: testosterone replacement therapy IM, gel, patch, or depot injection.

Bronchial carcinoma	*Suggested by:* smoking history, haemoptysis, weight loss, clubbing.
	Confirmed by: **CXR, bronchoscopy** with biopsy.
	Initial management: surgical referral for resection combined with radiotherapy or chemotherapy.
Klinefelter's syndrome	*Suggested by:* poor sexual development, infertility, eunuchoid.
	Confirmed by: **47, XXY karyotype**.
	Initial management: testosterone replacement therapy IM, gel, patch, or depot injection.
Obesity	*Suggested by:* no breast tissue, only mammary fat.
	Confirmed by: improvement with weight loss.
	Initial management: lifestyle changes; diet and exercise. Drug and surgical treatment, e.g. gastric banding, if intractable and life-threatening.

Axillary lymphadenopathy

Axillary lymphadenopathy ± tenderness. Initial investigations (other tests in **bold** below):

Main differential diagnoses and typical outline evidence, etc.	
Reaction to infection, e.g. viral prodrome, HIV infection, etc.	*Suggested by:* tender, solid nodular swelling(s).
	Confirmed by: clinical features.
	Initial management: identify underlying cause and treat if necessary.
Infiltration by tumour, e.g. breast	*Suggested by:* non-tender, solid nodular swelling(s).
	Confirmed by: excision biopsy.
	Initial management: identify underlying cause and treat as necessary.
Reticulosis or primary tumour	*Suggested by:* non-tender, solid nodular swelling(s).
	Confirmed by: excision biopsy.
	Initial management: identify underlying cause and treat if necessary.
Drug effect	*Suggested by:* drug history, e.g. phenytoin, retroviral drug.
	Confirmed by: improvement when drug withdrawn.
	Initial management: stop suspect drug.

Hirsutism in female

Upward extension of pubic hair in female. Hirsute upper lip, sideburns, chin. Initial investigations (other tests in **bold** below): plasma LH, FSH, testosterone, SHBG, ultrasound scan ovaries.

Main differential diagnoses and typical outline evidence, etc.	
Racial skin sensitivity	*Suggested by:* family history, normal menstrual periods (and fertility if applicable).
	Confirmed by: **LH** normal, **testosterone** normal.
	Initial management: explanation, recommend cosmetic measures.
Polycystic ovary syndrome	*Suggested by:* gradual increase in hirsutism since puberty, thin head hair, irregular periods, infertility.
	Confirmed by: ↑**testosterone**, ↓**SHBG**, ↑**LH** (tests done in follicular phase of menstrual cycle). **US scan** showing cystic ovaries.
	Initial management: metformin to reduce insulin resistance. Combined oestrogen 'pill' to ↑SHBG and ↓free androgen. Co-cyprindiol (contains cyproterone) for hirsutism. Clomifene to induce ovulation.
Ovarian or adrenal carcinoma	*Suggested by:* change in hair pattern over months, voice deeper, breast atrophy, no periods, cliteromegaly.
	Confirmed by: ↓**LH** and ↑↑**testosterone**. **US scan** and laparoscopy findings.
	Initial management: surgical removal of adrenal or ovary-containing tumour.
Cushing's syndrome pituitary-driven Cushing's disease, or autonomous adrenal Cushing's, or glucocorticoid therapy	*Suggested by:* round, florid face (and trunk with purple striae) with thinner arms and legs, hirsutism in females. Inability to rise from squatting position (due to proximal myopathy).
	Confirmed by: ↑**midnight cortisol** and/or failure to suppress on **dexamethasone suppression test** 0.5mg 6 hourly for 48h, or drug history of glucocorticoids.
	Initial management: treat any infection, DM, hypertension, and hypokalaemia. Consider metopirone for temporary control. Plan pituitary adenectomy if Cushing's disease or adrenalectomy for adrenal adenoma + radiotherapy for carcinoma.

Abdominal striae

White striae are healed pink or purple striae. Initial investigations (other tests in **bold** below): pregnancy test, 24 hour urinary free cortisol.

- Pink striae

Main differential diagnoses and typical outline evidence, etc.	
Pregnancy	*Suggested by:* no periods and obvious pregnant uterus.
	Confirmed by: **pregnancy test** +ve and **US scan abdomen/pelvis**.
	Initial management: explanation.
Simple obesity	*Suggested by:* large abdomen and usually rapid weight increase.
	Confirmed by: above clinical findings.
	Initial management: lifestyle changes, diet, and exercise.

- Purple striae

Main differential diagnoses and typical outline evidence, etc.	
Glucocorticoid steroid therapy	*Suggested by:* truncal obesity, purple striae, bruising, moon face, and buffalo hump.
	Confirmed by: drug history: taking high dose of glucocorticoid.
	Initial management: stop medications if appropriate.
Cushing's disease (ACTH driven)	*Suggested by:* truncal obesity, purple striae, bruising, moon face and buffalo hump. Pigmented creases (suggest ↑ACTH, especially in ectopic ACTH from a carcinoma or carcinoid tumour). **↑24h urinary free cortisol**.
	Confirmed by: 2x **↑midnight cortisol** and failure to suppress cortisol after dexamethazone 0.5mg 6 hourly for 48h and **↑midnight ACTH**, and bilaterally large adrenals on **CT or MRI** *scan*.
	Initial management: treat infections, electrolyte disturbances, DM, hypertension and psychiatric symptoms. Initial control with metopirone until response to surgery. Removal of pituitary adenoma or bilateral adrenalectomy if source not identified.
Cushing's syndrome due to adrenal adenoma or carcinoma	*Suggested by:* truncal obesity, purple striae, and bruising. No pigmentation in skin creases. **↑24h urinary free cortisol**.
	Confirmed by: 2x **↑midnight cortisol** and failure to suppress cortisol after **dexamethasone suppression test** 0.5mg 6 hourly for 48h and **↓midnight ACTH**, and unilateral large adrenal on **CT or MRI** *scan*.
	Initial management: treat infection, DM, hypertension and hypokalaemia. Initial control with metopirone until surgical treatment successful. Adrenalectomy for adenoma and carcinoma, also radiotherapy.

Obesity

Definition: BMI >30kgm^{-2}. Initial investigations (other tests in **bold** below):
TSH, FT4, 24 hour urinary free cortisol.

Main differential diagnoses and typical outline evidence, etc.	
Simple obesity	*Suggested by:* limb and truncal obesity.
	Confirmed by: TSH and FT4 normal. 24h urinary cortisol normal.
	Initial management: lifestyle changes, dieting, and exercise. Medical and surgical treatment for↑ appropriate candidates.
Hypothyroidism	*Suggested by:* cold intolerance, tiredness, ↑ constipation, bradycardia.
	Confirmed by: ↑**TSH**, ↓**FT4**.
	Initial management: levothyroxine 50mcg/d. Assess clinically and TSH after 4–8wk. Aim TSH to be normal (not suppressed). For elderly or in angina, start treatment with half the dose of levothyroxine.
Cushing's syndrome pituitary-driven Cushing's disease, or autonomous adrenal Cushing's, or glucocorticoid therapy	*Suggested by:* round, florid face (and trunk with purple striae) with thinner arms and legs, hirsutism in females. Inability to rise from squatting position (due to proximal myopathy).
	Confirmed by: ↑**midnight cortisol** and/or failure to suppress on **dexamethasone suppression test** 0.5mg 6 hourly for 48h, or drug history of glucocorticoids.
	Initial management: treat any infection, DM, hypertension, and hypokalaemia. Consider metopirone for temporary control. Plan pituitary adenectomy if Cushing's disease or adrenalectomy for adrenal adenoma + radiotherapy for carcinoma.

Pigmented creases and flexures (and buccal mucosa)

Suggests excess ACTH secretion. Initial investigations (other tests in **bold** below): U&E, 9am fasting cortisol, 24 hour urinary free cortisol.

Main differential diagnoses and typical outline evidence, etc.	
Addison's disease = 1° adrenal failure due to autoimmune destruction or TB	*Suggested by:* fatigue, ↓BP, and postural drop. *Confirmed by:* ↓9 a.m cortisol with poor response to **Synacthen stimulation test** and ↑**ACTH**. *Initial management:* hydrocortisone (e.g. 10mg mane and 5mg evening) and fludrocortisone 50–200mcg. Supply steroid deficiency warning card. Hydrocortisone IM if oral therapy is not possible.
Cushing's disease (ACTH-driven)	*Suggested by:* truncal obesity, purple striae, bruising, moon face, and buffalo hump. Pigmented creases (suggest ↑ACTH, especially in ectopic ACTH from a carcinoma or carcinoid tumour). ↑**24h urinary free cortisol**. *Confirmed by:* 2x ↑**midnight cortisol** and failure to suppress cortisol after dexamethazone 0.5mg 6 hourly for 48h, and ↑**midnight ACTH**, and bilaterally large adrenals on **CT or MRI** *scan*. *Initial management:* treat infections, electrolyte disturbances, DM, hypertension, and psychiatric symptoms. Initial control with metopirone until response to surgery. Removal of pituitary adenoma or bilateral adrenalectomy if source not identified.
Ectopic ACTH secretion	*Suggested by:* general weakness, proximal myopathy, usually evidence of lung cancer or other malignancy. *Confirmed by:* ↓serum potassium, 2x ↑**midnight cortisols**, and ↑**ACTH**. *Initial management:* medical treatment using Metopirone to reduce cortisol production. Surgical treatment if tumour source of ACTH can be localized or bilateral adrenalectomy if tumour source cannot be localized.

Spider naevi

Red, pinhead-sized spots with radiating blood vessels that empty when centre pressed by pinhead-sized object. Initial investigations (other tests in **bold** below): pregnancy test, LFTs.

Main differentials, typical outline evidence & initial management	
Normal	*Suggested by:* small numbers on chest (<3), usually in a young woman on chest and upper back.
	Confirmed by: no increase with time.
	Initial management: explanation and reassurance.
Taking oestrogens	*Suggested by:* small numbers on chest in a young woman on pill.
	Confirmed by: decrease when pill stopped in due course (no urgency).
	Initial management: explanation and reassurance.
Pregnancy	*Suggested by:* moderate numbers in a pregnant woman.
	Confirmed by: decrease when pregnancy over.
	Initial management: explanation and reassurance.
Liver failure	*Suggested by:* large numbers on chest, also on neck and face, jaundice, features of liver failure.
	Confirmed by: ↓**albumin**, ↑**prothrombin time**.
	Initial management: explanation, no alcohol, dietary advice, vitamin K *if* ↑prothrombin time, low salt diet if ascites, anti-flu and pneumococcal vaccination, colestyramine for pruritus.

Thin, wasted, cachectic

Initial investigations (other tests in **bold** below): FBC, TSH, FT4.

Main differential diagnoses and typical outline evidence, etc.	
Low calorie intake, e.g. anorexia nervosa, alcoholism, drug abuse, any prolonged systemic illness, e.g. severe **COPD**	*Suggested by:* dietary history.
	Confirmed by: dietitian's assessment, as inpatient if necessary.
	Initial management: controlled balanced diet with food chart to document intake, twice weekly weighing.
Thyrotoxicosis	*Suggested by:* normal appetite and adequate intake, frequent loose bowel movement, lid retraction and lag, sweats, tachycardia.
	Confirmed by: **↓TSH**, **↑FT4↑** and/or **↑FT3**.
	Initial management: propranolol to control symptoms. Medical treatments with antithyroid drugs, e.g. carbimazole; radioiodine for hot nodules or offer this or surgery if relapse after 6–18mo course.
AIDS	Suggested by: signs of opportunistic infection, e.g. oral candidiasis, oral hairy leukoplakia, Kaposi's sarcoma, lymphadenopathy.
	Confirmed by: detection of **HIV antibodies** in serum, **HIV RNA in plasma**.
	Initial management: chemotherapy using anti-retroviral therapy, chemoprophylaxis against opportunistic infections, e.g. TB, and general and sexual health advice.
Malignancy	*Suggested by:* progressive weight loss and malaise, poor appetite.
	Confirmed by: metastases in liver on **US scan**, bone 2° on **plain X-rays**, 1° tumour on **upper or lower GI endoscopy, bronchoscopy**, etc .
	Initial management: plan surgery or chemotherapy or radiotherapy depending on nature of 1° and staging of disease.
TB	*Suggested by:* cough, night sweats, haemoptysis, CXR: abnormal shadowing.
	Confirmed by: **AFB in sputum** on microscopy, **mycobacteria on culture**, response to antibiotics.
	Initial management: refer to TB specialist for provisional treatment pending result of culture and sensitivity with isoniazid, pyrazinamide, rifampicin for 2mo. If malnourished, add pyridoxine. Refer for contact tracing.

Purpura

Covers a spectrum from small pinpoint petechiae to large areas of 'bruising' in skin; do not blanch when compressed. Initial investigations (other tests in **bold** below): FBC, ESR, clotting (PT/INR)

Main differential diagnoses and typical outline evidence, etc.	
Thrombocytopenia due to autoimmune process or idiopathic **(ITP), SLE**	*Suggested by:* petechiae, haemorrhagic manifestations, e.g. epistaxis, and history of associated condition, e.g. viral illness. *Confirmed by:* ↓**platelet count** but *RBC* and *WCC* normal. No splenomegaly and normal bone marrow examination; **platelets antibodies** +ve. *Initial management:* for mild cases (e.g. platelets >20×10⁹ or no haemorrhagic manifestations): observe. Otherwise, oral steroids over 2wk, then tapered over months ± immunoglobulin, immunosuppressants, and splenectomy.
Pancytopenia due to aplastic anaemia, hypersplenism, myelodysplasia, disseminated intravascular coagulation	*Suggested by:* petechiae and history of associated condition. *Confirmed by:* ↓**platelet count**, ↓*WCC*, ↓*Hb*. *Initial management:* prompt treatment of infections, prophylactic antibiotics, and antifungal agents, try oral steroids and immunoglobulin IV.
Platelet dysfunction due to aspirin, NSAIDs, renal failure	*Suggested by:* bruising and drug history. *Confirmed by:* less bruising when suspected drug stopped or other cause removed. *Initial management:* stop suspected drug or treat potential cause.
Congenital vasculopathy due to Osler–Weber–Rendu syndrome, etc.	*Suggested by:* bruising from punctiform malformations on mucous membranes. Nose bleeds, gastrointestinal (GI) bleeding. *Confirmed by:* clinical findings, and normal **platelet count** and **clotting**. *Initial management:* topical oestrogen.
Acquired vasculopathy senile changes, autoimmune vasculitis (Henoch–Schönlein), steroids, scurvy	*Suggested by:* bruising into associated thin skin with atrophied subcutaneous tissue. *Confirmed by:* normal **platelet count** and **clotting**. *Initial management:* protection of skin from mechanical injury, treatment directed at cause, e.g. oral steroids for autoimmune conditions.

Acquired coagulopathy	*Suggested by:* bruising and history of associated condition.
due to liver disease, vitamin K deficiency, **DIC**	*Confirmed by:* prolonged **prothrombin time**.
	Initial management: protection of skin and joints from injury, treatment directed at cause, e.g. vitamin K injections for vitamin K deficiency.
Congenital coagulopathy	*Suggested by:* lifelong bruising and bleeding (after tooth extraction, heavy periods).
e.g. Von Willebrand's disease	*Confirmed by:* abnormal platelets function (count normal) and long **APTT**.
	Initial management: protection of skin and joints from injury, avoid NSAIDs. In Von Willebrand's, vasopressin for mild bleeding, rich Factor VIII prior to surgery.
Drug effect	*Suggested by:* drug history, e.g. warfarin, steroids.
	Confirmed by: improvement or drug withdrawal.
	Initial management: stop suspected drugs.

Generalized lymphadenopathy

Initial investigations (other tests in **bold** below): FBC

Main differential diagnoses and typical outline evidence, etc.	
Infectious mononucleosis (glandular fever) due to Epstein–Barr virus	*Suggested by:* very severe throat pain with enlarged tonsils covered with creamy membrane. Petechiae on palate. Profound malaise. Generalized lymphadenopathy, splenomegaly. *Confirmed by:* **Paul–Bunnel test** +ve. **Viral titres**: ↑Epstein–Barr titres. *Initial management:* analgesia, e.g. paracetamol, avoid antibiotics (amoxicillin may cause rash).
Hodgkin's lymphoma	*Suggested by:* anaemia, splenomegaly, multiple lymph node enlargement. *Confirmed by:* **lymph node histology** showing Reed–Sternberg cells. *Initial management:* radiotherapy for the early stage, for the more advanced chemotherapy (MOPP) alone or combined with radiotherapy.
Non-Hodgkin's lymphoma	*Suggested by:* anaemia, multiple lymph node enlargement. *Confirmed by:* **lymph node histology** with no Reed–Sternberg cells. *Initial management:* radiotherapy for localized disease, chlorambucil for systemic disease.
Chronic myeloid leukaemia (CML)	*Suggested by:* splenomegaly, variable hepatomegaly, bruising, anaemia. *Confirmed by:* presence of **Philadelphia chromosome**, ↑**WCC**, e.g. >100x10⁹/L. *Initial management:* allopurinol, imatinib, HLA typing, sibling-matched allogenic transplantation in the chronic phase.
Chronic lymphocytic leukaemia (CLL)	*Suggested by:* anorexia, weight loss, enlarged, rubbery, non-tender lymph nodes. Hepatomegaly, late splenomegaly. Bruising, anaemia. *Confirmed by:* **FBC**: marked lymphocytosis. **Bone marrow** infiltration with leukaemic cells. *Initial management:* monitor asymptomatic patients, chemotherapy for the symptomatic, allogenic, or autologous stem cell transplantation.
Acute myeloid leukaemia (AML)	*Suggested by:* generalized lymphadenopathy in adult patient, previous cytotoxics for myelodysplasia, variable hepatomegaly, bruising, anaemia. *Confirmed by:* blast cells in **bone marrow biopsy**. *Initial management:* explanation and counselling, prompt treatment of infection, supportive transfusions, allopurinol to prevent hyperuricaemia, plan for need of cranial irradiation and intrathecal chemotherapy, cytotoxics, stem cell transplantation.

Acute lymphoblastic leukaemia (ALL)	*Suggested by:* generalized lymphadenopathy in childhood or Down's patient, variable hepatomegaly, bruising, anaemia.
	Confirmed by: presence of **immunological marker** of common (CD10), T-cell, β-cell, null-cell, associated **chromosomal abnormalities**.
	Initial management: explanation and counselling, prompt treatment of infection, supportive transfusions, allopurinol to prevent hyperuricaemia, plan for need of cranial irradiation and intrathecal chemotherapy, cytotoxics, stem cell transplantation.
Sarcoidosis	*Suggested by:* dry cough, breathlessness, malaise, fatigue, weight loss, enlarged lacrimal glands, erythema nodosum.
	Confirmed by: **CXR** appearances (e.g. bilateral lymphadenopathy), and **tissue biopsy** showing non-caseating granuloma.
	Initial management: observe if asymptomatic, then NSAIDs for pains and erythema nodosum; if symptoms not mild or progression, oral steroids and immunosuppressive agents.
Drug effect	*Suggested by:* drug history, e.g. phenytoin, retroviral drug.
	Confirmed by: improvement when drug withdrawn.
	Initial management: stop suspected drug(s).

Localized groin lymphadenopathy

Non-specific finding. Initial investigations (other tests in **bold** below): FBC

Main differential diagnosis and typical outline evidence, etc.	
Infection somewhere in lower limb or pelvis (usually in past and node remained large)	*Suggested by:* enlarged nodes confined to groins.
	Confirmed by: local infection in foot or leg, or no symptoms or signs of generalized condition.
	Initial management: antibiotics if bacterial infection not resolving within days.

Pressure sores

Blisters or ulcers on heel or sacrum. Initial investigations (other tests in **bold** below): FBC, U&E

Main differential diagnoses and typical outline evidence, etc.	
Prolonged contact	*Suggested by:* history ± sensory loss, e.g. spinal cord injury, cerebrovascular accident.
	Confirmed by: response to frequent turning, dressings, and wound care.
	Initial management: frequent turning, dressings, and wound care. Swab wound and treat specific infections, e.g. MRSA.
Poor nutrition	*Suggested by:* weight falling, **↓Hb**, **↓total protein**, **↓potassium**.
	Confirmed by: formal dietary assessment, response to improved nutrition.
	Initial management: controlled diet, food diary, weigh 2x weekly, monitor FBC, serum protein, potassium, etc.

Skin symptoms and physical signs

Diagnosis in dermatology

Diagnosis is based on pattern recognition in a far more direct way in dermatology than in other specialties. The diagnosis becomes final with the response of the problem to treatment or by its long-term progress. Biopsy and histology are also used widely, especially when malignancy is suspected or the treatment involves prolonged use of toxic drugs. Identify one aspect of the skin appearance so that it can be used as a diagnostic lead, and scan the pages showing diagnoses linked to that lead to see if you can recognize the remainder of a pattern compatible only with one condition. By seeing many patients, you will learn to 'recognize' conditions more readily.

Brown macule

Flat, well-demarcated area of brown skin of any size. Main test is photography to assess change or biopsy usually to exclude malignancy. Initial investigations (others below in **bold**): FBC, digital photography of lesion.

Main differential diagnoses and typical outline evidence, etc.	
Flat mole (junctional naevus) (distinguish from malignant melanoma)	*Suggested by:* little variability of brown pigmentation, smooth outline—not irregular, multiple, no symmetry of lesions, not raised, or surrounded by erythema. *Confirmed by:* no change over weeks to months, benign **biopsy** appearance. *Initial management:* reassurance and review biopsy, in case of doubt or patient's anxiety.
Freckles and solar lentigines	*Suggested by:* small (<5mm), pale brown, asymmetrical macules, especially on face, red-haired, increased prominence after exposure to sun, asymmetrically distributed. *Confirmed by:* no change over months to years. *Initial management:* reassurance; if lentigine, responds to cryotherapy.
Chloasma	*Suggested by:* appearance of large (>5mm) areas of pigmentation during pregnancy. *Confirmed by:* resolution in months following delivery. *Initial management:* reassurance, sunscreens, and camouflage cosmetics.
Café-au-lait spot	*Suggested by:* one or more light brown, flat, sharply demarcated, evenly pigmented oval macules. *Confirmed by:* no change over months to years. *Initial management:* if >6 in number and >5mm in diameter, investigate for neurofibromatosis.
Pseudo-acanthosis nigricans (benign, no association with malignancy)	*Suggested by:* dark spots on the skin in the flexures, e.g. axillae of obese people, type 2 diabetics, or acromegalics. *Confirmed by:* no change over months or years. Diagnosis of underlying condition. *Initial management:* reassurance. Treat underlying condition.
Acanthosis nigricans (may be associated with malignancy)	*Suggested by:* skin thickening and pigmentation over months or years. *Confirmed by:* presence of pigmented, velvety, and papillomatous skin lesion of flexures, neck, nipples, and umbilicus. *Initial management:* advise weight reduction, and investigations for an underlying cause, e.g. diabetes mellitus, acromegaly, and malignancy.

Berloque dermatitis	*Suggested by:* red-brown macules on neck after exposure to sunlight. *Confirmed by:* history of bergamot-containing cosmetics applied to same area. *Initial management:* sunblock and avoidance of exposure to sun. Cosmetics to conceal pigmentation.
Plant chemical hyperphoto-sensitivity	*Suggested by:* red-brown macules on arms, hands, and face (blistering first) after exposure to sunlight. *Confirmed by:* history of cutting plants (e.g. giant hogweed) without skin covering. *Initial management:* sunblock and avoidance of exposure to sun. Cosmetics to conceal pigmentation.
Hutchinson's freckle (with risk of progression to malignant melanoma)	*Suggested by:* large, irregular macule developed from smaller one with variable expansion, regression, or coalescence to form irregular pigmented areas up to 10cm in diameter. *Confirmed by:* characteristic history and appearance. *Initial management:* regular follow-up, biopsy if features of malignancy appear.
Peutz-Jegher's syndrome (with risk of colonic and other neoplasms)	*Suggested by:* small (<5mm) macules on the lips, in the mouth, and around the eyes and nose; also around the anus, hands, and feet. Present since infancy or childhood and fade with age. *Confirmed by:* presence of *Polyposis coli* on **colonoscopy**. *Initial management:* refer for regular colonoscopy.

Red macule

Flat, well-demarcated area of red skin. Main test is photography to assess change or biopsy, usually to exclude malignancy. Initial investigations (others below in **bold**): digital photography of lesion.

Main differential diagnoses and typical outline evidence, etc.	
Drug reaction or allergy (e.g. due to penicillins, cephalosporins, antiepileptics)	*Suggested by:* red macular (or papular) rash up to 2wk after taking drug ± itching, burning, uniform pigmentation, symmetrical, on lower face or trunk ± fever, eosiniphilia.
	Confirmed by: resolution when drug removed and no recurrence if avoided.
	Initial management: emollient ± antihistamines, withdrawal of most recent drug, especially↑ antibiotics.
Viral exanthema from unknown agent	*Suggested by:* red, non-itchy rash with uniform pigmentation. Related systemic symptoms.
	Confirmed by: appearance, persistence, and resolution.
	Initial management: reassurance, antipyretic, and review for complications (e.g. check for pregnancy and potential malformation if rubella).
Measles	*Suggested by:* red, non-itchy rash with uniform pigmentation. Related systemic symptoms.
	Confirmed by: appearance, persistence, and resolution consistent with incubation period of 10 to 14 days.
	Initial management: reassurance, antipyretic, and review for complications (e.g. check for pregnancy and potential malformation if rubella).
Rubella	*Suggested by:* red, non-itchy rash with uniform pigmentation. Related systemic symptoms.
	Confirmed by: appearance, persistence, and resolution consistent with incubation period of 14 to 21 days.
	Initial management: reassurance, antipyretic, and review for complications (e.g. check for pregnancy and potential malformation)

Pale macule

Flat, well-demarcated, pale area. Initial investigations (others below in **bold**): digital photography of lesion.

Main differential diagnoses and typical outline evidence, etc.	
Post-inflammatory hypopigmentation	*Suggested by:* history of preceding red macule.
	Confirmed by: resolution when drug removed and no recurrence if avoided.
	Initial management: withdrawal of most recent drug, especially antibiotics.
Vitiligo	*Suggested by:* FH, non-itchy, white patches of the skin, usually sun-exposed areas, premature greying of hair, and symptoms of other associated autoimmune disorders, e.g. thyroid problems, pernicious anaemia, alopecia areata, and diabetes.
	Confirmed by: typical appearance, +ve **autoimmune profile**, **skin biopsy** shows absence of melanocytes.
	Initial management: treat underlying conditions. Reassurance, sunscreens, and cosmetics. Counselling in depressed patients (because of appearance), topical steroids, psoralen and UVA (PUVA), or depigmentation of normal skin to match affected one.
Pityriasis versicolor	*Suggested by:* history of excessive sweating or immunosupression. Appearance of well-defined, scaly, pale brownish, and uneven patches, usually on upper back and chest.
	Confirmed by: **microscopy**, **culture**, and **Wood's light examination** of skin scrapings show presence of *Pityrosporum orbiculare*.
	Initial management: local application of selenium sulphide or ketoconazole shampoos. In the more severe cases, advise systemic antifungals, e.g. itraconazole.
Pityriasis alba	*Suggested by:* young age, excessive dry skin, abrasive clothing, stress, and atopy. Skin lesions itchy and more apparent in summer.
	Confirmed by: presence of superficial, pale, slightly scaly, brown macules with irregular margins on face, neck, arms, and trunk, and the rash quickly becoming red in the sun.
	Initial management: reassurance, moisturizing creams, topical steroids, and oral antihistamines, e.g. chlorphenamine.

Papules

Raised lesion, <5mm diameter. Initial investigations (others below in **bold**): digital photography of lesion.

Main differential diagnoses and typical outline evidence, etc.	
Acne	*Suggested by:* young teen, oily skin.
	Confirmed by: multiple comedones, open (blackhead spots) or closed (whitehead spots), in addition to papules and pustules, cysts, and scarring depending on severity.
	Initial management: wash face gently with a gentle cleanser. Warn treatment may take up to many weeks, months, or even years. Topical and/or systemic treatment, depending on severity.
Scabies	*Suggested by:* severe itching, especially at night ± other members of family affected.
	Confirmed by: presence of burrows on sides of fingers, wrists, ankles, and nipples. **Microscopic examination**.
	Initial management: malathion lotion applied on the whole body for 24h ± reapplication after 2wk. Treat all close contacts. Wash all worn clothes and beddings.
Viral wart	*Suggested by:* history of contacts, use of swimming baths, immunosuppressant.
	Confirmed by: presence of dome- or flat-topped papules on hand, leg, and face, usually multiple.
	Initial management: may disappear spontaneously. Topical salicylic acid, cryotherapy, cautery, or curettage.
Molluscum contagiosum	*Suggested by:* affecting children or young adults, and history of contacts.
	Confirmed by: dome-shaped, umbilicated papules; if squeezed, produce a cheesy material.
	Initial management: resolve spontaneously, removal by expressing contents with forceps, curettage, or cryotherapy.
Orf	*Suggested by:* history of contact with sheep, e.g. farmers, vets. Bottle-feeding of a lamb. Presence of affected sheep.
	Confirmed by: solitary, rapidly growing, red papule, usually on a finger.
	Initial management: spontaneous resolution, topical and systemic antibiotics for 2° infections.
Campbell de Morgan spots	*Suggested by:* small, bright red papules on trunk of elderly or middle-aged people.
	Confirmed by: no change for months.
	Initial management: reassurance, can be removed by cautery, etc.
Skin tags	*Suggested by:* elderly or middle-aged, often obese.
	Confirmed by: pedunculated, usually neck, axilla, eyelids.
	Initial management: excision or cryotherapy.

Milia	*Suggested by:* age, usually a child. Mostly on face as small, white papules.
	Confirmed by: above typical appearance.
	Initial management: reassurance; no treatment needed.
Insect bite	*Suggested by:* history.
	Confirmed by: presence of a localized papule or blister, or a generalized allergic reaction. A sting mark in the centre.
	Initial management: if anaphylactic reaction, give adrenaline and oxygen, and admit. Advise carrying of EpiPen®. For local irritation, apply ice pack, and give local or systemic antihistamines.
Early seborrhoeic wart	*Suggested by:* patient is elderly or middle-aged. Pigmented, raised spot.
	Confirmed by: multiple lesions, mostly on trunk and face. Lesions have a 'stuck-on' appearance with keratin plugs and well-defined edges.
	Initial management: reassurance, liquid nitrogen, or cryotherapy.
Xanthomata	*Suggested by:* yellowish papules on the hands, tendons, and eyelids.
	Confirmed by: raised **fasting lipids**.
	Initial management: treat underlying disease. For local lesions, may consider cauterization or excision.
Guttate psoriasis	*Suggested by:* +ve FH. Sudden onset. History of a throat infection.
	Confirmed by: acute, symmetrical eruption of 'drop-like' and slightly scaly lesions on trunk and limbs.
	Initial management: antibiotics for streptococcal infections. Topical agents (e.g. using emollients), steroids, vitamin D analogues, dithranol. Systemic treatment, e.g. PUVA, methotrexate.
Lichen planus	*Suggested by:* very itchy, polygonal, flat-topped, violaceous papules affecting flexor surfaces, palms, soles, membrane, and genitalia. Recurrent and can affect mucous membranes like inside of mouth.
	Confirmed by: typical appearance of the rash. If necessary, **skin biopsy** with the typical telltale appearance under the microscope.
	Initial management: spontaneous resolution in most. Moderate to high potency topical steroids.
	Oral antihistamines, e.g. Piriton®. Mouthwashes for the oral lesions. Systemic oral steroids or PUVA for more severe cases.

(Continued)

Papules (continued)

Main differential diagnoses and typical outline evidence, etc.	
Pityriasis lichenoides chronica	*Suggested by:* chronic nature, scattered, small papules on limbs and trunk. *Confirmed by:* papules topped by a fine, single scale. *Initial management:* antibiotics for associated infections, antihistamines for itching, local steroids, or tacrolimus ointments, and sometimes UV treatment.
Prickly heat	*Suggested by:* history of travel to a high temperature area. *Confirmed by:* tiny red papules improving when back to colder environment. *Initial management:* cool bathing and avoidance of excessive temperatures.
Keratosis pilaris	*Suggested by:* papule in child or young adults, better during summer, worse in winter. *Confirmed by:* tiny, follicular, hyperkeratotic, non-itchy papules with erythema on upper arms with a typical gooseflesh or sandpaper appearance. *Initial management:* abrasive pad can smooth skin, exposure to sun to try to improve rash; local treatment, e.g. medium to high potency steroid, urea, and topical retinoids for more severe cases.
Blue naevus	*Suggested by:* solitary, blue, small papule on the dorsum of the foot or hand. *Confirmed by:* colour is a shade of blue. **Excision and histology.** *Initial management:* advise simple excision.
Basal cell carcinoma	*Suggested by:* history of chronic solar damage, in white-skinned, most commonly face and neck. Nodular, domed-shaped, necrozing in the centre, producing an ulcer with rolled edges. *Confirmed by:* **excision and histology.** *Initial management:* cryotherapy, excision, or radiotherapy.
Malignant melanoma	*Suggested by:* FH, fair skin, multiple moles. The mole itself is asymmetrical in shape, has an irregular border, is deep black or two colours and >7mm in diameter. *Confirmed by:* **excision and histology.** *Initial management:* referral to dermatology.
Darier's disease	*Suggested by:* usually teenagers or young adults, other members of the family may be affected, unpleasant smell from patient. *Confirmed by:* itchy, scaly, waxy, greasy papules, commonly affect the chest. *Initial management:* avoid sun exposure, heat, and humidity. Use of moisturizers and sunscreens. Tretinoin 0.1% cream under occlusion or a potent topical steroid.

Acanthosis nigricans	*Suggested by:* skin thickening and pigmentation over months or years.
	Confirmed by: presence of pigmented, velvety, and papillomatous skin lesion of flexures, neck, nipples, and umbilicus.
	Initial management: advise weight reduction; investigations for an underlying cause, e.g. diabetes mellitus, acromegaly, or internal malignancy.
Pseudoxanthoma elasticum	*Suggested by:* grouped, yellowish papules, mainly affecting neck and axillae.
	Confirmed by: presence of loose, wrinkled, and yellow skin. Involvement of arteries, e.g. presence of retinal angioid streaks.
	Initial management: reduce cardiovascular risks. Regular ophthalmology review.
Tuberous sclerosis	*Suggested by:* presence of skin lesions in a patient, usually a child with learning difficulties and epilepsy.
	Confirmed by: multiple, red-yellow papules on face, commonly on the nasal area and cheeks.
	Initial management: involvement of other specialties, genetic counselling, laser treatment for papules.

Nodules

Raised lesions >5mm diameter ± fixed to skin. Best viewed with magnifying glass. Patients usually report lesions because of unsightliness. Initial investigations (others below in **bold**): digital photography of lesion.

Main differential diagnoses and typical outline evidence, etc.	
Sebaceous cyst	*Suggested by:* a smooth, spherical, dermal nodule, usually on back of head and neck. *Confirmed by:* slowly growing over time. Sometimes a visible pole that periodically drains. *Initial management:* reassurance, excision if causing trouble.
Lipoma	*Suggested by:* soft, ill-defined lesion. *Confirmed by:* sometimes multiple in nature, soft consistency. *Initial management:* reassurance, excision if troublesome.
Basal cell carcinoma	*Suggested by:* history of chronic solar damage, white-skinned, most commonly face and neck. Nodular, domed-shaped, necrozing in the centre, producing an ulcer with rolled edges. *Confirmed by:* **histology.** *Initial management:* cryotherapy, excision, or radiotherapy.
Warts	*Suggested by:* soft, ill-defined lesion. *Confirmed by:* sometimes multiple in nature, soft consistency. *Initial management:* reassurance, excision if troublesome.
Xanthoma	*Suggested by:* yellowish papules on the hands, tendons, and eyelids. *Confirmed by:* ↑**fasting lipids**. *Initial management:* treat underlying disease. For local lesions, may consider cauterization or excision.
Acne	*Suggested by:* young teen, oily skin. *Confirmed by:* multiple comedones; open (blackhead spots) or closed (whitehead spots), in addition to papules and pustules, cysts, and scarring, depending on severity. *Initial management:* wash face gently with a gentle cleanser. Warn treatment may take up to many weeks, months, or even years. Topical and/or systemic treatment, depending on severity.
Dermatofibroma	*Suggested by:* solitary or multiple nodules—exposed sites in limbs. History of minor injury, thorn pricks, or an insect bite, may be some FH. *Confirmed by:* can hold the lesion between two fingers; feels like hard lump in dermis with the surface looking as if sucked in. *Initial management:* reassurance, excision biopsy.

Squamous cell carcinoma	*Suggested by:* background of solar damage. History of cumulative, previous skin lesion like Bowen's disease. A crusted, thick, eroded nodule, usually on exposed sites.
	Confirmed by: **biopsy histology.**
	Initial management: referral to dermatology. Excision or radiotherapy.
Keratoacanthoma	*Suggested by:* history of prolonged sun exposure, suggested by rapidly growing tumour reaching a larger size, present on face, ears, or dorsa of hands.
	Confirmed by: rapid growth for almost 2mo, followed by a static phase, and then involution—each stage lasting about 2mo. **Biopsy result**.
	Initial management: curettage and histology.
Gouty tophi	*Suggested by:* history of recurrent joint pain. Cutaneous nodules with stretched over and normal texture skin, on the fingers usually, occasionally the ear.
	Confirmed by: **aspiration from tophi**—uric acid crystals.
	Initial management: analgesics, allopurinol for long-term treatment. Excision.
Chondrodermatitis nodularis helicis externa	*Suggested by:* pressure effect on ear, especially when sleeping. Wakes patient up from sleep due to pain.
	Confirmed by: small, crusted nodule on the external ear.
	Initial management: sleeping on the other side. Local injection of triamcinolone or excision.
Rheumatoid nodules	*Suggested by:* previously well documented history of rheumatoid disease.
	Confirmed by: presence of painless, small lumps under the skin and over pressure points (e.g. elbow), knuckles nodule typical on elbow. Multiple joint swelling and deformities. **Rheumatoid factor** +ve.
	Initial management: analgesics, NSAIDs, avoid irritating trauma, local steroid injections, or excision of nodules.
Heberden's nodes	*Suggested by:* history of chronic osteoarthritis.
	Confirmed by: presence of painless, small nodes (bony growths) on the terminal interphalangeal joints.
	Initial management: no treatment.
Pyogenic granuloma	*Suggested by:* rapidly growing, vascular nodule, easily bleeds.
	Confirmed by: excision **biopsy, histology.**
	Initial management: arrest bleeding, shave biopsy, curettage, and electrocautery.
Malignant melanoma	*Suggested by:* FH, fair skin, multiple moles, by mole being asymmetrical in shape, irregular border, deep black or two colours, and >7mm in diameter.
	Confirmed by: excision + **histology.**
	Initial management: referral to dermatology for opinion ± biopsy.

(Continued)

Nodules (continued)

Main differential diagnoses and typical outline evidence, etc.

Erythema nodosum	*Suggested by:* red, tender, deeply placed nodules, usually on the shin. Multiple and bilateral. Associated fever and joint pain. *Confirmed by:* **↑ESR; CXR**: bilateral, hilar lymphadenopathy. *Initial management:* analgesics, NSAIDs ± systemic steroids.
Polyarteritis nodosa	*Suggested by:* tender nodules, fever, joint pain, neuropathic symptoms. *Confirmed by:* **↑ESR, +ve autoimmune profile, +ve PANCA**. *Initial management:* analgesics, NSAIDs.
Lepromatous leprosy	*Suggested by:* multiple nodules on face, ears, and other places. *Confirmed by:* **microbiology, biopsy.** *Initial management:* combination of rifampicin, clofazimine, and dapsone in specific doses for an average of 2y.
2° syphilis	*Suggested by:* history of ulcers in genitalia. Nodular scaly lesion on hands and soles. Constitutional symptoms. *Confirmed by:* **serological tests, microbiology.** *Initial management:* benzylpenicillin IM.
Lupus vulgaris	*Suggested by:* slow onset over months to years, hyperkeratotic, crusted nodule, usually at the site of accidental inoculation. *Confirmed by:* +ve **tuberculin test**. +ve **microbiology** for mycobacterium. *Initial management:* antituberculosis combination treatment. Surgical excision for early lesions.
Fish tank or swimming pool granuloma	*Suggested by:* occupation or hobbies bring the patient in contact with fish, or history of trauma treated in the past with antibiotics with no response. *Confirmed by:* +ve **microbiology** tests for mycobacterium. *Initial management:* antibiotics as per culture and sensitivity.

Blisters

Blisters <0.5cm diameter are vesicles, blisters >0.5cm are bullae. Initial investigations (others below in **bold**): digital photography of lesion.

Main differential diagnoses and typical outline evidence, etc.	
Skin friction	*Suggested by:* presence of blister friction marks on skin and a possible bruising. *Confirmed by:* history of traumatic friction. *Initial management:* keep clean, intact. If bursts, get rid of remaining fluid, then apply clean dressing.
Thermal burns	*Suggested by:* presence of blister possibly with some erythema. *Confirmed by:* history of burn. *Initial management:* relieve pain with waterproof antiseptic dressing (to prevent transpiration from damaged cells). Assess the degree of burn and treat accordingly.
Leg oedema	*Suggested by:* blister in the presence of swollen legs. *Confirmed by:* presence of severe pitting oedema, resolution when oedema treated. *Initial management:* diuretics, treat associated infections and cause of oedema.
Chemical burns	*Suggested by:* presence of blisters, possibly with traces of chemical. *Confirmed by:* history of contact with chemical. *Initial management:* pain control, assessment of degree of the burn, and treat accordingly.
Insect bites	*Suggested by:* history of contact with insect. *Confirmed by:* site of sting surrounded by redness. *Initial management:* paracetamol and antihistamines.
Chicken pox	*Suggested by:* contact with a case of chickenpox, a prodromal illness for 1–2d before the appearance of a rash. *Confirmed by:* erythematous lesions, rapidly changing to vesicles, then pustules, followed by crusts after 2–3d. Lesions itchy. *Initial management:* antipyretics, antihistamines, and calamine lotion to ease itching and irritability.
Herpes simplex	*Suggested by:* presence of contacts and occurring at a similar site each time, usually lips, face, or genitals, associated respiratory infection ('cold sore'). Lesions recurring. *Confirmed by:* presence of vesicles on the mouth or genitalia. Painful, later crusting with local lymphadenopathy. *Initial management:* paracetamol for pain. Aciclovir cream applied five times daily for recurrent mild facial and genital infections. Aciclovir PO for more severe infections. Confirmed genital herpes in a pregnant woman at the time of delivery is an indication for caesarean section.

Herpes zoster	*Suggested by:* pain, tenderness and paraesthesia in the affected area before the appearance of the rash. *Confirmed by:* presence of typical lesions which are usually unilateral. *Initial management:* for mild causes—analgesics, rest; local calamine lotion for more severe cases; and if seen within 72h of the rash appearance, give aciclovir 800mg five times daily for 1wk.
Herpetic whitlow	*Suggested by:* a painful lesion on finger, usually in a nurse or a dentist attending a patient with herpetic lesion, or in sportsmen like wrestlers (direct inoculation). *Confirmed by:* presence of a painful vesicular lesion on a finger. *Initial management:* paracetamol for pain. Aciclovir cream or tablets, depending on severity.
Hand, foot and mouth disease	*Suggested by:* presence of prodromal symptoms before the appearance of lesions restricted to the feet, hands, and mouth in a child or an adult. *Confirmed by:* presence of vesicles surrounded by an intense skin erythema on the palms, soles, and in the mouth. *Initial management:* analgesia, reassurance that condition is self-limiting.
Pompholyx	*Suggested by:* history of atopy, stress, allergic reactions to fungal infections elsewhere. *Confirmed by:* presence of persistent, itchy, clear blisters on fingers, sometimes palms. *Initial management:* symptomatic.
Acute eczema: contact dermatitis or atopic	*Suggested by:* acute onset affecting a particular site, suggesting contact with certain objects. History of occupation, hobbies, or nickel sensitivity can suggest a clue. *Confirmed by:* presence of vesicles, and sometimes large blisters with erythema, oedema, papules, and vesicles seen on the affected part. *Initial management:* avoid contact with allergens, if possible; moisturizers, creams and topical steroids. Topical or systemic antibiotic if there is infection.
Pemphigus	*Suggested by:* presence of superficial blisters on the scalp, face, back, chest, and flexures. These may be preceded by mouth erosions several weeks or months before. History of other autoimmune disease like hypothyroidism or myasthenia gravis. *Confirmed by:* presence of **IgG auto-antibodies** to epidermal components. Direct **immunofluorescence studies** show deposition of IgG antibodies in epidermis. *Initial management:* high dose of prednisolone PO (e.g. 1–1.5mg/kg/d) ± azathioprine or cyclophosphamide.

(Continued)

Blisters (continued)

Main differential diagnoses and typical outline evidence, etc.

Pemphigoid	*Suggested by:* tense, large blisters, arising on a red or a normal-looking skin, usually in an elderly patient, on the limbs, trunk and flexures, and very rarely, in the mouth. *Confirmed by:* specific **IgG antibodies** to the antigens BP230 and BP180 in subepidermal area. **Direct immunofluorescence studies** showing IgG and C3 antibodies in subepidermal area. *Initial management:* usually a low dose of prednisolone PO, e.g. 30–60mg daily with or without azathioprine.
Dermatitis herpetiformis associated with gluten enteropathy	*Suggested by:* a young adult male with gluten sensitivity, with small symmetrical, very itchy blisters on the extension surfaces. *Confirmed by:* **direct immunofluorescence** studies showing depositions and IgA antibodies in the dermis. *Initial management:* local and systemic antibiotics.
Bullous impetigo	*Suggested by:* presence of extensive, non-itchy golden or brown blisters, on face and limbs in children and adults. *Confirmed by:* **isolation of Staphylococcus** in the blister fluid. *Initial management:* local and systemic antibiotics.
Bullous drug eruption	*Suggested by:* use of a drug in the preceding 2–3 wk, e.g. barbiturates, furosemide. *Confirmed by:* accurate prescribing records of potential causal drug. +ve **patch or intradermal tests**. *Initial management:* withdrawal of the causative drug. Emollients and/or topical steroids.
Erythema multiforme A severe form involving mucous membranes called Stevens-Johnson syndrome.	*Suggested by:* presence of a potential cause like drug or infection. *Confirmed by:* presence of red rings with a central pale or purple area, giving the appearance of an 'iris' or a target lesion which then blisters. *Initial management:* identification and treatment of the underlying cause. Symptomatic treatment for mild cases and hospital admission, if severe.
Pemphigoid gestationis	*Suggested by:* presence of similar bullae lesions during previous pregnancies, subsided after delivery. *Confirmed by:* presence of intensely itchy bullae associated with pregnancy. *Initial management:* prednisolone PO, e.g. 30–60mg daily.
Porphyrias	*Suggested by:* presence of other affected members in the family. Lesions consist of painful red blistering eruptions. *Confirmed by:* presence of **porphyrins in blood and urine**, and **by gene studies**. *Initial management:* avoid sun exposure, alcohol, or aggravating drugs. Correct iron deficiency if present.

Toxic epidermal necrolysis	*Suggested by:* severe bullous eruption when taking an anticonvulsant, antibiotic, or allopurinol.
	Confirmed by: associated severe epidermal loss.
	Initial management: hospital admission, usually on an ITU ward.
Epidermolysis bullosa	*Suggested by:* blistering of skin after minimal trauma.
	Confirmed by: **genetic studies** (mapped to chromosomes 12 and 17). Prenatal diagnosis.
	Initial management: avoidance of trauma, supportive measures, and treatment of infection.

Erythema

Reddening of the skin which blanches on pressure. Initial investigations (others below in **bold**): digital photography of lesion.

Main differential diagnoses and typical outline evidence, etc.	
Cellulitis	*Suggested by:* painful red area on a limb, fever. An underlying condition, e.g. diabetes mellitus.
	Confirmed by: swelling, redness, localized pain, malaise.
	Initial management: antibiotic effective against Streptococcus or Staphylococcus, e.g. benzylpenicillin etc. and flucloxacillin IV initially.
Gout	*Suggested by:* severe joint redness, pain, and swelling, usually in one joint, commonly that of the big toe.
	Confirmed by: ↑**serum uric acid** and the presence of urate crystals in **joint fluid aspirate**.
	Initial management: indometacin or if contraindicated, colchicine to a maximum of 6mg until pain disappears or side effects appear. Allopurinol later.
Thermal burn	*Suggested by:* presence of blister, possibly with some erythema.
	Confirmed by: history of burn.
	Initial management: relieve pain with sterile waterproof dressing to prevent transpiration from damaged cells. Assess the degree of burn and treat accordingly.
Chemical burn	*Suggested by:* the presence of blisters, possibly with traces of chemical.
	Confirmed by: history of chemical burn.
	Initial management: pain control with sterile waterproof dressing to prevent transpiration from damaged cells, assessment of degree of the burn, and treat accordingly.
Sunburn	*Suggested by:* history of exposure to sun.
	Confirmed by: redness of exposed area.
	Initial management: no more sun. Soothing ointments, e.g. Sudocrem®; antihistamine if heat and cold intolerance due to loss of temperature regulation.
Drug eruption	*Suggested by:* intake of a drug in the preceding 2–3wk.
	Confirmed by: accurate prescribing records. **Patch skin testing.**
	Initial management: withdrawal of causative drug. Emollients and/or topical steroids.
Fixed drug eruptions	*Suggested by:* appearance of the rash at the same place every time the same drug taken.
	Confirmed by: **patch skin testing.**
	Initial management: avoiding the causative drug.
Viral toxic erythema	*Suggested by:* systemic symptoms with no obvious focus of infection in a child.
	Confirmed by: resolution when systemic symptoms resolve.
	Initial management: symptomatic.

Rosacea	*Suggested by:* facial erythema in middle-aged males or females.
	Confirmed by: presence of flushes, erythema, telangiectasis, papules, and pustules. Sometimes the presence of **rhinophyma** (a red lobulated nose). No comedones as in acne.
	Initial management: topical metronidazole 0.75% cream twice daily or tetracycline PO for 3–4wk, reduced dose for 2–3mo.
Palmar erythema	*Suggested by:* associated evidence of liver cirrhosis, pregnancy, and polycythaemia.
	Confirmed by: resolution with underlying condition.
	Initial management: treatment of underlying cause.
Drug phototoxicty	*Suggested by:* taking a drug and rash in areas exposed to sunlight.
	Confirmed by: disappearance of the rash after discontinuing the offending drug.
	Initial management: discontinuation of the offending drug. Emollients and/or topical steroids.
Erythema multiforme due to sarcoidosis	*Suggested by:* red, tender, deeply placed nodules, usually on the shin. Multiple and bilateral. Associated facet and joint pain.
	Confirmed by: ↑**ESR; CXR:** bilateral, hilar lymphadenopathy.
	Initial management: analgesics, NSAIDs ± systemic steroids.
Systemic lupus erythematosus (SLE)	*Suggested by:* facial butterfly eruptions commonly in females, with evidence of multisystem involvement.
	Confirmed by: **antinuclear auto-antibodies**.
	Initial management: sunscreens if multisystemic disease, steroids with or without immunosuppressive agents.
Erythema ab igne	*Suggested by:* history of an erythema as the shin of an elderly who sits before an open fire.
	Confirmed by: improving when avoiding sitting in front of a fire.
	Initial management: stop causative behaviour.
Livedo reticularis	*Suggested by:* cyanotic, net-like discoloration skin of legs.
	Confirmed by: presence of an underlying cause, e.g. exposure to cold, SLE, and polycythaemia.
	Initial management: treat underlying cause.
HIV seroconversion	*Suggested by:* fever, malaise, nausea, and vomiting with lymphadenopathy, erythematous rash in a homosexual or IV drug user.
	Confirmed by: detection of **P24 antigen or HIV RNA by PCR**.
	Initial management: of underlying disease.

(Continued)

Erythema (continued)

Main differential diagnoses and typical outline evidence, etc.	
Erythema nodosum (sarcoid, tuberculosis (TB), drugs, Streptococcus)	*Suggested by:* presence of tender, reddish-blue nodules, usually on the calves and shins, and presence of an underlying condition, e.g. bacterial, viral, fungal, drugs, and systemic disease. *Confirmed by:* **skin biopsy.** *Initial management:* pain relief by analgesics or NSAIDs.
Erythema induratum (TB: Bazin's disease)	*Suggested by:* presence of red, indurated lesions on the lower legs. *Confirmed by:* **biopsy** of lesion. *Initial management:* analgesia. Treat underlying cause.
Erythema chronicum migrans (Lyme disease)	*Suggested by:* slowly expanding erythematous ring at the site of a tic bite, on a limb usually ± multisystem symptoms. *Confirmed by:* **serology.** *Initial management:* doxycyline for 2–3wk. In children below 8y and in pregnancy: amoxicillin for a similar period.

Purpura and petechiae

Purplish lesions resulting from free red blood cells in the skin. They do not blanch on pressure. Purpurae are large (>5mm) and imply clotting defects or blood vessel fragility; petechiae are small (<5mm) and imply platelet defects or vasculitis. Initial investigations (others below in **bold**): digital photography of lesion, FBC, U&E, LFT.

Main differential diagnoses and typical outline evidence, etc.	
Trauma	*Suggested by:* history.
	Confirmed by: lesions matching site of trauma.
	Initial management: symptomatic treatment
Senile purpura	*Suggested by:* elderly patient.
	Confirmed by: atrophic small veins and skin.
	Initial management: none, reassurance.
Liver disease	*Suggested by:* jaundice, hepatomegaly, etc.
	Confirmed by: abnormal **LFT and ultrasound (US) scan of liver.**
	Initial management: treat underlying condition.
Raised venous pressure, e.g. vomiting	*Suggested by:* history of vomiting etc.
	Confirmed by: presence of purpuric spot, usually around the eyes.
	Initial management: none, reassurance.
Drugs (steroids, warfarin, aspirin)	*Suggested by:* intake of drugs.
	Confirmed by: disappearance when drug stopped.
	Initial management: treating underlying cause.
Vasculitis (Henoch–Schönlein, connective tissue)	*Suggested by:* purpurae on buttock and extensor surfaces, typically in a young male. Associated features of cause, e.g. proteinuria, hypertension, and abdominal pain of Henoch–Schönlein syndrome.
	Confirmed by: typical appearance of the rash.
	Initial management: treatment of underlying cause, e.g. with systemic steroids.
Thrombocyto-paenia (e.g. idiopathic thrombocytopaenic purpura (ITP), drug-induced, bone marrow replacement, aplastic anaemia)	*Suggested by:* features of the underlying cause.
	Confirmed by: FBC: ↓platelets etc.
	Initial management: of underlying cause.
Renal failure	*Suggested by:* symptoms and signs of renal impairment.
	Confirmed by: ↑urea, ↑creatinine.
	Initial management: of underlying condition.

Endocarditis	*Suggested by:* presence of fever, general malaise, heart murmur.
	Confirmed by: +ve **blood cultures** and an abnormal **ECG**.
	Initial management: benzylpenicillin IV + gentamicin.
Paraproteinaemia	*Suggested by:* back pain, loss of appetite, high temperature.
	Confirmed by: paraprotein on **electrophoresis.**
	Initial management: treatment of underlying cause.
Clotting disorder (haemophilia, Christmas, Von-Willebrand's)	*Suggested by:* easy bleeding and delayed clotting.
	Confirmed by: **clotting screen**.
	Initial management: vitamin K; treatment of clotting defect.
Meningoccocal septicaemia	*Suggested by:* rapidly progressive disease with headaches, neck stiffness, vomiting, and photophobia.
	Confirmed by: **blood culture and lumbar puncture.**
	Initial management: benzylpenicillin IM.
Vitamin K deficiency	*Suggested by:* disorder in a patient with malnutrition or malabsorption, Gastrointestinal (GI) bleeding.
	Confirmed by: reversal of bleeding when supplied with vitamin K.
	Initial management: vitamin K.
Vitamin C deficiency	*Suggested by:* anorexia, cachexia, gingivitis, loose teeth, and halitosis; pregnancy, poverty, odd diet.
	Confirmed by: low **vitamin C level.**
	Initial management: vitamin C supplement.
Disseminated intravascular coagulation (DIC)	*Suggested by:* severe bruising and failure to clot after starting to bleed. Features of a severe underlying condition such as malignancy, sepsis, trauma.
	Confirmed by: **FBC**: ↓platelets, ↑PT, ↑APTT, ↓fibrinogen.
	Initial management: treat the cause, and replace platelets and clotting factors.

Pustules

A well-defined, pus-filled lesion. Initial investigations (others below in **bold**): digital photography of lesion.

Main differential diagnoses and typical outline evidence, etc.	
Impetigo	*Suggested by:* presence of easily ruptured vesicles, leaving a yellow, crusted exudates, usually affect the face and extremities.
	Confirmed by: typical look and site of lesion.
	Initial management: local or systemic antibiotics, depending on severity.
Folliculitis	*Suggested by:* lesions being in hair-baring areas—in women, there might be a history of hair removal by shaving or waxing.
	Confirmed by: **swab**: isolation *S. aureus*.
	Initial management: local or systemic antibiotics.
Sycosis barbae	*Suggested by:* folliculitis in the beard area.
	Confirmed by: **swab** isolation of *S. aureus*.
	Initial management: local or systemic antibiotics.
Herpes simplex	*Suggested by:* presence of contacts and occurring at a similar site each time, usually lips, face, or genitals, and sometimes the presence of a respiration infection, therefore called a 'cold sore'. Lesions recurring.
	Confirmed by: presence of painful vesicles on the mouth or genitalia.
	Initial management: paracetamol for pain. Aciclovir cream applied five times daily for recurrent mild facial and genital infections, and aciclovir PO for more severe infections. Confirmed genital herpes in a pregnant woman at the time of delivery is an indication for caesarean section.
Herpes zoster	*Suggested by:* pain, tenderness, and paraesthesia in the affected area before the appearance of the rash.
	Confirmed by: presence of typical lesions which are normally unilateral.
	Initial management: for mild causes—analgesics, rest, local calamine lotion; for more severe cases and if seen within 72h of the rash appearance, give aciclovir 800mg five times daily for 1wk.
Acne vulgaris	*Suggested by:* presence of comedones, open (blackheads) or closed (whiteheads), papules, pustules, cysts, or scars depending on severity. Comedones appear first at around the age of 12y, then evolve into the different other lesion.
	Confirmed by: typical features of the skin lesions.
	Initial management: for mild acne, use local treatments (eg benzoyl peroxide cream or gel bd, tretinoin cream or gel) or local antibiotic gels like Zineryt® and Benzamycin® no larger available in UK, with or without antibiotic PO, e.g. minocycline.

Rosacea	*Suggested by:* facial erythema in middle-aged males or females. *Confirmed by:* flushes, erythema, telangiectasis, papules and pustules ± rhinophyma (a red lobulated nose). No comedones as in acne. *Initial management:* topical metronidazole or tetracycline PO for 3–4wk with lower dose for 2–3mo.
Hydranitis suppurativa	*Suggested by:* pustules in axilla, groin. *Confirmed by:* recurrent problem. *Initial management:* local or systemic antibiotics.
Candidiasis	*Suggested by:* itchy, symmetrical with 'satellite' pustules outside the outer edge of the skin rash. Underlying conditions, e.g. diabetes mellitus, AIDS or Cushing's. *Confirmed by:* **swabs and skin scrapings.** *Initial management:* local clotrimazole or miconazole for 2–4wk. Systemic treatment such as fluconazole for non-responding cases.
Localized pustular psoriasis	*Suggested by:* chronic nature of the illness in an elderly with psoriasis elsewhere. *Confirmed by:* presence of pustules surrounded by a scaly, erythematous skin on the palms and soles. *Initial management:* moderate to potent strength topical steroid.
Generalized pustular psoriasis	*Suggested by:* acute onset with fever, malaise, and general ill health with a psoriatic rash. *Confirmed by:* presence of sheets of small, yellowish pustules, on an erythematous background, which may spread rapidly. *Initial management:* rehydration IV ± antibiotics + local measures.
Dermatitis herpetiformis associated with gluten enteropathy	*Suggested by:* a young adult male with gluten sensitivity, with small, symmetrical, very itchy blisters in the extensor surfaces. *Confirmed by:* **direct immunofluorescence** studies showing depositions and IgA antibodies in the dermis. *Initial management:* local and systemic antibiotics.
Pseudomonas infection	*Suggested by:* history of long-term treatment of acne (if lesions are on face) or history of exposure to contaminated baths or whirlpools (if lesions are on body). *Confirmed by:* **swabs + isolation of organism, culture and sensitivity.** *Initial management:* with appropriate antibiotic based on culture and sensitivity.
Drug reactions	*Suggested by:* intake of a potentially causative drug in the preceding 2–3wk. *Confirmed by:* accurate prescribing records. Patch test. *Initial management:* withdrawal of the causative drug. Emollients and/or topical steroids.

Hyperkeratosis, scales, and plaques

Hyperkeratosis: thickening of the keratin layer; scale: fragment of dry skin; plaque: raised flat-topped lesion, usually over 2cm in diameter. Initial investigations (others below in **bold**): digital photography of lesion.

Main differential diagnoses and typical outline evidence, etc.	
Psoriasis	*Suggested by:* scaly, silvery scales on extensor surfaces and sites of minor trauma (Koebner's phenomenon); lesions usually clear after exposure to sun. *Confirmed by:* typical presence of plaques of scaly lesions covering extensor areas of trunk and limbs. *Initial management:* tar preparation, Dovobet®, short contact dithranol, or UVB. Immunosuppressants for extensive lesions.
Chronic eczema: atopic, contact	*Suggested by:* contact with certain objects or history of atopy. *Confirmed by:* improvement of condition after eliminating the offending subject. *Initial management:* removal of the cause; moisturizers, creams, and topical steroids. Antibiotics if there is infection.
Fungal infections	*Suggested by:* typical ring-like lesions (clearer centres) on the trunk and limbs in tinea corporis (ringworm) or lesions in the inner upper thigh, not involving the scrotum with an advancing scaly and pustular edge in tinea cruris. *Confirmed by:* **microscopy and culture of skin scrapings. Wood's UV light examination** for tinea capitis. *Initial management:* local or systemic antifungal agents.
Seborrhoeic dermatitis	*Suggested by:* scalp and facial involvement, excessive dandruff with an itchy and scaly eruption, affecting sides of nose, scalp margin, eyebrows, and ear. *Confirmed by:* typical skin lesions and distribution. *Initial management:* medicated shampoo alone or following the application of 2% sulphur ± preceding 2% salicylic acid for scalp lesions. Facial lesions treated with combined antimicrobial and steroid creams.
Lichen simplex chronicus	*Suggested by:* history of repeated rubbing or scratching of an area as a habit or caused by stress; typically Asian or Chinese patient. *Confirmed by:* presence of a single plaque on the back of the neck or in the perineum. *Initial management:* emollients and topical steroids.
Lichen planus	*Suggested by:* no FH, related to stress; presence of Koebner's phenomenon. *Confirmed by:* itchy, well-defined, raised, shiny-surfaced lesions with a violaceous colour divided by white streaks (Wickman's striae). *Initial management:* topical steroids, systemic steroids for very extensive lesions.

Solar keratosis	*Suggested by:* lesions on sites exposed to sun, patients work out of doors or history of excessive sunbathing, pipe smokers. *Confirmed by:* raised keratotic lesion <1cm in diameter with an irregular edge on face, back of the hands, arms and legs, and scalp in bald men. Lesions are pre-malignant. *Initial management:* cryotherapy for large and multiple lesion; trial of fluorouracil cream bd for 2weeks.
Pityriasis versicolor	*Suggested by:* chronic brown or pinkish oval or round scaly patches on trunk and limbs; hypopigmented spots in tanned or racially dark skin. *Confirmed by:* typical appearance on **microscopy of skin scrapings**. *Initial management:* clotrimazole or miconazole creams, or the use of topical selenium sulphide or ketoconazole shampoos applied for 30min, and then washed off tds for 2wk. If resistant, itraconazole PO for 1wk.
Pityriasis rosea	*Suggested by:* acute onset of scaly oval papules, mainly on trunk, preceded by a 2–8cm in diameter single lesion called the 'herald patch'. *Confirmed by:* typical appearance of the rash and the herald patch. *Initial management:* ease itching.
Juvenile plantar dermatosis	*Suggested by:* child <10y, wearing socks and shoes made of synthetic material. *Confirmed by:* presence of red, dry, fissured, and shiny skin, usually on the forefoot ± the whole sole. *Initial management:* emollients.
Guttate psoriasis	*Suggested by:* acute, symmetrical appearance of drop-like, scaly skin lesions, on trunk and limbs in an adolescent or young adult typically with sore throat. *Confirmed by:* typical appearance of the rash. *Initial management:* topical steroids, coal tar, or narrow band UV.
Bowen's disease	*Suggested by:* indurated, crusted, well-defined, erythematous macule trunk or limbs ± exposure to sheep dip or weed-killers. *Confirmed by:* **biopsy:** carcinoma *in situ*. *Initial management:* cryotherapy, topical fluorouracil cream, photodynamic therapy.
Mycosis fungoides (cutaneous T-cell lymphoma)	*Suggested by:* scaly, erythematous patches progressing over months to years to fixed infiltrated plaques, then cancerous nodules. *Confirmed by:* **biopsy**. *Initial management:* early lesion: topical steroids or PUVA, electron beam therapy.

(Continued)

Hyperkeratosis, scales and plaques (continued)

Main differential diagnoses and typical outline evidence, etc.	
Drug-induced (e.g. β-blockers, carbamazepine)	*Suggested by:* history of taking suspected drug in the preceding 2–3wk. *Confirmed by:* accurate prescribing records. **Patch test**. *Initial management:* withdrawal of causative drug. Emollients and/or topical steroids.
Ichthyois	*Suggested by:* mild to severe dry, scaly skin, seen mainly on the extensor surfaces with the flexures often spared ± FH. *Confirmed by:* typical appearance of skin and **biopsy**. *Initial management:* emollients and bath oils for mild cases.
Keratoderma	*Suggested by:* gradual onset in middle age, typically in post-menopausal female. *Confirmed by:* hyperkeratosis of palms and soles. *Initial management:* 5–10% salicylic acid ointment or 10% urea cream.
Erythroderma due to eczema, psoriasis, and lymphoma.	*Suggested by:* severe systemic symptoms with patchy, then generalized erythema followed by scaling days later ± features of an underlying cause. *Confirmed by:* **skin biopsy.** *Initial management:* hospital admission for fluids IV, steroids.
2° syphilis	*Suggested by:* history of previous chancre + presence of a non-itchy, pink-coloured, papular eruption, becoming scaly, on the trunk, limbs, palms, and soles. *Confirmed by:* +ve **serology for syphilis.** *Initial management:* procaine, penicillin IM for 14d (or doxycycline, erythromycin).

Itchy scalp

Initial investigations (others below in **bold**): digital photography of lesion.

Main differential diagnoses and typical outline evidence, etc.	
Head lice	*Suggested by:* intense itching of scalp, typically in a school child ± poor social and hygienic conditions.
	Confirmed by: seeing nits or lice on hair shafts.
	Initial management: malathion applied to scalp and left for 12h before being washed out, to be repeated in a week's time. Nits can be removed with a comb.
Seborrhoeic eczema	*Suggested by:* scalp and facial involvement, excessive dandruff with an itchy and scaly eruption, affecting sides of nose, scalp margin, eyebrows, and ear.
	Confirmed by: the above typical skin lesions and distribution.
	Initial management: medicated shampoo alone or 2% sulphur or 2% salicylic acid for scalp lesions. Facial lesions: combined antimicrobial and steroid creams.
Psoriasis	*Suggested by:* onset after period of stress, lesions at sites of minor trauma (Koebner's phenomenon) clearing after exposure to sun.
	Confirmed by: well-defined, raised, scaly, disc-shaped plaques on scalp hair margin.
	Initial management: 3% salicylic acid in a cream base applied daily in combination with a tar-containing shampoo. Trial of coconut oil compound.
Lichen simplex chronicus	*Suggested by:* history of repeated rubbing or scratching of an area habitually or during stress; typically Asian or Chinese.
	Confirmed by: single plaque on the back of the neck or in the perineum.
	Initial management: emollients and topical steroids.
Allergic contact dermatitis	*Suggested by:* exposure to suspect precipitant, e.g. hair dye.
	Confirmed by: improvement on removal of the offending agent.
	Initial management: avoid causative agent. Local steroid lotions.
Fungal infection (complicated by possible irreversible hair loss, if untreated)	*Suggested by:* mild, scaly, inflammatory areas with alopecia and broken hair shafts or an inflamed boggy pustular swelling called kerion.
	Confirmed by: **microscopy and culture of skin scrapings**.
	Initial management: griseofulvin for 1–2mo.

Herpes zoster	*Suggested by:* pain, tenderness, and paraesthesia in the affected area before the appearance of rash.
	Confirmed by: presence of typical unilateral lesions.
	Initial management: mild—analgesics, rest; local calamine lotion; if severe and seen within 72h of rash appearing: acyclovir e.g. 800mg five times daily for 1wk.
Anxiety and depression	*Suggested by:* history of low mood, anxiety.
	Confirmed by: normal appearance of scalp initially and on follow-up.
	Initial management: explanation, psychotherapy.

Itchy skin with lesions but no wheals

Skin scratched or rubbed ± a number of secondary skin signs: excoriations (scratch marks), lichenification (skin thickening), papules (localized skin thickening), or nodules. Initial investigations (others below in **bold**): digital photography of lesion.

Main differential diagnoses and typical outline evidence, etc.	
Allergic contact dermatitis	*Suggested by:* exposure to a potential allergen, e.g. hair dye.
	Confirmed by: improvement on removal of the offending agent.
	Initial management: avoid causative agent. Local steroid lotions.
Candidiasis e.g. due to diabetes mellitus, AIDS, or Cushing's syndrome.	*Suggested by:* itchy, symmetrical with 'satellite' pustules outside the outer edge of the skin rash. Symptoms and signs of underlying condition.
	Confirmed by: +ve swabs and **skin scrapings for yeasts**.
	Initial management: local clotrimazole or miconazole for 2–4wk. Systemic treatment for non-responding cases.
Discoid eczema	*Suggested by:* recurring itchy lesion in a middle-aged or an elderly man.
	Confirmed by: presence of coin-shaped lesions on the limbs with a symmetrical distribution.
	Initial management: potent steroid cream combined with an antibiotic.
Drug-induced eczema	*Suggested by:* itchy skin with a history of recent drug ingestion.
	Confirmed by: improvement on withdrawal of offending agent.
	Initial management: removal of the offending agent. Topical emollients and steroids.
Varicose eczema	*Suggested by:* associated varicose veins and swollen oedematous leg.
	Confirmed by: presence of the eczematous patch on the medial aspect of leg.
	Initial management: diuretics, leg elevation, compression bandage, emollient, and steroid creams.
Scabies	*Suggested by:* severe itching, especially at night; other member of family affected.
	Confirmed by: presence of burrows on sides of fingers, wrists, ankles, and nipples. **Microscopic examination** showing the mites.
	Initial management: malathion lotion applied on whole body for 24h ± reapplication after 2wk. Treat all close contacts. Wash all clothes and bedding.

Seborrhoeic dermatitis	*Suggested by:* scalp and facial involvement, excessive dandruff with an itchy and scaly eruption affecting sides of nose, scalp margin, eyebrows, and ear. *Confirmed by:* typical skin lesions and distribution. *Initial management:* medicated shampoo alone ± preceding 2% sulphur or 2% salicylic acid. Facial lesions treated with combined antimicrobial and steroid creams.
Asteatotic eczema	*Suggested by:* history of dryness and itching in elderly patient, excessive use of central heating, and washing. *Confirmed by:* presence of a scaly, red rash; in severe forms, fissuring and inflammation on leg. *Initial management:* emollients ± topical steroids.
Dermatitis herpetiformis associated with gluten enteropathy	*Suggested by:* a young adult male with gluten sensitivity, with small symmetrical, very itchy blisters in the extensor surfaces. *Confirmed by:* **direct immunofluorescence studies** showing depositions and IgA antibodies in the dermis. *Initial management:* local and systemic antibiotics.
Lichen planus	*Suggested by:* related to stress and the presence of Koebner's phenomenon. *Confirmed by:* presence of itchy, well-defined, and raised, shiny-surfaced lesions with a violaceous colour interpreted by white streaks (Wickman's striae). *Initial management:* topical steroids; systemic steroids for very extensive lesions.
Psoriasis	*Suggested by:* scaly, silvery scales on extensor surfaces and sites of minor trauma (Koebner's phenomenon); lesions usually clear after exposure to sun. *Confirmed by:* typical presence of plaques of scaly lesions covering extensor areas of trunk and limbs. *Initial management:* tar preparation, Dovobet®, short contact dithranol or UVB. Immunosuppressants for extensive lesions.
Eczema herpeticum	*Suggested by:* previous history of atopic eczema in a child who is generally unwell. *Confirmed by:* presence of herpetic lesions on a background of eczematous skin. *Initial management:* admission to hospital for fluids IV + aciclovir.
Lichen sclerosus	*Suggested by:* presence of lesion on the genitals and perineum in a female. History of autoimmune conditions, e.g. vitiligo and pernicious anaemia. *Confirmed by:* itchy, atrophic patches of skin in the genital area. *Initial management:* moderate to potent local skin steroid cream.

(Continued)

Itchy skin with lesions but no wheals (continued)

Main differential diagnoses and typical outline evidence, etc.	
Lichen simplex chronicus	*Suggested by:* history of habitual rubbing or scratching associated with stress and typically in Asian or Chinese patient.
	Confirmed by: presence of a single plaque on the back of the neck or in the perineum.
	Initial management: emollients and topical steroids.
Pellagra associated with carcinoid syndrome or antiTB drugs.	*Suggested by:* diarrhoea, dementia, and dermatitis. May be history of associated condition.
	Confirmed by: response to nicotinic acid treatment.
	Initial management: correction of fluid and electrolyte imbalance + nicotinamide.
Polymorphic light eruption	*Suggested by:* recurrent lesions on exposure typically in a female.
	Confirmed by: presence of an eruption which may range from a few inflamed papules to severely inflamed and oedematous skin.
	Initial management: avoid exposure to sun, use of sunscreens, topical and/or systemic steroids for the acute rash.
Pompholyx	*Suggested by:* history of atopy, stress, allergic reactions to fungal infections elsewhere.
	Confirmed by: presence of persistent, itchy, clear blisters on fingers and sometimes palms.
	Initial management: symptomatic with antihistamines, antibiotics, and local creams.

Itch with wheals

Initial investigations (others below in **bold**): digital photography of lesion.

Main differential diagnoses and typical outline evidence, etc.	
Chronic idiopathic urticaria	*Suggested by:* recurrent nature and by the appearance of wheals variable in size, shape, and number anywhere on skin with no obvious triggering factors.
	Confirmed by: disappearance of wheals in <24h and possible spontaneous resolution after 6mo.
	Initial management: cetirizine and systemic steroids for severe cases, anaphylactic shock treated with adrenaline.
Acute urticaria	*Suggested by:* sudden urticarial rash after the introduction of the known offending agent, e.g. eggs, fish, peanuts, antibiotics, or latex.
	Confirmed by: improvement after eliminating the offending agent.
	Initial management: avoid the offending agent, cetirizine and systemic steroids for severe cases, anaphylactic shock treated with adrenaline.
Physical urticaria	*Suggested by:* appearance of wheals after exposure to cold, sun, pressure water, and stress.
	Confirmed by: dermographism and improvement when excluding the offending agent.
	Initial management: avoid offending agents for the acute condition; cetirizine or fexofenadine and systemic steroid for more severe reaction. Adrenaline for anaphylaxis.
Hereditary angioedema	*Suggested by:* +ve FH and an onset from childhood of episodes of angioedema affecting the larynx, impairing respiration and GI system, causing abdominal pain and vomiting.
	Confirmed by: low levels of **C1-esterase inhibitor** and **complement studies** during the acute episode.
	Initial management: as for urticaria plus IV infusion of C1-esterase inhibitor.
Linear IgA disease	*Suggested by:* blisters and urticarial rash on back and extensor surfaces.
	Confirmed by: **direct immunofluorescence studies** revealing linear IgA at basement membrane.
	Initial management: symptomatic.

Itch with no skin lesion

Initial investigations (others below in **bold**): digital photography of lesion. FBC, U&E, LFT.

Main differential diagnoses and typical outline evidence, etc.	
Chronic liver disease	*Suggested by:* jaundice, spider naevi, enlarged liver.
	Confirmed by: **LFT**: ↑bilirubin and ↑alkaline phosphatase, prolonged prothrombin time, and low albumin.
	Initial management: colestyramine.
Chronic renal failure	*Suggested by:* dry, sallow skin itching.
	Confirmed by: ↑**urea and creatinine**, and ↓**Hb.**
	Initial management: dietary advice; salt and water management. Regular follow-up. When advanced, plan dialysis or renal transplant.
Iron deficiency	*Suggested by:* pale complexion and skin, koilonychias, angular stomatitis.
	Confirmed by: ↓**Hb**, ↓**MCV**, and ↓**ferritin.**
	Initial management: iron replacement, e.g. ferrous sulphate; investigate and treat underlying cause.
Hyperhidrosis	*Suggested by:* excessive sweating, itching, obesity.
	Confirmed by: typical features and no other features on follow-up.
	Initial management: topical aluminium chloride; if intractable, sympathectomy.
1° hypothyroidism	*Suggested by:* dry skin, fatigue, slow-relaxing ankle jerk.
	Confirmed by: ↑**TSH**, ↓**T4.**
	Initial management: thyroxine replacement.
Lymphoma (Hodgkin's or non-Hodgkin's)	*Suggested by:* loss of weight, night sweat, lymphadenopathy, hepatosplenomegaly.
	Confirmed by: **biopsy**: Reed–Sternberg cells in Hodgkin's, not in non-Hodgkin's lymphoma, etc.
	Initial management: refer to oncology for staging etc.
Malignancy	*Suggested by:* general ill health, loss of weight, hepatomegaly, clubbing of fingers, shadow in a **CXR**.
	Confirmed by: **CT scan** of suspect organ(s).
	Initial management: refer to specialist for staging, selection for potentially curative or palliative care.
1° biliary cirrhosis	*Suggested by:* non-tender hepatomegaly and splenomegaly, xanthoma, arthralgia, abnormal LFT.
	Confirmed by: +ve **anti-mitochondrial, US examination and liver biopsy**.
	Initial management: colestyramine; ursodeoxycholic acid (may increase life expectancy and avoid transplant).

Skin ulceration

Initial investigations (others below in **bold**): digital photography of lesion.

Main differential diagnoses and typical outline evidence, etc.	
Staphylococcal infection	*Suggested by:* thin-walled blisters, rupturing easily to leave a yellow, crusted area spreading rapidly, usually on face.
	Confirmed by: above typical appearance and site.
	Initial management: systemic antibiotic, avoiding local antibiotic due to risk of bacterial resistance.
Basal cell carcinoma	*Suggested by:* small, pearly nodule progressing to central necrosis, producing a crusted ulcer with a rolled edge or a large plaque with a central depression.
	Confirmed by: **histology.**
	Initial management: excision.
Squamous cell carcinoma	*Suggested by:* persistently ulcerated or crusted, firm, irregular lesion, usually on sun-exposed areas, e.g. ears, back of hands, bald scalp; in pipe smokers, and patients with leg ulcers.
	Confirmed by: **biopsy.**
	Initial management: excision.
Dermatomyositis	*Suggested by:* purple rash on eyelid/face, associated with muscle weakness.
	Confirmed by: +ve **auto-antibodies, skin and muscle biopsy.**
	Initial management: systemic steroids.
Pyoderma gangrenosum	*Suggested by:* recurring nodule, pustular ulcers, about 10cm wide, with a tender, red, necrotic edge, healing with pitted scars on legs, abdomen, and face.
	Confirmed by: dramatic response to dapsone.
	Initial management: saline cleansing and dapsone.
Rheumatoid arthritis with vasculitis	*Suggested by:* vasculitic ulcer ± purpura, swollen and deformed phalyngeal joints with ulnar deviation. Rheumatoid nodules.
	Confirmed by: +ve **rheumatoid factor**, erosive appearance on **joint X-ray.**
	Initial management: NSAIDs, steroids, disease-modifying drugs, skin grafting.
Syphilis	*Suggested by:* an isolated, painless genital ulcer (primary chancre).
	Confirmed by: **serology, histology** and typical appearance.
	Initial management: benzylpenicillin IM.

SLE	*Suggested by:* associated facial butterfly rash, photosensitivity (face, dorsum of hands, neck), red scaly rashes.
	Confirmed by: +ve and high titre **antinuclear auto-antibodies, immunofluorescence studies**.
	Initial management: symptomatic treatment, systemic steroids.
Wegener's granuloma	*Suggested by:* skin and mouth ulcers, nasal ulceration with epistaxis, cranial nerve lesions, haemoptysis.
	Confirmed by: **cANCA** +ve. **Biopsy** showing granulomatous vasculitis.
	Initial management: high dose systemic steroids.

Photosensitive rash

The initial management of all these conditions will clearly involve avoidance of exposure to sunlight and use of sun block creams. Initial investigations (others below in **bold**): digital photography of lesion.

Main differential diagnoses and typical outline evidence, etc.	
Polymorphic light eruptions	*Suggested by:* recurrent rash on exposure to sun, typically in a female patient.
	Confirmed by: presence of an eruption which may range from a few inflamed papules to severely inflamed and oedematous skin.
	Initial management: avoid exposure to sun, use of sunscreen. topical and/or systemic steroids for the acute rash.
Plant chemical hyperphotosensitivity	*Suggested by:* red-brown macules on arms, hands, and face (blistering first) after exposure to sunlight.
	Confirmed by: history of cutting plants (e.g. giant hogweed) without skin covering.
	Initial management: sunblock and avoidance of exposure to sun. Cosmetics to conceal pigmentation.
Actinic prurigo	*Suggested by:* presence since childhood with papules appearing on sun-exposed sites.
	Confirmed by: improvement after protecting the exposed site.
	Initial management: sunblock and avoidance of exposure to sun. Cosmetics to conceal pigmentation.
Drug-induced photosensitivity	*Suggested by:* intake of a drug or the application of a cream which are known to cause photosensitivity, e.g. amiodarone, furosemide, tetracycline, and sunscreen agents.
	Confirmed by: improvement after eliminating the offending agent.
	Initial management: emollients and steroid creams, and avoidance of exposure to sun.
Pellagra associated with carcinoid syndrome or antiTB drugs	*Suggested by:* diarrhoea, dementia, and dermatitis. History of predisposing condition.
	Confirmed by: response to treatment with nicotinic acid.
	Initial management: correction of fluid and electrolyte imbalance + nicotinamide.
Solar urticaria Idiopathic or drug-induced, e.g. aspirin or opiates	*Suggested by:* urticarial rash appearing after exposure to sun.
	Confirmed by: no other features on follow-up.
	Initial management: avoidance of exposure, cetirizine, local emollients.

SLE	*Suggested by:* facial butterfly rash, photosensitivity (face, dorsum of hands, neck), red scaly rashes.
	Confirmed by: +ve and high titre **antinuclear auto-antibodies. Direct skin immunoflorescence studies**.
	Initial management: avoid exposure to sun, systemic steroids.
Subacute cutaneous lupus erythematosus	*Suggested by:* symmetrical, scaly plaques on sun-exposed areas of face and forearm.
	Confirmed by: presence of **anti-Ro antibodies. Biopsy**.
	Initial management: avoid exposure to sun and sunscreen. Local steroid creams.
Pemphigus associated with autoimmune thyroiditis, hypothyroidism or myasthenia gravis	*Suggested by:* presence of superficial blisters on the scalp, face, back, chest, and flexures ± preceding mouth erosions. History of other autoimmune disease.
	Confirmed by: **IgG autoantibodies** to epidermal components. **Direct immunofluoresence studies** showing deposition of IgG antibodies.
	Initial management: avoid exposure to sun, High dose of prednisolone PO ± azathioprine or cyclophosphamide.

Pigmented moles

A flat or raised pigmented spot in the skin. Initial investigations (others below in **bold**): digital photography of lesion.

Main differential diagnoses and typical outline evidence, etc.	
Blue melanocytic naevus	*Suggested by:* solitary with colour commonly on hands and feet. *Confirmed by:* above appearance with no change on follow-up over weeks to months. Biopsy, if in doubt. *Initial management:* reassurance.
Splitz melanocytic naevus	*Suggested by:* fleshy, firm, reddish-brown, round papule or nodule, usually on face or leg of a child. *Confirmed by:* above appearance with no change on follow-up over weeks to months. *Initial management:* reassurance.
Halo melanocytic naevus	*Suggested by:* presence of a white halo of depigmentation surrounding the original naevus, usually on trunk of a child or an adolescent. May be history of vitiligo. *Confirmed by:* above appearance with no change on follow-up over weeks to months. *Initial management:* reassurance.
Becker's melanocytic naevus	*Suggested by:* large, hairy, pigmented area. Present unilaterally in an adolescent male on the upper back, shoulders, or chest. *Confirmed by:* above appearance with no change on follow-up over weeks to months. *Initial management:* reassurance.
Freckles	*Suggested by:* presence of small, pigmented macules <5mm in diameter on sun-exposed area of a fair-skinned person. *Confirmed by:* above appearance with no change on follow-up over weeks to months. *Initial management:* reassurance.
Seborrhoeic wart	*Suggested by:* presence of round or oval pigmented spot on the trunk or face in an elderly or middle-aged person. Progression from small papule into a pigmented warty nodule. *Confirmed by:* 'stuck-on' appearance and multiplicity of lesions. *Initial management:* cryotherapy, curettage, or shave biopsy.
Chloasma	*Suggested by:* appearance of large (<5mm) areas of pigmentation during pregnancy. *Confirmed by:* resolution in months following delivery. *Initial management:* reassurance, sunscreens, and camouflage cosmetics.

Peutz–Jegher's syndrome (with risk of colonic and other neoplasms)	*Suggested by:* small (<5mm) macules on the lips, in the mouth, and around the eyes and nose; also around the anus, hands, and feet. Present since infancy or childhood and fade with age.
	Confirmed by: presence of *Polyposis coli* on **colonoscopy**.
	Initial management: refer for regular colonoscopy to remove suspicious polyps.
Dysplastic naevi	*Suggested by:* irregular outline and deep pigmentation.
	Confirmed by: **biopsy.**
	Initial management: surgical excision.
Malignant melanoma 'Superficial spreading', 'lentigo', 'acral lentiginous', 'nodular'	*Suggested by:* recent increase in the size of a naevus, irregular outline, variation of colour, itchiness, and oozing or bleeding. 'Superficial spreading' (up to 50%, typically on leg, female), 'lentigo' (up to 50%); acral lentiginous (10%) on palms, soles, and nailbed of dark-skinned); 'nodular' (25%, typically on trunk).
	Confirmed by: **biopsy.**
	Initial management: referral to dermatologist or for surgical intervention. Prognosis is related to tumour thickness: 5-y survival rate: <1mm=95%; 1–2mm=90%; 2.1–4mm=77%; >4mm=65%.

Tumour on the skin

Initial investigations (others below in **bold**): digital photography of lesion.

Main differential diagnoses and typical outline evidence, etc.	
Seborrhoeic wart	*Suggested by:* a round or oval pigmented spot on the trunk or face in an elderly or middle-aged person, starting as a small papule, progressing to a pigmented warty nodule.
	Confirmed by: 'stuck-on' appearance and multiplicity of lesions.
	Initial management: cryotherapy, curettage, or shave biopsy.
Epidermal cyst	*Suggested by:* a cystic swelling on scalp, face, or trunk, with a firm consistency and skin-coloured.
	Confirmed by: typical appearance and little progression over weeks to months.
	Initial management: excision.
Milium	*Suggested by:* small, white cysts around the eyelids and on the cheeks, usually seen in children.
	Confirmed by: typical appearance.
	Initial management: reassurance or extraction by a sterile needle.
Dermatofibroma	*Suggested by:* a nodular lesion in a young adult, typically on the lower leg of a female.
	Confirmed by: **biopsy.**
	Initial management: reassurance or excision.
Pyogenic granuloma	*Suggested by:* a rapidly growing, easily bleeding, bright red, and may be pedunculated nodule, usually on a finger.
	Confirmed by: **excisional biopsy.**
	Initial management: excision.
Keloid	*Suggested by:* irregular and excessive skin growth at the site of a trauma, producing nodules or plaques on the upper back, neck, chest, and ear lobes.
	Confirmed by: typical appearance with failure to resolve.
	Initial management: steroid injections.
Campbell-de-Morgan spot	*Suggested by:* presence of small red papules on the trunk in elderly.
	Confirmed by: typical appearance with little change over months.
	Initial management: acceptance or cauterization.
Lipoma	*Suggested by:* soft, subcutaneous, fatty mass, usually multiple, and commonly found on trunk of neck.
	Confirmed by: above appearance, and slow or no progression over months to years.
	Initial management: reassurance or excision, if unsightly.

Chondrodermatitis nodularis	*Suggested by:* a painful nodule on the sun-exposed helix of the pinna in an elderly.
	Confirmed by: typical appearance and site.
	Initial management: excision.
Keratoacanthoma	*Suggested by:* a rapidly forming nodule on a sun exposed area. The centre falls leaving a crater.
	Confirmed by: **biopsy.**
	Initial management: excision.
Basal cell carcinoma	*Suggested by:* presence of a nodule, usually started as a papule, developing central necrosis and producing an ulcer with rolled edges, usually on sun-exposed sites, eg. by the nose and on the temple.
	Confirmed by: **excisional biopsy.**
	Initial management: excision.
Squamous cell carcinoma	*Suggested by:* history of chronic sun exposure, pipe smoking, chronic ulceration, e.g. a burn or renal transplant.
	Confirmed by: **biopsy.**
	Initial management: surgical excision.
Malignant melanoma	*Suggested by:* recent increase in the size of itchiness, and oozing or bleeding naevus, irregular outline, variation of colour.
	Confirmed by: **biopsy.**
	Initial management: referral to dermatology for surgical intervention.

Hyperpigmented skin

Initial investigations (others below in **bold**): digital photography of lesion.

Main differential diagnoses and typical outline evidence, etc.	
Freckles	*Suggested by:* brown macules, in face usually, and become darker on sun exposure. *Confirmed by:* above appearance and no progression over months to years. *Initial management:* reassurance.
Lentigines	*Suggested by:* brown macules, not affected by exposure to sun, usually seen in elderly. *Confirmed by:* above appearance and no progression over months to years. *Initial management:* reassurance.
Drug-induced	*Suggested by:* intake of a drug, e.g amiodarone, phenothiazine, minocycline, and oestrogen. *Confirmed by:* improvement on removing the drug. *Initial management:* eliminate offending agent.
Addison's disease,	*Suggested by:* pigmentation in palmar creases and buccal mucosa. Nausea, weight loss, ↓BP, etc. *Confirmed by:* ↑**ACTH** with ↓**cortisol,** and poor response to **Synacthen® stimulation test**. *Initial management:* replacement hydrocortisone and fludrocortisone.
Cushing's disease,	*Suggested by:* pigmentation in palmar creases and buccal mucosa. *Confirmed by:* ↑**ACTH** with ↑**cortisol** with failure to suppress normally in **dexamethasone test**. *Initial management:* metyrapone initially, then plan for pituitary adenectomy.
Biliary cirrhosis	*Suggested by:* non-tender hepatomegaly, splenomegaly, xanthelasmatosis, xanthoma, arthralgia. *Confirmed by:* +ve **anti-mitochondrial antibodies and liver biopsy**. *Initial management:* colestyramine.
Pemphigoid	*Suggested by:* presence of tense, large blisters arising on a red or a normal-looking skin, usually in an elderly patient, on the limbs, trunk and flexures, or mouth. *Confirmed by:* specific **IgG antibodies to the antigens BP230 and BP180, and direct immunofluorescence studies** show IgG and C3 antibodies in the subepidermis. *Initial management:* low dose of prednisolone PO ± azathioprine.

Pellagra	*Suggested by:* presence of diarrhoea, dementia, and dermatitis. History of carcinoid syndrome or antiTB drugs.
	Confirmed by: response to nicotinic acid.
	Initial management: correction of fluid and electrolyte imbalance + nicotinamide.
Carotenaemia	*Suggested by:* eating many carrots or dye-containing foods.
	Confirmed by: dietary history and response to advice.
	Initial management: dietary advice.
Lichen planus	*Suggested by:* associated Koebner's phenomenon.
	Confirmed by: presence of itchy, well-defined, and raised, shiny-surfaced lesions with a violaceous colour interpreted by white streaks (Wickman's striae).
	Initial management: topical steroids; systemic steroids for extensive lesions.
Acanthosis nigricans	*Suggested by:* skin thickening and pigmentation.
	Confirmed by: presence of pigmented, velvety, and papillomatous skin lesion of flexures, neck, nipples, and umbilicus.
	Initial management: treatment of underlying problem, e.g. diabetes mellitus.

Hypopigmented skin

Initial investigations (others below in **bold**): digital photography of lesion.

Main differential diagnoses and typical outline evidence, etc.	
Vitiligo	*Suggested by:* presence of symmetrical, non-scaly, white macules ± history of injury or sun exposure, usually on hand, neck, and around mouth.
	Confirmed by: above appearance and little or no change over months or years.
	Initial management: camouflage cosmetics, sunscreens, PUVA.
Albinism	*Suggested by:* FH, white or pink skin, white hair, poor sight.
	Confirmed by: above appearance and little or no change over months or years.
	Initial management: advise to avoid sun exposure (risk of cancer).
Phenylketonuria	*Suggested by:* fair skin, learning difficulties.
	Confirmed by: **↑phenylalanine in blood.**
	Initial management: low phenylalanine diet.

Cardiovascular symptoms and physical signs

Chest pain—alarming and increasing over minutes to hours

There will be a limited number of differential diagnoses for chest pain that is not sharp and is not an easily recognized pattern by the patient (e.g. as predicably familiar angina). Ideally, the detailed history and examination is taken where resuscitation facilities are available. Early non-specific ECG changes will suggest an acute coronary syndrome—a blanket term that includes angina or myocardial infarction (MI); serial ECG or enzyme changes may be needed to differentiate between them.

- Normal troponin 12h after pain: probability of MI <0.3%.
- ↑troponin indicates episode of muscle necrosis up to 2wk before.
- Initial investigations (other tests in bold below): FBC, U&E, ECG, troponin I 12h after onset of the pain.

Main differential diagnoses and typical outline evidence, etc.	
Angina (new or unstable) or acute coronary syndrome-ACS	*Suggested by:* central pain ± radiating to jaw and either arm (left typically). Intermittent, relieved by rest or nitrates, and lasting <30min.
	Confirmed by: no ↑**troponins** after 12h, and no T wave or ST segment changes on **serial ECG**.
	Initial management: O₂, high dose aspirin, nitrates IV and/or oral, β-blockers, statins. LMW heparin.
ST elevated myocardial infarction (STEMI)	*Suggested by:* central chest pain ± radiating to jaw and either arm (left typically). Continuous, typically over 30min, not relieved by rest or nitrates.
	Confirmed by: ↑ST 1mm in limb leads or 2mm in chest leads on **serial ECG**.
	Initial management: O₂, high dose aspirin, nitrates IV and/or oral, β-blockers, statins, and ACE inhibitor. Urgent thrombolysis and/or primary angioplasty.
Non-ST elevation myocardial infarction (NSTEMI)	*Suggested by:* central chest pain ± radiating to jaw and either arm (left typically). Continuous, typically over 30min, not relieved by rest or nitrates.
	Confirmed by: ↑**troponin** after 12h. T wave or ST segment depression but no ↑ST on **serial ECG**.
	Initial management: O₂, high dose aspirin, nitrates, IV and/or oral, β-blockers, statins and ACE inhibitor. LMW heparin. Consider early angiogram ± primary angioplasty.
Oesophagitis and oesophageal spasm	*Suggested by:* past episodes of pain when supine, after food, alcohol, NSAIDs. Relieved by antacids.
	Confirmed by: no ↑**troponin** after 12h and no serial changes on **ECG**. Oesophagitis on **endoscopy**.
	Initial management: PPI medication and lifestyle modification. Calcium antagonist, e.g. nifedipine, if spasm.

Pulmonary embolus/ infarction (arising from deep veins or in right atrium) fibrillating	*Suggested by:* sudden breathlessness, pleural rub, cyanosis, tachycardia, loud P2, associated DVT, or risk factors such as recent surgery, immobility, previous emboli, malignancy, etc.
	Confirmed by: **CT pulmonary angiogram** shows clot in pulmonary artery.
	Initial management: LMW heparin (treatment dose), then warfarin. Thrombolysis if ↓BP, large bilateral clots, or acutely dilated right ventricle on **echocardiogram**.
Pneumothorax ('tension', mod- erate, or mild)	*Suggested by:* pain in centre or side of chest with abrupt breathlessness, diminished breath sounds, and hyper- resonance to percussion.
	Confirmed by: above with tracheal deviation and distress, suggesting tension pneumothorax or **expiration CXR** showing loss of lung markings outside sharp line ('moderate' if >5cm gap from lung edge to chest wall; 'mild' if <5cm).
	Initial management: if tension pneumothorax, insert large Venflon into 2nd intercostal (IC) space, mid- clavicular line. Give O_2 if breathless. Analgesia. Aspirate if 'moderate'; if this is unsatisfactory or prior lung disease, insert IC drain into 'triangle of safety'. If 'mild' (<5cm gap) and not breathless, observe.
Dissecting thoracic aortic aneurysm	*Suggested by:* 'tearing' pain, often radiating to back, abnormal or absent peripheral pulses, early diastolic murmur, low BP, and widened mediastinum on **CXR**.
	Confirmed by: loss of single, clear lumen on **CT scan** or **MRI**.
	Initial management: O_2, analgesia, large bore IV access, crossmatch 6 units, and urgent surgical referral.
Chest wall pain (e.g. Tietze's syndrome.)	*Suggested by:* chest pain and tenderness of chest wall on twisting of neck or thoracic cage.
	Confirmed by: normal (or no changes in) **troponin**, **ECG**, and **CXR**. Good response to simple analgesia.
	Initial management: simple analgesia (e.g. NSAIDs) and avoidance of strenuous activity until ↓pain.

Severe lower chest or upper abdominal pain

Upper abdominal pain may also be difficult for the patient to separate from lower chest pain, so the causes of chest pain also have to be borne in mind. Initial investigations (other tests in **bold** below): FBC, U&E, LFT, CRP, D-dimer, troponin, ECG, CXR.

Main differential diagnoses and typical outline evidence, etc.	
Gastro-oesophageal reflux/gastritis	*Suggested by:* central or epigastric burning pain, onset over hours, dyspepsia, worse on lying flat, worsened by food, alcohol, NSAIDs.
	Confirmed by: **troponin** normal after 12h and no ↑ ST segments on **ECG**. Oesophagitis on **endoscopy**. Improvement with antacids.
	Initial management: antacid, e.g. PPI. Calcium antagonist, e.g. nifedipine, if spasm.
Biliary colic	*Suggested by:* post-prandial chest pain over minutes to hours (after fatty foods), severe, colicky, central, right upper quadrant, radiation to right scapula.
	Confirmed by: **US scan** showing gallstones and biliary dilatation and also on **ERCP**.
	Initial management: analgesia (e.g. pethidine IM). Nil by mouth. Fluids IV. Antibiotics, e.g. IV cefuroxime/metronidazole, if fever or ↑WCC. Avoid fatty foods.
Pancreatitis (often due to gallstone impacted in common bile duct; often complicated by chronic pancreatitis.)	*Suggested by:* mid-epigastric pain radiating to back, associated with nausea and vomiting, gallstones. Onset over hours.
	Confirmed by: ↑**serum amylase** (normal if gland destruction), pancreatic pseudocyst on **CT abdomen.**
	Initial management: opiate analgesia, e.g. pethidine IM, nil by mouth, Fluids IV, monitor glucose and Ca^{2+}, NG tube if ileus ± colloid and blood. Antibiotics, e.g. IV cefuroxime + metronidazole. Chronic: analgesics, pancreatic supplements, monitor blood glucose.
Myocardial infarction (often inferior MI)	Suggested by: continuous pain, onset over minutes to hours, not relieved by rest or GTN.
	Confirmed by: T waves inversion ± ↑STof 1mm in limb leads or 2mm in chest leads on **serial ECG**, or ↑**troponin**.
	Initial management: O_2, high dose aspirin, nitrates, IV and/or oral, β-blockers, statins, and ACE inhibitor. If ↑ST of 1mm in limb leads or 2mm in chest leads, thrombolysis. Primary angioplasty for any MI.

Sudden breathlessness, onset over seconds

This situation may be life-threatening; the severity of the underlying condition often creates helpful diagnostic information. Initial investigations (other tests in **bold** below): FBC, U&E, ABG, ECG, CXR.

Main differential diagnoses and typical outline evidence, etc.	
Pulmonary embolus/ infarction (arising within the lung or from deep veins or right atrium) fibrillating	*Suggested by:* sudden breathlessness, pleural rub, cyanosis, tachycardia, loud P2, associated DVT, or risk factors such as recent surgery, immobility, previous emboli, malignancy, etc. *Confirmed by:* **CT pulmonary angiogram** shows clot in pulmonary artery. *Initial management:* LMW heparin (treatment dose), then warfarin. Thrombolysis if ↓BP, large bilateral clots, or acutely dilated right ventricle on **echocardiogram**.
Pneumothorax ('tension', moderate, or mild)	*Suggested by:* pain in centre or side of chest with abrupt breathlessness, diminished breath sounds, and hyperresonance to percussion. *Confirmed by:* above with tracheal deviation and distress, suggesting tension pneumothorax or **expiration CXR** showing loss of lung markings outside sharp line ('moderate' if >5cm gap from lung edge to chest wall; 'mild' if <5cm.) *Initial management:* if tension pneumothorax, insert large Venflon into 2nd intercostal (IC) space, mid-clavicular line. Give O_2 if breathless. Analgesia. Aspirate if 'moderate'; if this is unsatisfactory or prior lung disease, insert IC drain into 'triangle of safety'. If 'mild' (<5cm gap) and not breathless, observe.
Anaphylaxis ?precipitant	*Suggested by:* dramatic onset over minutes, recent allergen exposure. Flushing, sweating facial oedema, urticaria, warm but clammy extremities, tachypnoea, bronchospasm, and wheeze. Tachycardia and hypotension. *Confirmed by:* precipitant identification and response to adrenaline (epinephrine) IM. *Initial management:* remove antigen (e.g. bee sting, medication). Adrenaline IM 1 in 10,000. High flow O_2, fast fluids IV, steroids IV, and antihistamines IV. If stridor, secure airway early as laryngeal oedema may progress, and transfer to HDU/ITU.
Inhalation of foreign body	*Suggested by:* history of putting an object in mouth, e.g. peanut. Sudden stridor, severe cough, low-pitched, monophonic wheeze, and reduced breath sounds, more typically on the right. *Confirmed by:* If not *in extremis*, **CXR/CT thorax** or **bronchoscopy** to see foreign body. *Initial management:* if *in extremis*, slap back between the shoulder blades with patient leaning forward; if fails, do Heimlich manoeuvre.

Orthopnoea and paroxysmal nocturnal dyspnoea (PND)

Orthopnoea is shortness of breath when lying flat. (Try to confirm by observing what happens when patient lies flat.) This can be explained by oedema gathering along the posterior length of the lungs or less efficient lung movement when the abdominal contents press against the diaphragm. PND can happen when the patient slides down in bed at night or by bronchospasm due to night-time asthma. Initial investigations (other tests in **bold** below): FBC, U&E, ECG, and CXR.

Main differential diagnoses and typical outline evidence, etc.	
Pulmonary oedema (due to congestive (chronic) heart failure or left ventricular failure—due to ischaemic heart disease, mitral stenosis.)	*Suggested by:* background fatigue and exertional breathless, cardiac risk factors. Displaced apex beat, 3rd heart sound, bilateral basal fine crackles. Raised JVP and leg swelling.
	Confirmed by: **CXR** fluffy opacification, especially near hila. Loss of costophrenic angle. Impaired left ventricular function on **echocardiogram**.
	Initial management: sit patient up, controlled O2, diuretics IV. nitrates IV if very breathless and systolic BP >90. *Chronic:* thiazide or loop diuretic, ACE inhibitor (or angiotensin receptor blocker). β-blocker and spironolactone (monitor potassium).
COPD	*Suggested by:* long history of cough ± sputum, >10-pack year smoking, recurrent 'exacerbations'. **CXR** radiolucent lungs.
	Confirmed by: **spirometry:** FEV$_1$ <80% predicted and FEV/FVC ratio <0.7. <15% reversibility. Emphysema on **CT chest** ± reduced **α1-antitrypsin** levels.
	Initial management: Controlled O2, prednisolone 7–10d, and nebulized bronchodilators. If worsening breathlessness, cough and mucopurulent sputum, antibiotics (e.g. amoxicillin/clarithromycin or tetracycline or trimethoprim). No smoking. Trials of bronchodilators prn, then regular long-acting bronchodilators. Regular inhaled steroids if FEV<50% predicted and three exacerbations per year.
Asthma	*Suggested by:* wheeze, chronic cough worse at night/early morning, specific triggers. Family history or childhood history of asthma or atopy.
	Confirmed by: reduced **peak flow**. **FEV$_1$** that improves by >15% with treatment.
	Management: acute: high flow O2, prednisolone PO or hydrocortisone IV. Nebulized salbutamol and ipratropium ± magnesium IV + aminophylline IV; chronic: identify precipitants, smoking cessation, trial of bronchodilator prn, and inhaled steroids, long-acting β-agonist/steroid combinations, leukotriene inhibitors/antihistamines.

Cardiac arrhythmia	*Suggested by:* palpitations, chest pain, dizziness, cardiac risk factors, pallor, hypotension, tachycardia (occasionally bradycardia), may have low BP. No wheeze, but may have bibasal crackles from associated left ventricular failure.
	Confirmed by: **ECG** (pulse typically >140 or <40) and improvement in symptoms/signs as pulse rate improves.
	Initial management: controlled O_2; if tachycardia (pulse often >140), consider vasovagal manoeuvres and rate-lowering medications, or electric cardioversion if adverse signs (e.g. confusion, hypotension, chest pain); if bradycardia (pulse typically <40 to cause compromise), give controlled O_2, atropine IV, or pacing (external, temporary internal) if adverse signs. Thereafter should be managed in a CCU.

Palpitations

Very subjective and a poor lead (with many self-limiting undiagnosable causes) unless forceful, fast, prolonged, and associated with chest pain, dizziness, or loss of consciousness. Initial investigations (other tests in **bold** below): FBC, U&E, ECG, CXR.

Main differential diagnoses and typical outline evidence, etc.	
Runs of SVT ?exercise-induced due to IHD ?due to electrolyte abnormalities	*Suggested by:* abrupt onset, sweats, and dizziness.
	Confirmed by: baseline **ECG** or **24-h ECG** normal QRS complexes with absent or abnormal P waves >140/min. **Exercise ECG** to see if precipitated by exercise.
	Initial management: O₂, vasovagal manoeuvres, trial of adenosine IV, verapamil, or amiodarone. If adverse signs (↓BP, LVF, ↓consciousness, chest pain), DC cardioversion.
Episodic heart block	*Suggested by:* onset over minutes or hours, slow and forceful beats. Pallor or loss of consciousness.
	Confirmed by: fixed or progressive prolonged PR interval, A-V dissociation, and slow QRS rate on baseline or **24-h ECG**.
	Initial management: O₂, correct electrolyte abnormalities, stop β-blockers/verapamil/digoxin. Temporary pacing wire if compromised, otherwise permanent pacemaker.
Sinus tachycardia (multitude of causes, anxiety, caffeine, febrile illness, hypovolaemia, pulmonary embolism, hyperventilation, nebulizers, etc.)	*Suggested by:* gradual onset over minutes of regular palpitations. Typically clear history of precipitating cause.
	Confirmed by: basal **ECG.** Resolution by stopping precipitating factors.
	Initial management: controlled O₂ and address underlying cause. Unlikely cardiac cause if pulse <150. If believed to be primary cardiac conduction, treat as SVT.
AF (acute (<24h) may have precipitating cause, e.g. MI, infection, electrolyte imbalance, thyrotoxicosis.)	*Suggested by:* irregularly irregular pulse.
	Confirmed by: **ECG** showing no P waves and irregularly irregular normal QRS complexes.
	Initial management: If new onset (<24h) and/or HR >130: treat cause, anticoagulate, and chemically cardiovert (digoxin/verapamil/amiodarone). **Cardiac monitor.**
	NB. DC shock if unstable. If rate <50, anticoagulate and treat as bradycardia. If rate 50–100 and duration unknown, rate control and anticoagulate. Referral for **echocardiogram** and consider outpatient cardioversion.

Ventricular ectopics unifocal (benign) or multifocal (may have underlying pathology)	*Suggested by:* palpitations, noted over hours or days, associated anxiety. *Confirmed by:* premature wide QRS complexes on **baseline ECG** or **24-h ECG**. *Initial management:* **echocardiogram**. Consider β-blockers, verapamil, and ACE inhibitors (if left ventricular dysfunction).
Menopause	Suggested by: irregular or no more periods, worse over weeks or months. Confirmed by: ↓**serum oestrogen**, ↑**FSH/LH**. Initial management: consider combined oestrogen/ progesterone HRT.
Thyrotoxicosis	Suggested by: onset over weeks or months. Irritability, weight loss, loose frequent stools, goitre, lid retraction and lag, brisk reflexes. Confirmed by: ↑**FT4** and/or ↑**FT3** and ↓**TSH**. Initial management: propranolol tds prn, if required for symptoms control. Carbimazole/ propylthiouracil daily to treat thyroid overactivity.
Phaeochromocytoma (rare)	Suggested by: abrupt episodes of anxiety, fear, chest tightness, sweating, headaches, and marked rises in BP. Confirmed by: catecholamines (**VMA, HMMA**) or ↑**free metadrenaline** in urine and blood soon after episode. Initial management: α- and β-blockers IV, then orally until vascular volume restored (monitor Hb/haematocrit for fall). Surgical referral for excision.

Acute breathlessness, wheeze ± cough

This symptom suggests airway narrowing. The commonest cause is bronchospasm (constriction of the smooth muscle in the distal bronchioles); less common causes are wheeze due to inhalation of a foreign body or hydrostatic pulmonary oedema, i.e. 'cardiac wheeze.' Initial investigations (other tests in **bold** below): FBC, U&E, CRP, ABG, ECG, and CXR.

Main differential diagnoses and typical outline evidence, etc.	
Exacerbation of asthma	*Suggested by:* widespread polyphonic wheeze with exacerbations over hours. Silent chest if severe. Anxiety, tachypnoea, tachycardia, and use of accessory muscles.
	Confirmed by: reduced peak flows. **FEV$_1$** that improves by >15% with treatment.
	Initial management: high flow O$_2$, prednisolone PO or hydrocortisone IV. Nebulized salbutamol and Atrovent® ± magnesium IV and aminophylline IV. NB. Keep hydrated and monitor ABG and serum K$^+$. Refer to HDU if drowsy, ↑CO$_2$.
Exacerbation of COPD	*Suggested by:* long history of cough ± sputum, >10-pack year smoking, recurrent 'exacerbations'. **CXR:** radiolucent lungs.
	Confirmed by: **spirometry:** FEV$_1$ <80% predicted and FEV/FVC ratio <0.7. <15% reversibility. Emphysema on **CT chest**. ± reduced α -1 antitrypsin levels.
	Initial management: controlled O$_2$, prednisolone 7–10d, and nebulized bronchodilators. Antibiotics if worsening breathlessness, cough, *and* mucopurulent sputum. Stop smoking. Trials of bronchodilators prn, then regular long-acting bronchodilators. Regular inhaled steroids if FEV<50% predicted and three exacerbations per year.
Acute viral or bacterial bronchitis	*Suggested by:* onset of wheeze over days. No dramatic progression. Fever, mucopurulent sputum, dyspnoea.
	Confirmed by: **sputum culture** and sensitivities. No consolidation on **CXR**.
	Initial management: simple analgesia and antibiotics, if continued purulent sputum.
Acute left ventricular failure due to ?cardiac event ?valvular disease ?electrolyte imbalance ?arrhythmia	*Suggested by:* onset over minutes to hours. Breathless, distressed, and clammy; displaced tapping apex beat, 3rd heart sound, bilateral basal late fine inspiratory crackles. Often also signs of right ventricular failure (↑JVP, swollen legs).
	Confirmed by: **CXR:** fluffy opacification (greatest around the hila), horizontal linear opacities peripherally, bilateral effusions, large heart. Impaired left ventricular function on **echocardiogram**.
	Initial management: sit patient up, controlled O$_2$, diuretics IV. nitrates IV if very breathless and systolic BP >90. Identify and treat potential causes. *Chronic:* thiazide or loop diuretic, ACE inhibitor (or angiotensin receptor blocker). β-blocker and spironolactone (monitor K$^+$).

Anaphylaxis
?precipitant

Suggested by: dramatic onset over minutes, recent allergen exposure. Flushing, sweating, facial oedema, urticaria, warm but clammy extremities, tachypnoea, bronchospasm, and wheeze. Tachycardia and hypotension.

Confirmed by: precipitant identification and response to IM adrenaline (epinephrine).

Initial management: remove antigen (e.g. bee sting, medication). Adrenaline IM 1 in 10,000. High flow O_2, fast fluids IV, steroids IV, and antihistamines IV. If stridor, secure airway early as laryngeal oedema may progress, and transfer to HDU / ITU.

Cough and pink frothy sputum

This is due to a combination of frothy sputum of pulmonary oedema mixed with blood from haemoptysis from pulmonary hypertension, causing distension and congestion of the pulmonary vasculature bed. Initial investigations (other tests in **bold** below): FBC, U&E, CRP, D-dimer, troponin, ECG, CXR.

Main differential diagnoses and typical outline evidence, etc.	
Acute pulmonary oedema due to left ventricular failure (due to ischaemic heart disease, mitral stenosis)	*Suggested by:* background fatigue and exertional breathless, cardiac risk factors. Displaced apex beat, 3rd heart sound, bilateral basal fine crackles. Raised JVP and leg swelling. *Confirmed by:* **CXR:** fluffy opacification, especially near hila. Loss of costophrenic angle. Impaired left ventricular function on **echocardiogram**. *Initial management:* sit patient up, controlled O_2, diuretics IV. nitrates IV if very breathless and systolic BP >90. *Chronic:* thiazide or loop diuretic, ACE inhibitor (or angiotensin receptor blocker). β-blocker and spironolactone (monitor K^+).
Mitral stenosis (± dilated left atrium ± atrial fibrillation)	*Suggested by:* months to years of orthopnoea, mitral facies, tapping, displaced apex, loud 1st heart sound, diastolic murmur, fine bibasal crackles. AF on **ECG**. Enlarged left atrial shadow (behind heart) and splayed carina on **CXR**. *Confirmed by:* large left atrium and mitral stenosis on **echocardiogram**. *Initial management:* aspirin and or warfarin if AF. Valvotomy/valve replacement if patient fit enough and high pressure gradient (>30mmHg) or very small valve area (<1.5cm²).

Syncope

This is sudden loss of consciousness over seconds. Think of abnormal 'electrical' activity in the central nervous system or a temporary drop in cardiac output and BP that improves as soon as the patient is in a prone position. Fits can occur due to a profound fall in BP so they are not specific of epilepsy. Initial investigations (other tests in **bold** below): FBC, U&E, CRP, glucose, ECG, and CXR.

Main differential diagnoses and typical outline evidence, etc.	
Vasovagal attack—simple faint ? precipated by emotion, pain, fear, prolonged standing etc.	*Suggested by:* syncope within seconds or minutes of preceding precipitant. Nausea, sweating, and darkening of vision. Recovery within minutes. No incontinence. *Confirmed by:* history. No abnormal physical signs. *Initial management:* reassurance.
Postural hypotension (often due to BP-lowering drugs, hypovolaemia)	*Suggested by:* sudden loss of consciousness after getting up from sitting or lying position. *Confirmed by:* >20mmHg fall in BP from reclining to standing. *Initial management:* minimize/avoid precipitants. Advice on posture and prolonged standing. Support stockings. Fludrocortisone PO or midodrine, if symptoms persist and disabling.
Stokes–Adams attack	*Suggested by:* sudden loss of consciousness with no warning. Pallor, then recovery within seconds or minutes, often with flushing. *Confirmed by:* **24-h ECG** showing episodes of asystole or heart block, SVT or VT. *Initial management:* correct electrolyte disturbances, temporary/permanent pacemaker.
Aortic stenosis	*Suggested by:* syncope on exercise. Slow rising pulse, low BP and pulse pressure, and heaving apex. Mid-systolic crescendo murmur, soft S2. **ECG**: tall R waves, left ventricular hypertrophy, left axis deviation, ST/T wave changes of 'strain'. *Confirmed by:* **echocardiogram** and **cardiac catheter**: stenosed valve. *Initial management:* aspirin, keep on cardiac monitor if syncope as could be due to ventricular fibrillation. Refer for consideration of valve replacement.
Hypertrophic cardiomyopathy (HOCM)	*Suggested by:* syncope. Family history of sudden death or HOCM. Angina, breathless, jerky pulse, high JVP with 'a' wave, double apex beat, thrill and murmur best at left sternal edge. *Confirmed by:* **echocardiogram** showing hypertrophied septum and ventricular walls with small ventricular cavities, especially on left. *Initial management:* β-blockers, aspirin. Keep on cardiac monitor if syncope as could be due to ventricular fibrillation. Refer to specialist centre.

Micturition syncope	*Suggested by:* sudden loss of consciousness after micturating. Often nocturnal and associated prostatism.
	Confirmed by: history. Normal examination.
	Initial management: advice. Treat prostatism, e.g. with α-blocker.
Cough syncope	*Suggested by:* sudden loss of consciousness after severe bout of coughing.
	Confirmed by: history. Normal examination.
	Initial management: treat cause of cough.
Carotid sinus syncope	*Suggested by:* sudden syncope on turning head (e.g. while shaving)
	Confirmed by: history and reproducible symptoms on movement.
	Initial management: aspirin, carotid Doppler scans, surgical referral if >70% stenosis.
Hypoglycaemia ?insulin intake mismatch (e.g. meals, alcohol, etc.)	*Suggested by:* preceded by seconds or minutes of hunger, sweating, and darkening of vision. Typically known diabetes.
	Confirmed by: **blood sugar** <2mmol/L and exclusion of associated cardiac condition.
	Initial management: give glucose (IV or oral 'hypostop'/ glucagon. Reassess insulin requirements and lifestyle.
Epilepsy ?precipitant (e.g.alcohol, infection, electrolyte abnormalities, BP drop)	*Suggested by:* preceding aura for few minutes, then tonic phase with cyanosis, clonic jerks of limbs, incontinence of urine and/or faeces.
	Confirmed by: history from witness. **EEG** changes, e.g. 'spike and wave'.
	Initial management: BLS algorithm. Rectal or diazepam IV. phenytoin IV. Address precipitants.
Cerebrovascular accident	*Suggested by:* residual sensorimotor deficit, may have pre-aura.
	Confirmed by: **CT head** will show infarct or bleed.
	Initial management: nil by mouth and fluids IV if dysphagia. SALT assessment. DVT prophylaxis: stockings/ LMW heparin (if no bleed). If infarct: stat high dose and daily regular dose aspirin. Start dipyridamole if stroke occurred whilst on aspirin. If haemorrhage: treat severe hypertension (systolic >200mmHg), refer to neurosurgeons.
Pulmonary embolus/ infarction (arising within the lung or from deep veins or right atrium) fibrillating	*Suggested by:* sudden breathlessness and sharp or central chest pain, recent surgery, immobility, previous emboli, malignancy, etc. Cyanosis, tachycardia, loud P2, pleural rub. Associated DVT or risk factors.
	Confirmed by: **CT pulmonary angiogram** showing clot in pulmonary artery.
	Initial management: LMW heparin (treatment dose) then ≥3mo warfarin. Thrombolysis if ↓BP, large and bilateral clots, no response to anticoagulation, or acutely dilated right ventricle on **echocardiogram**.

Leg pain on walking—intermittent claudication

This is analogous to angina, but pain comes on in the legs, instead of the chest, on exercise. Quantify the effect on daily activity (especially distance walked) and ability to cope at home, work, recreation, and rest. Initial investigations (other tests in bold below): FBC, U&E, D-dimer, CRP.

Main differential diagnoses and typical outline evidence, etc.	
Arterial disease in legs (if associated impotence=Leriche's syndrome) Risk factors (e.g. smoking, poor diabetes control)	*Suggested by:* predictable claudication distance. Worse on exertion, relieved with rest. Worse uphill, better downhill. Pain at rest implies incipient gangrene. Sleeps with leg hanging over edge of bed or in chair. Poor peripheral pulses and perfusion of skin and toes. *Confirmed by:* **Doppler ultrasound** or **arteriogram** showing stenosis and poor flow. *Initial management:* regular aspirin 150mg od. Address risk factors. Check skin and feet↑ viability. Refer to vascular surgeon.
Spinal claudication	*Suggested by:* weakness associated with pain. Improves slowly with rest but variable. Worse downhill. Brisk/reduced reflexes. Sensory↑ deficits according to level of compression. *Confirmed by:* **MRI spine** showing canal stenosis or disc compression of cord or cauda equina. *Initial management:* analgesia, e.g. NSAIDs, carbamazepine. Refer to neurosurgeons.

Leg pain on standing—relieved by lying down

Think of something relieved by reducing 'pressure' on lying down. Two possibilities are relief of the pressure transmitted down to leg tissues by incompetent venous valves or relief of pressure by the spinal column on a damaged disc, aggravating its protrusion and pressure on adjacent nerve roots. Initial investigations (other tests in **bold** below): FBC, CRP, thoracic/lumbar spine X-rays.

Main differential diagnoses and typical outline evidence, etc.	
Peripheral venous disease and varicose veins	*Suggested by:* generalized ache, itching, varicose veins and venous eczema ± ulcers. Cough impulse. **Trendelenberg test** shows filling down along extent of communicating valve leaks.
	Confirmed by: clinical findings or **Doppler ultrasound** to confirm any incompetence in sapheno-femoral junction or short saphenous vein.
	Initial management: advice to avoid prolonged standing and keep leg(s) elevated when sitting. Compression bandages and support stockings. Surgical referral.
Disc protrusion ('slipped disc')	*Suggested by:* severe referred ache or shooting pains, affected by position. Neurological deficit in root distribution.
	Confirmed by: **MRI spine** showing disc impinging on nerve roots.
	Initial management: analgesia. Bed rest. Surgical referral.

Unilateral calf or leg swelling

Swelling is explained as fluid gathering in the extravascular space. Think of this possibly being due to increased pressure within the veins or lymphatic vessels. It can also be due to unilateral damage to the local small veins and capillaries due to local inflammation. Unilateral swelling thus implies local inflammation, damage or obstruction to a vein or lymphatic duct. The speed of onset allows one to imagine what process might be taking place—traumatic, thrombotic, or infective. Initial investigations (other tests in **bold** below): FBC, CRP, D-dimer.

Main differential diagnoses and typical outline evidence, etc.	
Deep venous thrombosis Risk Factors (e.g. obesity, immobility, malignancy, contraceptive, smoking, previous clots)	*Suggested by:* onset over hours. Legs tense, tender, and warm. Risk factors (see over left). *Confirmed by:* poor flow on **Doppler ultrasound scan**, filling defect on **venogram**. *Initial management:* analgesia, treatment dose heparin until therapeutic warfarin. Anticoagulate at least 3mo. Address risk factors. Compression stockings reduce risk of post-thrombotic syndrome.
Ruptured Baker's cyst (leaking synovial fluid, sometimes no cyst)	*Suggested by:* onset sudden over seconds, e.g. when walking up a step. Typically arthritic knee. *Confirmed by:* normal flow on **Doppler ultrasound** and extravascular collection of fluid. No filling defect on **venogram**. Leakage of contrast from joint capsule if **arthrogram** done soon after the event. *Initial management:* analgesia, rest, and leg elevation.
Cellulitis	*Suggested by:* onset over days. Warm, tender erythema, tracking (red lines), fever, ↑**WBC**. *Confirmed by:* **skin swabs** if discharge from skin, **blood cultures**, response to antibiotics. *Initial management:* analgesia. Leg elevation. High dose benzylpenicillin IV + flucloxacillin for 10–14d. Consider fusidic acid + vancomycin if penicillin allergy. Prophylactic heparin.
Abnormal lymphatic drainage caused by lymphoma or malignant infiltration (or **trypanosomiasis** in tropics). Rarely, a hereditary in young women.	*Suggested by:* onset over years, firm, non-tender, non-pitting oedema. *Confirmed by:* obstruction to flow on↑ **lymphangiogram**. *Initial management:* compression stockings and leg elevation. Often difficult to treat and needs specialist nursing input.

Congenital oedema (Milroy's syndrome)	*Suggested by:* presence since childhood. worse pre-menstrually, in warm weather.
	Confirmed by: history and **lymphangiogram** showing primary lymphatic hypoplasia.
	Initial management: compression stockings and leg elevation. Often difficult to treat and needs specialist nursing input.

Bilateral ankle swelling

Think of increased pressure within the veins or lymphatic vessels or low albumin in the vascular space, bilateral damage to veins, lymphatics or capillaries due to local inflammation. Initial investigations (other tests in **bold** below): FBC, U&E, LFT, CRP.

Main differential diagnoses and typical outline evidence, etc.	
Right ventricular failure due to pulmonary hypertension or congestive cardiac failure	*Suggested by:* ↑JVP, liver enlargement and pulsation, right ventricular heave, loud S2. Onset over months typically.
	Confirmed by: dilated right ventricle on **echocardiogram**.
	Initial management: thiazide or loop diuretics, O₂ if hypoxic. Metolazone and fluid restriction in resistant cases.
Poor venous return due to abdominal or pelvic masses, post-phlebitic or thrombotic venous damage at inferior vena cava level or bilateral deep veins	*Suggested by:* onset over months. Worse on prolonged standing or sitting, varicosities, venous eczema, pigmentation, or ulceration.
	Confirmed by: clinical findings or **Doppler ultrasound** to determine incompetence in sapheno-femoral junction or short saphenous vein.
	Initial management: avoid prolonged standing and keep leg(s) elevated when sitting. Compression bandages/ stockings. **CT abdomen and pelvis**. Long-term warfarin if clot. Refer to vascular surgeons if symptoms worsen.
Low albumin states due to liver failure, nephrotic syndrome, malnutrition.	*Suggested by:* onset over months. Generalized oedema, often including face after lying down.
	Confirmed by: ↓**serum albumin**.
	Initial management: diuretics, correct serum albumin with quality diet.
Bilateral cellulitis often associated with diabetes mellitus	*Suggested by:* onset over days. warm, red, and tender legs, thrombophlebitis and tracking, ulcers, etc..
	Confirmed by: ↑**WBC** positive **blood cultures/skin swabs** (typically streptococcal or staphylococcal). ↑**blood sugar** in diabetes.
	Initial management: analgesia, leg elevation, high dose benzylpenicillin IV + flucloxacillin for 10–14d. Consider fusidic acid + vancomycin if penicillin allergy. Prophylactic heparin.

Inferior vena cava (IVC) obstruction due to prolonged immobility, carcinoma, and oral combined contraceptive use	*Suggested by:* bilateral leg swelling, onset over hours, associated risk factors. May have symptoms/signs of pulmonary embolism (PE).
	Confirmed by: **CT abdomen**, low flow on **Doppler ultrasound**, or filling defect on **venogram**.
	Initial management: analgesia, treatment dose heparin until warfarin dose is therapeutic. Anticoagulate for at least 3mo and address underlying risk factors. Consider IVC filter if large thrombus or recurrent PE despite anticoagulation.
Drugs	*Suggested by:* onset over days to weeks since starting calcium channel blocker.
	Confirmed by: symptom improves when calcium channel blocker stopped.
	Initial management: stop or substitute drug.
Bilateral thromboses	*Suggested by:* onset over hours. Legs firm, warm, tender. Presence of risk factors.
	Confirmed by: poor flow on **Doppler ultrasound scan**, filling defect on **venogram**.
	Initial management: analgesia, treatment dose heparin until warfarin provides therapeutic INR. Anticoagulate for at least 3mo and address underlying risk factors. Compression stockings reduce the risk of post-thrombotic syndrome.
Impaired lymphatic drainage	*Suggested by:* firm, non-tender, non-pitting oedema of gradual onset over months to years.
	Confirmed by: obstruction to flow on **lymphangiogram**.
	Initial management: compression stockings, e.g. elevation. Often needs specialist nursing input.

Thoughts on interpreting cardiovascular signs

The findings are described in a sequence of the cardiovascular examination, thinking of cardiac output, beginning with hand warmth, checking the radial pulse, measuring the BP. Continuing to think of cardiac output, examine the carotids. Next, think of venous return by inspecting the JVP. Finally, inspect, palpate, percuss, and auscultate the heart. Examine the legs and again think of cardiac output (e.g. temperature of skin and peripheral pulses), venous return (e.g. pitting oedema, leg veins, and liver enlargement).

Peripheral cyanosis

Cyanosis of hands but not tongue. Initial investigations (other tests in **bold** below): FBC, CRP, blood cultures, ABG, CXR.

Main differential diagnoses and typical outline evidence, etc.	
Raynaud's phenomenon due to exposure of hands to cold or vibration	*Suggested by:* blue hands after exposure to cold, vibrating tools, connective tissue disease. *Confirmed by:* symptoms improve with warmth. *Initial management:* avoid precipitating factors. Calcium channel blockers. Ilioprost infusions in a specialist setting if connective tissue disease.
Arterial obstruction due to atheroma or small vessel disease in diabetics	*Suggested by:* absent or poor pulsation of radial or dorsalis pedis. Absent hair and skin atrophy. *Confirmed by:* **Doppler ultrasound** (reduced blood flow) and **angiography**. *Initial management:* stop smoking, optimize blood sugar control. Aspirin. Refer to vascular surgeon.
Haemorrhage due to external or internal bleeding	*Suggested by:* low BP, high pulse rate, poor peripheral perfusion and urine output. *Confirmed by:* low **Hb** (although initial Hb is often normal) and **response to volume replacement**. *Initial management:* **blood transfusion** or plasma expander, and control of bleeding. Locate source of bleeding. Consider **CT abdomen** if no identifiable source of bleeding.
Low cardiac output due to large myocardial infarction, severe valvular stenosis or incompetence, arrhythmia or electrolyte imbalance.	*Suggested by:* onset over minutes or hours of breathlessness, distressed and clammy, displaced tapping apex beat, 3rd heart sound, bilateral basal late fine inspiratory crackles. Often also signs of right ventricular failure (↑JVP, swollen legs). Poor urine output. *Confirmed by:* **CXR:** fluffy opacification (greatest around the hila), horizontal linear opacities peripherally, bilateral effusions, large heart. Response to diuretics. Impaired left ventricular function on **echocardiogram**. *Initial management:* sit patient up, controlled O_2. diuretics IV and nitrates IV (if systolic BP>80mmHg). Identify and treat cause.
Septicaemia due to Gram –ve organisms commonly	*Suggested by:* warm, well-perfused peripheries, bounding pulse, low BP, tachycardia. Poor urine output. *Confirmed by:* +ve **blood cultures,** and response to plasma expanders and control of infection. *Initial management:* push fluids IV, e.g. normal saline stat and 2–4 hourly. Cefuroxime + metronidazole IV or co-amoxiclav/piperacillin with tazobactam according to likely source.

Central cyanosis

Cyanosis of tongue and hands. Significant hypoxia is present to cause this sign, so higher flow O_2 and close monitoring of saturations with ABG is needed. Initial investigations (confirmatory tests in **bold** below): FBC, CRP, blood cultures, ABG, ECG, CXR.

Main differential diagnoses and typical outline evidence, etc.	
Right-to-left cardiac shunt due to congenital heart disease, e.g. Tetralogy of Fallot, Eisenmenger's syndrome, tricuspid atresia, Ebstein's anomaly, pulmonary AV fistula, transposition of the great vessels	*Suggested by:* breathlessness, clubbing, systolic or continuous murmur, right ventricular heave. *Confirmed by:* **echocardiogram** and **cardiac catheterization**. *Initial management:* antibiotic prophylaxis for procedures and refer to paediatric cardiologist.
Right-to-left pulmonary shunt due to no perfusion of lung tissue from extensive collapse or con-solidation due to alveolar infection or bronchial obstruction	*Suggested by:* breathlessness, poor chest movement, dullness to percussion, and absent breath sounds over a large area of the chest. *Confirmed by:* **CXR** and **bronchoscopy**. *Initial management:* high flow O_2. See also management of: Inhaled foreign body, see 🔲p.328 Extensive consolidation, see 🔲p.314 Large/bilateral pulmonary embolus, see 🔲p.338 Pneumothorax, see 🔲p.316 Severe COPD (cor pulmonale), see 🔲p.292
Haemoglobin abnormalities due to congenital NADH diaphorase, Hb M disease or acquired meth-aemo-globinaemia or sulfhaemo-globinaemia	Exacerbation of severe asthma, see 🔲p.328 Severe pulmonary fibrosis, see 🔲p.293 Neuromuscular disease, see 🔲p.293 Pulmonary hypertension, see 🔲p.293 *Suggested by:* no clubbing, no murmurs, normal chest movement, no chest signs. History from childhood or exposure to toxic drugs, e.g. aniline dyes, phenacatin, etc. *Confirmed by:* **Hb electrophoresis**. *Initial management:* high flow O_2. O_2 saturations may be unreliable. Refer to haematologist for long-term management.

Pulse rate >120bpm

Initial investigations (other tests in **bold** below): FBC, U&E, CRP, D-dimer, troponin, ABG, ECG, CXR.

Main differential diagnoses and typical outline evidence, etc.	
Fever	*Suggested by:* warm skin, erythema, sweats, temperature >38°C.
	Confirmed by: temperature chart, fever pattern.
	Initial management: **blood/sputum/urine/skin swab cultures**. Antipyrectics. Provisional antibiotics: amoxicillin (chest/skin source), cefuroxime/metronidazole/trimethoprim (bowel/ urinary source). Antibiotics IV if severe infection. Fluids IV/plasma expanders if ↓BP, poor urine output.
Haemorrhage	*Suggested by:* pallor, sweats, ↓BP, poor urine output, and peripheral perfusion.
	Confirmed by: ↓**Hb** (can be normal initially), low central venous pressure.
	Initial management: identify and control bleeding source. Multiple large bore IV access, fluids IV resuscitation until blood available.
Hypoxia	*Suggested by:* cyanosis, distress.
	Confirmed by: ↓**P_aO_2**.
	Initial management: controlled O_2 aiming to keep saturations above 92%. Address underlying cause. (see p.242)
Thyrotoxicosis	*Suggested by:* sweating, fine tremor, weight loss, lid lag, frequent bowel movements.
	Confirmed by: ↑FT4 ± ↑FT3 and ↓TSH.
	Initial management: propranolol for symptoms. Carbimazole/propylthiouracil for thyrotoxicosis.
Severe anaemia ?due to acute blood loss or chronic pathology/deficiencies (e.g. folate/iron/B_{12})	*Suggested by:* subconjunctival and nail-bed pallor.
	Confirmed by: ↓**Hb**.
	Initial management: resuscitate with fluids/blood. Identify and treat cause, e.g. start supplements for deficiencies or treat chronic pathology.

Heart failure (left ventricular, right ventricular, congestive) associated with ischaemic heart disease, myocarditis, valvular disease, arrhythmias.	*Suggested by:* onset over minutes or hours of breathlessness, often distressed and clammy, displaced tapping apex beat, 3rd heart sound, bilateral basal late fine inspiratory crackles. Often also signs of right ventricular failure (↑JVP, swollen legs). Poor urine output. *Confirmed by:* **CXR:** fluffy opacification (greatest around the hila), horizontal linear opacities peripherally, bilateral effusions, large heart. Response to diuretics. Impaired left ventricular function on **echocardiogram**. *Initial management:* sit patient up, controlled O_2, diuretics IV. nitrates IV if very breathless and systolic BP >90. Identify and treat causes. (eg. myocardial infarction, valve disease, arrhythmia). *Chronic:* thiazide or loop diuretic, ACE inhibitor (or angiotensin receptor blocker). β-blocker and spironolactone (monitor K^+).
Pulmonary embolus/infarction arising within the lung or from deep veins or left atrium	*Suggested by:* sudden breathlessness and sharp or central chest pain, recent surgery, immobility, previous emboli, malignancy, etc. Cyanosis, tachycardia, loud P2, pleural rub. ↑D-dimers, S1,Q3,T3 on **ECG**. *Confirmed by:* **CT pulmonary angiogram** showing clot in pulmonary artery. *Initial management:* LMW heparin (treatment dose), then ≥3 months warfarin. Thrombolysis if ↓BP, large and bilateral clots, no response to anticoagulation or acutely dilated right ventricle on **echocardiogram**.
Drugs e.g. amphetamines, beta-agonists	*Suggested by:* drug history. *Confirmed by:* normal heart rate when drug stopped. *Initial management:* stop drug, **ECG monitor**, **check electrolytes**; if adverse signs, then give antidote or consider cardioversion.
Severe electrolyte disturbances e.g. K^+	Suggested by: drug history, renal failure. Confirmed by: normal heart rate when electrolyte corrected. ECG. Initial management: fluids IV and correct electrolyte imbalance, e.g. ↑K^+: calcium gluconate IV, dextrose-insulin IV, consider calcium resonium PO/PR. ↓K^+: potassium chloride IV and stop K^+ loss (typically diuretics).

Bradycardia (<60bpm)

Initial investigations (other tests in **bold** below): FBC, U&E, TFT, CRP.

Main differential diagnoses and typical outline evidence, etc.	
Athletic heart	*Suggested by:* young/fit, asymptomatic.
	Confirmed by: normal history/examination.
	Initial management: reassure.
Drugs	*Suggested by:* history, e.g. beta-blockers, digoxin. Look for 'reverse tick' sign, and check serum levels if suspect digoxin toxicity.
	Confirmed by: normal heart rate when drug stopped.
	Initial management: check electrolytes. **Cardiac monitor**. Atropine or pacing when unstable.
Sinoatrial disease	*Suggested by:* elderly, known ischaemic heart disease.
	Confirmed by: **ECG**—abnormal P wave or P–R interval.
?myocardial ischaemia	*Initial management:* check electrolytes. Cardiac monitor. Atropine or pacing when unstable. **Echocardiogram** for left ventricular function if history of syncope.
Ventricular or supraventricular bigemini	*Suggested by:* known ischaemic heart disease.
	Confirmed by: **ECG** and **24-h ECG** premature ectopics **with and** compensatory pause.
?myocardial ischaemia	*Initial management:* check electrolytes. Keep on cardiac monitor. Atropine or pacing when unstable. **Echocardiogram** for left ventricular function if history of syncope.
Myocardial infarction	*Suggested by:* central chest pain ± radiating to jaw and either arm (left typically). Continuous, typically over 30 minutes, not relieved by rest or nitrates.
	Confirmed by: ↑ST of 1mm in limb leads or 2mm in chest leads on **serial ECG**. Troponin↑.
	Initial management: O$_2$, high dose aspirin, nitrates IV and/or oral, β-blockers, statins, and ACE inhibitor. Urgent thrombolysis and/or primary angioplasty.
Hypothyroid	*Suggested by:* constipation, weight gain, dry skin, dry hair, reduced reflexes/energy.
	Confirmed by: ↑**TSH**, ↓**T4**.
	Initial management: thyroxine supplements.
Hypothermia	*Suggested by:* history of exposure to cold temperature and/or prolonged immobility.
	Confirmed by: core temperature <35°C.
	Initial management: gentle rewarming (space blanket, warmed fluids IV, bladder irrigation).

Severe electrolyte disturbances e.g. K^+	*Suggested by:* drug history, renal failure.
	Confirmed by: normal heart rate when electrolyte corrected. **ECG**: T wave changes
	Initial management: fluids IV and correct electrolyte imbalance, e.g. ↑K^+: calcium gluconate IV, dextrose-insulin IV, consider calcium resonium PO/PR. ↓K^+: potassium chloride IV and stop K^+ loss (typically diuretics).

Pulse irregular

Initial investigations (other tests in **bold** below): FBC, U&E, CRP, ECG, CXR.

Main differential diagnoses and typical outline evidence, etc.	
AF Acute (<24h) may have precipitating cause (e.g. myocardial infarction, infection, electrolyte imbalance, thyrotoxicosis)	*Suggested by:* irregularly irregular pulse. *Confirmed by:* **ECG** showing no P waves, and irregularly irregular normal QRS complexes. *Initial management:* if new onset (<24h) and/or heart rate >130: treat cause, anticoagulate, and chemically cardiovert (digoxin/verapamil/amiodarone). **Cardiac monitor.** DC shock if unstable. If rate <50, anticoagulate and treat as bradycardia. If rate 50–100 and duration unknown, anticoagulate. Referral for echocardiogram and consider outpatient cardioversion.
Atrial flutter with variable heart block caused by ischaemic heart disease, etc.	*Suggested by:* irregularly irregular pulse. *Confirmed by:* **ECG** showing 'saw tooth' F waves, and irregularly irregular normal QRS complexes. *Initial management:* as AF above.
Atrial or ventricular ectopics caused by ischaemic heart disease, etc.	*Suggested by:* regular rate with irregular dropped beat. *Confirmed by:* **ECG** showing normal sinus rhythm with irregular QRS complexes not preceded by P wave, and then compensatory absence of subsequent QRS. *Initial management:* **cardiac monitor.** Treat cause (e.g. myocardial infarction, ↑K$^+$, etc.). If prolonged PR (>200ms) and/or syncope, consider pacemaker. Consider β-blockers if multiple ectopics and ACE inhibitors if left ventricular dysfunction.
Wenkenbach heart block caused by ischaemic heart disease, etc.	*Suggested by:* regular rate with regular dropped beat. *Confirmed by:* **ECG** showing progressive prolongation of PR interval with normal QRS complex, followed by an eventually 'dropped' absent QRS complex. *Initial management:* **cardiac monitor.** Treat cause (e.g. myocardial infarction, ↑K$^+$, etc.). If prolonged PR and/or syncope, consider pacemaker. Consider ACE inhibitors if left ventricular dysfunction.

Pulse volume high

This is an indication of the width of the pulse pressure. It can be confirmed by a large difference between the systolic and diastolic blood pressure. Initial investigations (other tests in **bold** below): FBC, U&E, CRP, ECG, CXR.

Main differential diagnoses and typical outline evidence, etc.	
Aortic incompetence	*Suggested by:* striking 'water hammer' radial pulse. Systolic BP high (e.g. >160mmHg) and diastolic BP very low (e.g. <50mmHg), early diastolic murmur.
	Confirmed by: **echocardiogram** and **cardiac catheterization** showing aortic regurgitation.
	Initial management: If acute/signs of sepsis or vegetations on the valve, treat as bacterial endocarditis with high dose antibiotics. If acute and severe chest/back/abdominal pain and low BP, consider aortic dissection. If otherwise stable, start aspirin and refer for cardiology opinion and longer term follow-up for consideration of valve replacement.
Arteriosclerosis	*Suggested by:* history of thrombi/emboli. Systolic hypertension (>160mmHg) without diastolic hypotension (>80mmHg).
	Confirmed by: palpable thickening of small arteries, e.g. radial and/or absence of some peripheral pulses, absence of features of differential diagnoses of high pulse pressure, **echocardiogram** to exclude aortic incompetence.
	Initial management: start aspirin, treat risk factors (smoking, cholesterol, BP, diabetes).
Severe anaemia ?due to acute blood loss or chronic pathology/deficiencies (e.g. folate/iron/B_{12})	*Suggested by:* subconjunctival and nail bed pallor.
	Confirmed by: **Hb↓**.
	Initial management: identify and treat cause, e.g. start supplements for deficiencies or treat chronic pathology. Fluids IV/blood resuscitation if unstable.
Bradycardia of any cause with normal myocardium	*Suggested by:* slow heart rate (e.g <50bpm).
	Confirmed by: **ECG** showing slow rate and type of rhythm.
	Initial management: see 'differential diagnosis of bradycardia on □p.242.
Hyperkinetic circulation e.g. due to hypercapnia, thyrotoxicosis, fever, Paget's disease, AV fistula	*Suggested by:* warm peripheries and features of cause, e.g. cyanosis, tremor, lid lag, fever, skull deformity, etc.
	Confirmed by: **ABG**—↑P_aCO_2 (if hypercapnia) or TFT—↑FT4 ± ↑FT3 and ↓TSH (if thyrotoxic), or **septic screen** positive or ↑**hydroxyproline** (Paget's).
	Initial management: controlled O_2. IV access, check electrolytes, find and treat cause.

Pulse volume low

This is an indication of the width of the pulse pressure. It can be confirmed by a small difference between the systolic and diastolic blood pressure. Initial investigations (other tests in **bold** below): FBC, U&E, CRP, ECG, CXR.

Main differential diagnoses and typical outline evidence, etc.	
Poor cardiac contractility due to ischaemic heart disease, cardiomyopathy, cardiac tamponade, constrictive pericarditis	*Suggested by:* quiet heart sounds, ↑JVP, peripheral oedema, basal lung crackles. Poor R wave progression, low amplitude complexes on **ECG**. *Confirmed by:* **echocardiogram** confirm poor left ventricular contractility. *Initial management:* sit patient up, controlled O₂, diuretics IV. nitrates IV if very breathless and systolic BP >90. Treat reversible causes. ACE inhibitor/angiotensin receptor blocker, β-blocker, and spironolactone (monitor K⁺).
Hypovolaemia due to blood loss, dehydration	*Suggested by:* cold peripheries, thirst, dry skin, low urine output. ↑**urea**, ↑**creatinine**. *Confirmed by:* ↓**Hb** (in loss) or ↑ (if haemo-concentrated). Response to fluids. *Initial management:* large bore IV access, fast IV resuscitation with fluids/blood transfusion if anaemic. Catheterize and hourly urine output. Identify and treat any blood loss.
Relative hypovolaemia due to poor vascular tone (vasodilation) typically due to septicaemic shock	*Suggested by:* warm peripheries, thirst, dry skin, ↓urine output. Symptoms/signs of infection. ↑**urea**, ↑**WCC**. *Confirmed by:* **positive blood cultures**, response to antibiotics. *Initial management:* fluids IV and antibiotics IV, e.g. cefuroxime and metronidazole (for gastrointestinal tract), benzylpenicillin and flucloxacillin (for skin), co-amoxiclav or cefuroxime (for chest).
Aortic stenosis	*Suggested by:* slow rising pulse, narrow pulse pressure, soft S2, systolic murmur. *Confirmed by:* **echocardiogram** and **cardiac catheterization**. *Initial management:* aspirin, and if moderate to severe, refer to cardiology for assessment for possible surgery.

Blood pressure high—hypertension

(Systolic >150mmHg and diastolic >90mmHg)

The level treated depends on the presence of risk factors. Generally, any sustained systolic BP >150 is treated, but in diabetics, >135 systolic or >80 diastolic. Initial investigations (other tests in **bold** below): FBC, U&E, CRP.

Main differential diagnoses and typical outline evidence, etc.	
Temporary hypertension with no risk factors	*Suggested by:* normal BP <150mmHg systolic and <90mmHg diastolic, when repeated.
	Confirmed by: **24-h ambulatory blood pressure monitoring.**
	Initial management: reassure and repeat BP check in 2–3mo.
Essential hypertension 95% cases	*Suggested by:* sustained hypertension. If well established, then AV nipping present.
	Confirmed by: **24-h ambulatory blood pressure** monitoring. No symptoms or signs of cause, normal urea and electrolytes, and prompt control on treatment.
	Initial management: thiazide diuretic or calcium channel blocker or ACE inhibitor. Increase dose as tolerated before adding additional antihypertensives.
Hypertension of pregnancy (pre-eclampsia sometimes progressing to eclampsia)	*Suggested by:* only occurring during pregnancy, oedema, and proteinuria. Fits in eclampsia. Additionally, Haemolysis, Elevated Liver enzymes and Low Platelets in HELLP syndrome
	Confirmed by: resolution or improvement when pregnancy over or brought to an early end.
	Initial management: β-blockers IV, hydralazine, methyl-dopa to bring diastolic BP <100mmHg. Refer to specialist centre, consider delivery if >30–34wk gestation.
Obstructive sleep apnoea	*Suggested by:* daytime somnolence, witnessed apnoeas whilst asleep. Collar size >17 inches.
	Confirmed by: **apnoea-hypoapnoea index >15 events per h** on sleep study.
	Initial management: weight loss and continuous positive airways pressure (CPAP) whilst asleep.
Renal hypertension due to renovascular stenosis or 1° renal disease	*Suggested by:* chronic renal impairment. ↑urea and ↑**creatinine**, low Hb.
	Confirmed by: **renal ultrasound** and **renogram** of renal vasculature.
	Initial management: treat cause (e.g. diabetes, autoimmune disease). Calcium channel blockers and β-blockers before ACE inhibitors (which precipitate renal failure if renovascular) and diuretics if severe renal impairment.

Endocrine hypertension due to primary hyperaldosteronism (Conn's syndrome if tumour too), Cushing's syndrome, phaeochromocytoma, acromegaly, etc	*Suggested by:* proximal muscle weakness in Cushing's syndrome or severe aldosteronism. Paroxysms of vascular symptoms in 'phaeo'. *Confirmed by:* ↑**aldosterone** and ↓**renin**, (in primary hyperaldosteronism) ↑**24-h urinary free cortisol**, etc. in Cushing's syndrome. ↑**VMA** and ↑**metadrenaline** in phaeochromocytoma. *Initial management:* spironolactone in primary hyperaldosteronism. β-blockers and α-blockers in phaeochromocytoma.
Vascular hypertension due to coarctation of the aorta, subclavian artery stenosis	*Suggested by:* upper body hypertension (right arm) and diminished pulses in legs (and left arm in subclavian artery stenosis). Radio-radial/femoral delay. *Confirmed by:* **echocardiography** *(also measure pressure gradients)*, **MR angiogram/angiography**. *Initial management:* aspirin, refer to cardiology/surgery.
Drug-induced due to NSAIDs, oestrogen pill, steroids, erythropoeitin	*Suggested by:* drug history. *Confirmed by:* re↑ Solution or improvement when drug stopped. *Initial management:* stop drug

Blood pressure very low

Initial investigations (other tests in **bold** below): FBC, U&E, CRP, ECG.

Main differential diagnoses and typical outline evidence, etc.	
Cardiogenic—low output due to poor myocardium, stenosis or regurgitation, etc.	*Suggested by:* very low BP, fast or slow heart rate, peripheral and central cyanosis, displaced apex beat, quiet heart sounds ± abnormal murmur. ↑JVP, crepitations at lung bases. *Confirmed by:* ↑central venous pressure, ECG abnormal ± rhythm abnormalities, cardiomegaly ± 'pulmonary oedema' on CXR. Abnormal myocardium ± valvular lesions on **echocardiogram**. *Initial management:* sit patient up, controlled O₂, diuretics IV and nitrates IV (if systolic BP >80mmHg). Treat any identified causes.
Low circulating blood volume due to haemorrhage (GI etc.), dehydration, etc.	*Suggested by:* very low BP, fast heart rate, cold peripheries often with peripheral cyanosis, ↓JVP, thirst, dry skin, low urine output. ↑urea, ↑creatinine. Background evidence of cause. *Confirmed by:* ↓Hb (in loss) or ↑ (if haemo-concentrated), ↓central venous pressure, improvement with fluid resuscitation. *Initial management:* resuscitate with fluids/transfusions. Catheterize and hourly urine output. Identify and treat source of bleeding.
Loss of vascular tone due to septicaemia, anaphylaxis, adrenal failure, etc.	*Suggested by:* fever, warm peripheries, shock, ↓JVP, ↓urine output, signs of anaphylaxis. *Confirmed by:* +ve **blood cultures**, response to plasma expanders/fluids and antibiotics, identified allergen. *Initial management:* fluids IV with central venous pressure monitoring and hourly urine output. Adrenaline IM/ steroids IV if anaphylaxis. Antibiotics IV for infection.
Addison's disease	*Suggested by:* ↑K⁺, ↓Na⁺, ↓glucose, pallor with hyperpigmentation skin/palmar creases. *Confirmed by:* ↓serum cortisol, poor cortisol response to **Synacthen® test.** *Initial management:* hydrocortisone IV or prednisolone. Consider fludrocortisone.
Spinal cord injuries/ disease	*Suggested by:* sensorimotor deficits. *Confirmed by:* **MRI spine.** *Initial management:* hydrocortisone IV, fluids IV, strict immobilization, and transfer to specialist unit.

Postural fall in blood pressure

To be a strong diagnostic lead, the systolic blood pressure must fall >20mmHg (or15%) and stay down for at least 1 minute and be accompanied by dizziness/syncope; otherwise many of the 'causes' will be self-limiting, and no diagnosis will be confirmed. Initial investigations (other tests in **bold** below): FBC, U&E, CRP, ECG, CXR.

Main differential diagnoses and typical outline evidence, etc.	
Drug-induced due to excessive dose of any hypotensive agent	*Suggested by:* drug history (e.g. antihypertensives, L-dopa, carbidopa, phenothiazines, tricyclic antidepressants). *Confirmed by:* by resolution or improvement after stopping or reducing drug. *Initial management:* stop/reduce drug.
Autonomic neuropathy typically secondary to other diseases	*Suggested by:* long-standing diabetes, alcoholism, hypovolaemia (e.g. diarrhoea, vomiting, over diuresis.) *Confirmed by:* **ECG monitor of beat-to-beat variation:** <10 beats per min change in heart rate on deep breathing at 6 breaths per min or getting up from lying. *Initial management:* treat cause and stop any contributing drugs. Advice on posture, e.g. get up slowly. TED stockings, and in severe cases, fludrocortisone or sympathomimetics, e.g. midodrine.
Idiopathic orthostatic hypotension (due to blunting of autonomic tone, sino-atrial node, and vascular responses)	*Suggested by:* normal history. Typically elderly. Probably a combination of blunting of autonomic tone, sino-atrial node and vascular responses. *Confirmed by:* postural hypotension with no other associated features. *Initial management:* advice on posture, e.g. stand slowly. Consider TED stockings, and in severe cases, fludrocortisone or sympathomimetics, e.g. midodrine.
Cardiogenic—low output due to poor myocardium, stenosis or regurgitation, etc.	*Suggested by:* ↑JVP, cyanosis, displaced apex beat, quiet heart sounds ± abnormal murmur, crepitations at lung bases. *Confirmed by:* ↑central venous pressure, ECG abnormal ± rhythm abnormalities, cardiomegaly ± 'pulmonary oedema' on CXR. Abnormal myocardium ± valvular lesions on **echocardiogram**. *Initial management:* controlled O_2, diuretics IV and nitrates IV. Treat any identified causes.

Low circulating blood volume due to haemorrhage (GI etc.) dehydration etc.	*Suggested by:* very low BP, fast heart rate, cold peripheries, peripheral cyanosis, ↓JVP, thirst, dry skin, low urine output. ↑**urea and creatinine**. Background evidence of cause. *Confirmed by:* ↓Hb (in loss) or ↑ (if haemo-concentrated), ↓central venous pressure, improvement with fluid resuscitation. *Initial management:* resuscitate with fluids/transfusions. Catheterize and hourly urine output. Identify and treat any bleeding or negative fluid balance.
Loss of vascular tone due to septicaemia, adrenal failure, etc.	*Suggested by:* fever, warm peripheries, shock, ↓JVP, ↓urine output, signs of anaphylaxis. *Confirmed by:* +ve **blood cultures**, response to plasma expanders/fluids and antibiotics, identified allergen. *Initial management:* fluids IV with central venous pressure monitoring and hourly urine output. Adrenaline IM/steroids IV if anaphylaxis. Antibiotics IV for infection.
Central nervous system diseases, e.g. multiple sclerosis, Parkinson's disease	*Suggested by:* history. *Confirmed by:* **abnormal neurological signs consistent with disease**. *Initial management:* advice on posture, e.g. stand slowly. Consider TED stockings, and in severe cases, consider fludrocortisone or sympathomimetics, e.g. midodrine.
Also	Primary autonomic neuropathies (e.g. Shy–Drager syndrome), B_{12} deficiency and subacute combined degeneration of the spinal cord, amyloidosis, porphyria, Guillain–Barré, phaeochromocytoma, myelopathies.

BP/pulse difference between arms

Right > left by 15mmHg. Initial investigations (other tests in **bold** below): FBC, U&E, ECG, CXR.

Main differential diagnoses and typical outline evidence, etc.	
Old or acute thrombosis in atheromatous artery or aneurysm or dissection of ascending aorta	*Suggested by:* associated peripheral vascular disease. *Confirmed by:* **CT chest** and arms with contrast in arterial phase, **MRA/angiography**. *Initial management:* resuscitate with fluids IV/transfusions. Surgical referral for correction.
Supravalvular aortic stenosis (congenital)	*Suggested by:* 'elfin-like' facies, ejection systolic murmur, angina, and syncope. *Confirmed by:* **echocardiography** and **angiography**. *Initial management:* monitor BP, refer for surgery.
Subclavian steal syndrome	*Suggested by:* associated neurological symptoms. Exercising right arm induces cerebral ischaemia. *Confirmed by:* **Doppler scans** and **angiography** showing abnormal subclavian artery. *Initial management:* refer for surgery.
Thoracic inlet syndrome	*Suggested by:* bracing shoulder aggravates BP difference. *Confirmed by:* **MR angiogram/angiography** showing abnormal subclavian artery. **CT thoracic inlet** also needed to view external occluding structure. *Initial management:* surgical referral. May need vein bypass graft and offending structure (e.g. aneurysm, congenital band, accessory rib) removed at the same time.
Aortic arch syndrome, Takayasu's syndrome	*Suggested by:* typically young Asian female with cerebral and peripheral ischaemic symptoms. Fever, weight loss, fatigue, and arthralgia often precede these symptoms. Vascular bruits and pulseless extremities. ↑↑ESR. *Confirmed by:* **angiography** showing abnormal subclavian artery. *Initial management:* corticosteroids.

BP/pulse difference between arm and legs

Right > left by 15mmHg. Need wide cuff for thigh. NB. Patient arms and legs must be level. Initial investigations (other tests in **bold** below): FBC, U&E, ECG, CXR.

Main differential diagnoses and typical outline evidence, etc.	
Old or acute thrombosis in atheromatous artery	*Suggested by:* associated peripheral vascular disease. Atrophic skin and hair loss on lower legs.
	Confirmed by: **Doppler ultrasound** of legs to try to find remediable flow reduction. **Angiography** to try to identify surgically remediable arterial stenosis.
	Initial management: aspirin. Urgent surgical referral if acute thrombosis and signs of ischaemic leg.
Aneurysm or dissection of descending thoracic or abdominal aorta or iliac arteries, especially in diabetics	*Suggested by:* associated peripheral vascular disease, severe abdominal/back/groin pain. Signs of shock.
	Confirmed by: **CT abdomen and pelvis**.
	Initial management: large bore IV access. Resuscitate with fluids IV/transfusions. Urgent surgical review.
Coarctation of aorta	*Suggested by:* ejection systolic murmur, presenting in childhood or early adult life.
	Confirmed by: rib notching on **CXR** and↑ stenosis on **CT angiography**.
	Initial management: refer for specialist surgery.

Prominent leg veins ± unilateral leg swelling

Initial investigations (other tests in **bold** below): FBC, U&E, CRP, D-dimer.

Main differential diagnoses and typical outline evidence, etc.	
Varicose veins ± competent communicating valves	*Suggested by:* generalized ache, itching, varicose veins, and venous eczema ± ulcers. Cough impulse. **Trendelenberg test** shows filling down along extent of communicating valve leaks.
	Confirmed by: clinical findings or **Doppler ultrasound** to confirm any incompetence in sapheno-femoral junction or short saphenous vein.
	Initial management: advice to avoid prolonged standing and keep leg(s) elevated when sitting. Compression bandages and support stockings. Refer to vascular surgeons if symptoms debilitating.
Thrombophlebitis	*Suggested by:* tender, hot veins with redness of surrounding skin.
	Confirmed by: history. Resolution on antibiotics.
	Initial management: NSAIDs and amoxicillin.
Deep vein thrombosis	*Suggested by:* immobility, prominent dilated veins, warm and tender swollen calf.
	Confirmed by: reduced flow on compression **Doppler**, filling defect seen on **venography.**
	Initial management: analgesia, treatment dose heparin until therapeutic warfarin. Anticoagulate for at least 3mo.

Unilateral leg and ankle swelling

Initial investigations (other tests in **bold** below): FBC, U&E, CRP, D-dimer.

Main differential diagnoses and typical outline evidence, etc.	
Deep vein thrombosis	*Suggested by:* immobility, prominent dilated veins, warm and tender swollen calf. *Confirmed by:* reduced flow on compression **Doppler**, filling defect seen on **venography.** *Initial management:* analgesia, treatment dose heparin until therapeutic anticoagulation on warfarin acheived. Anticoagulate for at least 3mo.
Ruptured Baker's cyst	*Suggested by:* onset sudden over seconds, e.g. when walking up a step. Typically arthritic knee. *Confirmed by:* normal flow on **Doppler ultrasound** and extravascular collection of fluid. No filling defect on **venogram**. Leakage of contrast from joint capsule if **arthrogram** done soon after the event. *Initial management:* analgesia, rest, and leg elevation.
Cellulitis from infection secondary or primarily due to insect bites	*Suggested by:* onset over days. Warm and tender erythema, tracking (red lines), fever, ↑**WBC**. *Confirmed by:* **skin swabs** if discharge from skin, **blood cultures**, response to antibiotics. *Initial management:* analgesia. Leg elevation. High dose benzylpenicillin IV + flucloxacillin for 10–14d. Fusidic acid and vancomycin if penicillin allergy. Prophylactic heparin.
Unilateral varicose veins	*Suggested by:* distended and tortuous veins made worse when standing. *Confirmed by:* **Doppler ultrasound probe** to confirm where incompetence is present. *Initial management:* advice not to do prolonged standing and keep leg(s) elevated when sitting. Compression bandages and support stockings. Refer to vascular surgeons if symptoms worsen.
Chronic venous insufficiency from old deep vein thromboses (e.g. post-thrombotic syndrome)	*Suggested by:* past history, veins distended and made worse on standing. *Confirmed by:* **Doppler ultrasound** probe to where incompetence is present. *Initial management:* advice not to do prolonged standing and keep leg(s) elevated when sitting. Compression bandages and support stockings.
Venous insufficiency from obstruction by tumour or lymph node	*Suggested by:* onset over weeks, veins distended. *Confirmed by:* **Doppler ultrasound. CT abdomen/pelvis** and **venography** to explore where obstruction is present. *Initial management:* relief of obstruction.

Immobility (e.g. disabling cerebrovascular accident, hemiplegia, trauma)	*Suggested by:* history of immobility. *Confirmed by:* response to elevation legs and mobilization. *Initial management:* TED stockings, physiotherapy as able.
Abnormal lymphatic drainage caused by lymphoma or malignant infiltration (or trypanosomiasis in tropics).	*Suggested by:* onset over years, firm, non-tender, non-pitting oedema. *Confirmed by:* obstruction to flow on **lymphangiogram.** *Initial management:* compression stockings and leg elevation, specialist nursing input.
Congenital oedema (Milroy's syndrome)	*Suggested by:* presence since childhood. worse pre-menstrually, in warm weather. *Confirmed by:* history and **lymphangiogram** showing primary lymphatic hypoplasia. *Initial management:* compression stockings and leg elevation, specialist nursing input.
Acute lymphatic obstruction due to streptococcal lymphangitis	*Suggested by:* sudden, unilateral swelling developing over hours. No venous dilatation but lymphangitic streaks. *Confirmed by:* clinical features and response to penicillin. **Doppler ultrasound** to show normal venous flow. *Initial management:* penicillin and leg elevation. Prophylactic heparin to cover immobility.

Bilateral leg and ankle swelling

Initial investigations (other tests in **bold** below): FBC, U&E, LFT, CRP, ECG, CXR.

Main differential diagnoses and typical outline evidence, etc.	
Bilateral varicose veins or old deep vein thromboses	*Suggested by:* veins distended and tortuous made worse when standing. *Confirmed by:* **Doppler ultrasound** probe to confirm where incompetence is present. *Initial management:* mobilize. Avoid prolonged standing. Compressions stockings, anticoagulate if clots.
Low albumin due to poor nutrition, malabsorption, liver failure, nephrotic syndrome, protein-losing enteropathy	*Suggested by:* history of facial puffiness in morning and evidence of possible cause of low albumin. *Confirmed by:* ↓**serum albumin** (<30g/L to be significant). *Initial management:* treat cause, oral dietary supplements, consider NG/PEG feeding.
Congestive cardiac failure due to ischaemic heart disease, mitral stenosis, cardiomyopathy, etc.	*Suggested by:* breathlessness, fatigue, orthopnoea. ↑JVP, liver large, fine bibasal crackles at bases, 3rd heart sound. *Confirmed by:* **CXR**: cardiomegaly, upper lobe vascular prominence, pleural effusions. **Echocardiogram**: ventricular dysfunction. *Initial management:* sit patient up, controlled O_2, diuretics IV. nitrates IV if very breathless and systolic BP >90. Treat reversible causes. Consider ACE inhibitor/angiotensin receptor blocker, β-blocker and spironolactone (monitor K$^+$).
Cor pulmonale (right heart failure due to pulmonary hypertension) due to long-standing lung disease, old pulmonary emboli, etc.)	*Suggested by:* chronic hypoxia, ↑JVP, hepatomegaly, loud pulmonary 2nd sound, and right ventricular heave. Signs of chronic lung disease. *Confirmed by:* **CXR** showing pulmonary disease, **ECG** showing right axis deviation. **Echocardiogram:** high estimated pulmonary artery pressures, right ventricular dysfunction. *Initial management:* treat hypoxia. Diuretics.
Immobility	*Suggested by:* history of immobility. *Confirmed by:* response to elevation legs and mobilization. *Initial management:* TED stockings, physiotherapy as able.

Abnormal lymphatic drainage caused by lymphoma or malignant infiltration (or trypanosomiasis in tropics).	*Suggested by:* onset over years, firm, non-tender, non-pitting oedema. *Confirmed by:* obstruction to flow on **lymphangiogram.** *Initial management:* compression stockings and leg elevation. Often difficult to treat and needs specialist nursing input.
Congenital oedema (Milroy's syndrome)	*Suggested by:* presence since childhood. worse pre-menstrually, in warm weather. *Confirmed by:* history and **lymphangiogram** showing primary lymphatic hypoplasia. *Initial management:* compression stockings and leg elevation. Often difficult to treat and needs specialist nursing input.
Acute lymphatic obstruction due to streptococcal lymphangitis	*Suggested by:* sudden, unilateral swelling developing over hours. No venous dilatation but lymphangitic streaks. *Confirmed by:* clinical features and response to penicillin. **Doppler ultrasound** to show normal venous flow. *Initial management:* penicillin and leg elevation. Prophylactic heparin to cover immobility.

Raised jugular venous pressure

Measured with patient lying at 45°. Undetectably low if external jugular empties when compressing finger released. Initial investigations (other tests in **bold** below): FBC, U&E, CRP, ECG, CXR.

Main differential diagnoses and typical outline evidence, etc.	
Fluid volume overload	*Suggested by:* history of high input of fluids IV. Pulsatile. JVP with 'a' waves. Normal left ventricular function in echocardiogram.
	Confirmed by: drop in JVP with fluid management.
	Initial management: fluid restriction/diuretics.
Congestive cardiac failure	*Suggested by:* breathlessness, fatigue, orthopnoea. ↑JVP, liver large, fine bibasal crackles at bases, 3rd heart sound.
	Confirmed by: **CXR:** cardiomegaly, upper lobe vascular prominence, pleural effusions. **Echocardiogram:** ventricular dysfunction.
	Initial management: sit patient up, controlled O_2, diuretics IV, nitrates IV if very breathless and systolic BP >90. Treat reversible causes. Consider ACE inhibitor/angiotensin receptor blocker, β-blocker and spironolactone (monitor K^+).
Cor pulmonale due to high right atrial pressure	*Suggested by:* large 'a' waves present.
	Confirmed by: **ECG** showing tall P wave, right axis deviation, right heart strain pattern.
	Initial management: treat hypoxia. Diuretics.
AF Acute (<24h) may have precipitating cause (e.g. myocardial infarction, infection, electrolyte imbalance, thyrotoxicosis)	*Suggested by:* irregularly irregular pulse.
	Confirmed by: **ECG** showing no P waves, and irregularly irregular normal QRS complexes.
	Initial management: if new onset (<24h) and/or HR >130: treat cause, anticoagulate, and chemically cardiovert (e.g. digoxin/verapamil/amiodarone). Cardiac monitor. DC shock if unstable. If rate <50, anticoagulate and treat as bradycardia. If rate 50–100 and duration unknown, anticoagulate. Referral for echocardiogram and consider outpatient cardioversion.
Complete heart block	*Suggested by:* intermittent giant 'v' waves. Bradycardia.
	Confirmed by: **ECG** showing no association between P waves and QRS complex.
	Initial management: **Cardiac monitor.** Temporary pacing if symptomatic. Treat identifiable cause. Assess for permanent pacemaker.

Tricuspid regurgitation ?right ventricular dilatation due to pulmonary embolus, endocarditis, cor pulmonale	*Suggested by:* large 'v' waves. Pansystolic murmur present. *Confirmed by:* **echocardiogram** showing large right atrium and tricuspid incompetence. *Initial management:* diuretics. Treat identifiable cause.
Pericardial effusion ?due to myocardial infarction, haemorrhagic, infective, inflammation, malignant, autoimmune	*Suggested by:* pulsatile JVP with 'a' wave and rapid descent. Very breathless. Quiet heart sounds. globular heart shadow on **CXR**. Low voltage QRS complexes on **ECG**. *Confirmed by:* significant effusion on **echocardiogram**. *Initial management:* diagnostic/therapeutic pericardiocentesis. Treat identifiable cause.
Constrictive pericarditis ?due to myocardial infarction, infection, uraemia, hypothyroidism, trauma, autoimmune	*Suggested by:* rapid descent of 'a' waves. Quiet heart sounds. Pericardial rub. Chest pain relieved on sitting forward. **ECG** shows widespread concave 'saddle-shaped' ↑ST except in AVR and V1–2 which have ↓ST. *Confirmed by:* **echocardiogram** shows small cavity and little contraction. *Initial management:* analgesia, steroids, pericardiocentesis if significant effusion or signs of tamponade. Treat identifiable cause.
Jugular vein obstruction ?luminal (e.g. thrombus) or extraluminal (e.g. tumour)	*Suggested by:* no JVP pulsation, external jugular vein also distended. *Confirmed by:* **US** or **CT scan** to explore site of obstruction. *Initial management:* treat obstruction.

Abnormal apex impulse

Look for displacement from normal site in mid-clavicular line, heave, and character of impulse (tapping, double). Initial investigations (other tests in **bold** below): FBC, CRP, ECG, CXR.

Main differential diagnoses and typical outline evidence, etc.	
Fat, fluid, or air between the apex and palpating hand	*Suggested by:* impalpable apex.
	Confirmed by: evidence of obesity, emphysema, pneumothorax, pleural effusion, pericardial effusion.
	Initial management: pneumothorax (see ▢p.321), pericardial effusion (see ▢p.307), emphysema (see ▢p.346)
Dextrocardia	*Suggested by:* apex on the right side of chest.
	Confirmed by: **CXR**.
	Initial management: look for associated congenital cardiac abnormalities, bronchiectasis (Kartagener's syndrome and situs inversus).
Large left ventricle due to ischaemic cardiomyopathy, mitral incompetence, aortic incompetence, right-to-left ventral septal defect shunt	*Suggested by:* apex heaving and displaced.
	Confirmed by: **echocardiogram** shows left ventricular dysfunction and cause.
	Initial management: O_2 and diuretics ± ACE inhibitors and β-blockers. Investigation of underlying cause.
Hypertrophied left ventricle due to hypertension, aortic stenosis	*Suggested by:* apex heaving but not displaced.
	Confirmed by: **echocardiogram** shows left ventricular dysfunction and cause.
	Initial management: treat BP (aim for <140/80mmHg). Consider aspirin and ACE inhibitors. Investigation of underlying cause.
Hypertrophic cardiomyopathy (HOCM)	*Suggested by:* double apex beat, angina, jerky pulse, ↑JVP with 'a' wave, thrill and murmur at left sternal edge.
	Confirmed by: **echocardiogram** showing hypertrophied septum and ventricular walls with small ventricular cavities, more on left side.
	Initial management: β-blockers (main risk is ventricular fibrillation) and aspirin. Refer for cardiac investigation and genetic counselling.

Ventricular aneurysm	*Suggested by:* double impulse. Persistently raised ST segments on **ECG**. *Confirmed by:* paradoxical movement of ventricular wall on **echocardiogram**. *Initial management:* aspirin/anticoagulation for at least 3mo, if associated thrombus. ACE inhibitor. Refer to cardiologist for assessment for possible surgery.
Mitral stenosis	*Suggested by:* tapping left ventricular impulse (palpable 1st heart sound) and rumbling diastolic murmur. *Confirmed by:* **ECG** findings, **echocardiogram** and **cardiac catheterization**. *Initial management:* aspirin, anticoagulate if AF. Refer to cardiologist for assessment for possible surgery.
Right ventricular hypertrophy due to pulmonary hypertension or pulmonary stenosis	*Suggested by:* left parasternal heave. *Confirmed by:* **ECG** findings and **echocardiogram**. *Initial management:* correct hypoxia, anticoagulate if clot/pulmonary hypertension. Diuretics.

Extra heart sounds

Initial investigations (other tests in **bold** below): FBC, CRP, ECG, CXR, echocardiogram.

Main differential diagnoses and typical outline evidence, etc.	
Normal young heart	*Suggested by:* 4th heart sound.
	Confirmed by: normal **CXR** and **echocardiogram**.
	Initial management: reassure.
Heart failure, cardiomyopathy, constrictive pericarditis	*Suggested by:* onset over minutes or hours of breathlessness, often distressed and clammy, displaced tapping apex beat, 3rd heart sound, bilateral basal late fine inspiratory crackles. Often also signs of right ventricular failure (↑JVP, swollen legs). Poor urine output.
	Confirmed by: **CXR**: fluffy opacification (greatest around the hila), horizontal linear opacities peripherally, bilateral effusions, large heart. Response to diuretics. Impaired left ventricular function on **echocardiogram**.
	Initial management: sit patient up, controlled O_2, diuretics IV. nitrates IV if very breathless and systolic BP >90. Identify and treat causes. (e.g. myocardial infarction, valve disease, arrhythmia).
	Chronic: thiazide or loop diuretic, ACE inhibitor (or angiotensin receptor blocker). β-blocker and spironolactone (monitor K^+).

Diastolic murmur

Find where it is heard best (e.g. apex or left sternal edge). For any significant valvular heart disease, antibiotic prophylaxis should be considered for procedures that carry a risk of bacteraemia. Monitor for resulting ventricular compromise. Initial investigations (other tests in **bold** below): FBC, CRP, ECG, CXR, echocardiogram.

Main differential diagnoses and typical outline evidence, etc.	
Mitral stenosis	*Suggested by:* tapping left ventricular impulse (palpable 1st heart sound) and rumbling diastolic murmur.
	Confirmed by: ECG findings, **echocardiogram,** and **cardiac catheterization**.
	Initial management: aspirin, anticoagulate if AF. Prophylactic antibiotics for surgical procedures. Refer to cardiologist for assessment for possible surgery.
Mitral stenosis with pliable valve	*Suggested by:* opening snap.
	Confirmed by: **echocardiogram**.
	Initial management: aspirin, anticoagulate if AF. Prophylactic antibiotics for surgical procedures. Refer to cardiologist for assessment for possible surgery.
Aortic incompetence ?due to aortic dissection, endocarditis, Marfan's, connective tissue disease.	*Suggested by:* ↑BP, collapsing pulse, displaced apex beat, early diastolic murmur best heard at left sternal edge.
	Confirmed by: **echocardiogram** and **cardiac catheter** displaying valve lesion.
	Initial management: if acute onset and unstable—O$_2$, diuretics, blood cultures ×3, and monitor ABG and serial ECG. Prophylactic antibiotics for surgical procedures. Identify and treat cause. Liaise early with cardiology/cardiothoracics for aortic valve replacement. May need HDU/ITU if severe.

Mid-systolic murmur

Mid-systolic murmur means that the 1st and 2nd heart sounds can be heard clearly. Monitor for any resulting ventricular compromise. Initial investigations (other tests in **bold** below): FBC, CRP, ECG, CXR, echocardiogram.

Main differential diagnoses and typical outline evidence, etc.	
Aortic stenosis	*Suggested by:* cool extremities, slow rising pulse, low BP and pulse pressure, heaving apex, and soft or absent aortic component of 2nd heart sound (A_2). **ECG**: tall R waves and left axis deviation. *Confirmed by:* **echocardiogram** and **cardiac catheter** stenosed valve. *Initial management:* aspirin. Treat any ischaemic heart disease. Prophylactic antibiotics for surgical procedures. Refer to cardiologist for assessment for possible surgery.
Hypertrophic cardiomyopathy (HOCM)	*Suggested by:* double apex beat, angina, jerky pulse, ↑JVP with 'a' wave, thrill and murmur at left sternal edge. *Confirmed by:* **echocardiogram** showing hypertrophied septum and ventricular walls with small ventricular cavities, more on left side. *Initial management:* β-blockers (main risk is ventricular fibrillation) and aspirin. Refer to cardiology and genetic counselling.
Aortic sclerosis	*Suggested by:* normal pulse and BP ± no heaving apex. Typically elderly and evidence of atherosclerosis, e.g. palpably thickened arteries or absent pulses. Aortic calcification on CXR. *Confirmed by:* normal **ECG** and sclerotic valve on **echocardiogram.** *Initial management:* aspirin, keep BP <140/80mmHg and treat associated risk factors/ischaemia. Repeat echocardiogram every 12mo.
Pulmonary high flow	*Suggested by:* normal pulse and BP, normal JVP, and no left parasternal heave. Typically in young woman. *Confirmed by:* normal **ECG** and **echocardiogram**. *Initial management:* reassure if no pulmonary hypertension or other lesion.
Atrial septal defect (rare) causing high pulmonary flow	*Suggested by:* normal pulse and BP, normal JVP, and left parasternal heave present. **ECG**: peaked P waves, right axis deviation in secundum defect, left axis deviation in primum defect. *Confirmed by:* **echocardiogram** and **cardiac catheter**. *Initial management:* refer to cardiology for assessment for possible surgery.
Pulmonary stenosis	*Suggested by:* low pulse, ↑JVP, and left parasternal heave. Right bundle branch block and right axis deviation on **ECG**. *Confirmed by:* **echocardiogram** and **cardiac catheter**. *Initial management:* aspirin, consider angioplasty/surgical repair.

Pansystolic murmur

Pansystolic murmurs mean that the 1st and 2nd heart sounds cannot be heard in all areas. Initial investigations (other tests in bold below): FBC, CRP, ECG, CXR, echocardiogram.

Main differential diagnoses and typical outline evidence, etc.	
Mitral incompetence due to rheumatic heart disease, valve dysfunction after myocardial infarction	*Suggested by:* pansystolic murmur at apex with radiation to axilla. No large JVP, 'V' waves. Displaced heaving apex beat. **CXR:** large round opacity 'behind heart' (big left atrium). **ECG:** 'M' shaped P wave. *Confirmed by:* **echocardiogram** and **cardiac catheter**. *Initial management:* aspirin/anticoagulate if AF. Treat left ventricular dysfunction. Prophylactic antibiotics for surgical procedures. Refer to cardiology for assessment for possible surgery.
Tricuspid incompetence (rarely alone, e.g. severe cor pulmonale or after pulmonary embolus)	*Suggested by:* pansystolic murmur at left sternal edge. Large JVP 'V' waves. Left parasternal heave. **ECG:** tall peaked 'P' waves, right axis deviation and right bundle branch block. *Confirmed by:* **echocardiogram** and **cardiac catheter** show incompetence. *Initial management:* treat primary causes. O$_2$ and diuretics if associated cor pulmonale.
Ventricular septal defect typically congenital, sometimes rupture of septum after infarction	*Suggested by:* pansystolic murmur loud and rough. ↑JVP. Central cyanosis if right-to-left shunt. Displaced heaving apex beat. Right bundle branch block and right axis deviation in **ECG**. *Confirmed by:* **echocardiogram** and **cardiac catheter** show defect. *Initial management:* aspirin/anticoagulate if AF. Treat left ventricular dysfunction. Prophylactic antibiotics for surgical procedures. Refer to cardiology for assessment for possible surgery.

Murmurs not entirely in systole or diastole

Initial investigations (other tests in **bold** below): FBC, CRP, ECG, CXR, echocardiogram.

Main differential diagnoses and typical outline evidence, etc.	
Patent ductus arteriosus	*Suggested by:* newborn infant, high pulse volume, diastolic and systolic murmur to give continuous murmur.
	Confirmed by: **echocardiogram** and **cardiac catheter**.
	Initial management: aspirin/anticoagulate if AF. Refer to cardiology for assessment for possible surgery.
Pericarditis with pericardial friction rub ?due to myocardial infarction, infection, uraemia, hypothyroidism, trauma, autoimmune	*Suggested by:* rapid descent of 'a' waves. Quiet heart sounds. Pericardial rub. Chest pain relieved on sitting forward. **ECG** shows widespread concave 'saddle-shaped' ↑ST except in AVR and V1–2 which have ↓ST.
	Confirmed by: **echocardiogram** shows small cavity and little contraction.
	Initial management: analgesia, steroids, pericardiocentesis if significant effusion or signs of tamponade. Treat identifiable causes.

Respiratory symptoms and physical signs

Chest pain—sharp and aggravated by breathing or movement

This is a common symptom that is experienced in mild or transient forms by many in the population and resolves with no cause being discovered. It frightens a patient into seeking advice when it is severe or accompanied by other symptoms such as breathlessness. Initial investigations (other tests in **bold** below): FBC, U&E, ECG, troponin I 12h after onset of the pain.

Main differential diagnoses and typical outline evidence, etc.	
Musculoskeletal injury or inflammation	*Suggested by:* associated focal tenderness ± history of trauma or lying awkwardly. *Confirmed by:* normal (or no changes in) troponins, ECG, and CXR. Good response to simple analgesia. *Initial management:* simple analgesia (e.g. NSAIDs) and avoidance of strenuous activity until pain improves.
Chest wall pain e.g. Tietze's syndrome	*Suggested by:* chest pain and tenderness of chest wall on twisting of neck or thoracic cage. *Confirmed by:* normal (or no changes in) troponins, ECG, and CXR. Good response to simple analgesia. *Initial management:* simple analgesia (e.g. NSAIDs) and avoidance of strenuous activity until pain improves.
Pneumonia with pleurisy	*Suggested by:* onset over hours or days, rusty brown sputum ± blood. Sharp pain worse on inspiration, fever, cough, crackles, dullness to percussion, bronchial breathing, **WCC**: ↑neutrophils, ↑**CRP**. *Confirmed by:* patchy shadowing on **CXR** and organisms grown in **sputum/blood culture**. *Initial management:* analgesia and provisional antibiotic, e.g. amoxicillin/clarithromycin PO for 5d. If >2 features of <u>C</u>onfusion, <u>R</u>esp rate >30/min, <u>BP</u> <90/60, age >65y), then antibiotic IV, e.g. amoxicillin/co-amoxiclav or cefuroxime + controlled O_2 and fluids. If suspected aspiration, then anti-anaerobics, e.g. cefuroxime/metronidazole IV. If hospital/nursing home acquired, cefuroxime or piperacillin with tazobactam IV.
Pulmonary embolus/ infarction arising from deep veins or in left atrium	*Suggested by:* sudden breathlessness, pleural rub, cyanosis, tachycardia, loud P2, associated DVT or risk factors such as recent surgery, immobility, previous emboli, malignancy, etc. *Confirmed by:* **CT pulmonary angiogram** showing clot in pulmonary artery. *Initial management:* LMW heparin (treatment dose), then warfarin. Thrombolysis if ↓BP, large bilateral clots, or acutely dilated right ventricular on echocardiogram.

Pneumothorax ('tension', moderate, or mild)	*Suggested by:* pain in centre or side of chest with abrupt breathlessness, diminished breath sounds, and hyper-resonance to percussion.
	Confirmed by: above findings, tracheal deviation, and distress suggesting tension pneumothorax, or **expiration CXR** showing loss of lung markings outside sharp line ('moderate' if >5cm gap from lung edge to chest wall; 'mild' if <5cm).
	Initial management: if tension pneumothorax, insert large Venflon into 2nd intercostal (IC) space, midclavicular line. Give O₂ if breathless. Analgesia. Aspirate if moderate; if this is unsatisfactory or prior lung disease, insert IC drain into 'triangle of safety'. If 'mild' (<5cm gap) and not breathless, observe.
Pericarditis caused by myocardial infarction, infection (especially viral), malignancy, uraemia, connective tissue diseases	*Suggested by:* sharp pain worse lying flat, but relieved by leaning forward. Pericardial rub.
	Confirmed by: ECG: concave ↑ST, 'bright' pericardial signal on **echocardiogram. CXR** showing cardiomegaly and globular heart shadow if significant pericardial effusion.
	Initial management: close cardiac monitoring, NSAIDs and treat cause (e.g. viral—typically self-limiting; if uraemic, treat renal failure; steroids if autoimmune).
Referred cervical root pain	*Suggested by:* previous minor episodes of exacerbation of chest pain by neck movement (producing closure of nerve root foramina related to area of pain).
	Confirmed by: clinical features and **MRI scan.**
	Initial management: analgesia, trial of neck collar, and physiotherapy.
Shingles	*Suggested by:* pain (often burning in nature) in a dermatomal distribution, recent exposure to chicken pox, or previous shingles attacks.
	Confirmed by: vesicles appearing within days in the same dermatome.
	Initial management: NSAIDs ± co-analgesics, e.g. carbamazepine/gabapentin. Aciclovir if severe/immunosuppressed.

Sudden breathlessness, onset over seconds

This situation may be life-threatening. Initial investigations (other tests in **bold** below): FBC, U&E, CXR, ECG, D-dimer.

Main differential diagnoses and typical outline evidence, etc.	
Pulmonary embolus/ infarction arising from deep veins or in left atrium	*Suggested by:* sudden breathlessness, pleural rub, cyanosis, tachycardia, loud P2, associated DVT, or risk factors such as recent surgery, immobility, previous emboli, malignancy, etc.
	Confirmed by: **CT pulmonary angiogram** showing clot in pulmonary artery.
	Initial management: LMW heparin (treatment dose), then warfarin. Thrombolysis if ↓BP, large bilateral clots or acutely dilated right ventricular on echocardiogram.
Pneumothorax ('tension', moderate, or mild)	*Suggested by:* pain in centre or side of chest with abrupt breathlessness, diminished breath sounds and hyper-resonance to percussion.
	Confirmed by: tracheal deviation and distress suggesting tension pneumothorax, or **expiration CXR** showing loss of lung markings outside sharp line ('moderate' if >5cm gap from lung edge to chest wall; 'mild' if <5cm).
	Initial management: if tension pneumothorax, insert large Venflon into 2nd intercostal (IC) space, mid-clavicular line. Give O₂ if breathless and analgesia. Aspirate if moderate; if this is unsatisfactory or prior lung disease, insert IC drain into 'triangle of safety'. If 'mild' (<5cm gap) and not breathless, observe.
Anaphylaxis	*Suggested by:* onset over minutes, history of recent allergen exposure, feeling of dread, flushing, sweating, facial oedema, urticaria, warm clammy extremities, dyspnoea and tachypnoea, wheeze. Tachycardia and ↓BP.
	Confirmed by: clinical presentation and response to adrenaline (epinephrine) IM. Results of controlled allergen exposure.
	Initial management: remove antigen (e.g. bee sting, medication). Adrenaline IM 1 in 10,000. Secure airway early if stridor. High flow O2, fast fluids IV, steroids IV and antihistamines IV. Transfer to HDU/ITU.
Inhalation of foreign body	*Suggested by:* history of putting an object in mouth, e.g. peanut. Sudden stridor, severe cough, low-pitched, monophonic wheeze, and reduced breath sounds, typically on the right.
	Confirmed by: if not *in extremis*, **CXR/CT thorax** or **bronchoscopy** to show foreign body.
	Initial management: if *in extremis*, slap back between the shoulder blades with patient leaning forward. If fails, perform Heimlich manoeuvre.

Cardiac arrhythmia	*Suggested by:* palpitations, chest pain, dizziness, pallor, hypotension, tachycardia or ± ↓BP.
	Confirmed by: **ECG** (pulse typically >140 or <40) and improvement in symptoms/signs as pulse rate improves.
	Initial management: controlled O_2. If pulse >140, vasovagal manoeuvres or rate-lowering medication or electric cardioversion. If pulse <40, atropine IV or pacing (external, temporary internal), transfer to CCU.

Acute breathlessness, wheeze ± cough

This symptom suggests airway narrowing. The commonest cause is bronchospasm (constriction of the smooth muscle in the distal bronchioles); less common causes are wheeze due to inhalation of a foreign body or hydrostatic pulmonary oedema, i.e. 'cardiac wheeze.' Initial investigations (other tests in **bold** below): FBC, U&E, CRP, ABG, ECG, CXR.

Main differential diagnoses and typical outline evidence, etc.	
Exacerbation of asthma	*Suggested by:* widespread polyphonic wheeze with exacerbations over hours. Silent chest if severe. Anxiety, tachypnoea, tachycardia, and use of accessory muscles.
	Confirmed by: reduced peak flows. **FEV$_1$** that improves by >15% with treatment.
	Initial management: high flow O_2, prednisolone PO or hydrocortisone IV. Nebulized salbutamol and Atrovent® ± magnesium IV and aminophylline IV. NB. Keep hydrated, and monitor ABG and serum K^+. Refer to HDU if drowsy, ↑CO_2.
Exacerbation of COPD	*Suggested by:* long history of cough ± sputum, many pack years of smoking, recurrent 'exacerbations'. **CXR:** radiolucent lungs.
	Confirmed by: **spirometry:** FEV$_1$<80% predicted and FEV/ FVC ratio <0.7. <15% reversibility. Emphysema on **CT chest** ± reduced α1-antitrypsin levels.
	Initial management: controlled O_2, prednisolone 7–10d, and nebulized bronchodilators. Antibiotics if worsening breathlessness, cough, and mucopurulent sputum. Stop smoking. Trials of bronchodilators prn, then regular long-acting bronchodilators. Regular inhaled steroids if FEV<50% predicted and three COPD exacerbations per year.
Acute viral or bacterial bronchitis	*Suggested by:* onset of wheeze over days. No dramatic progression. Fever, mucopurulent sputum, dyspnoea.
	Confirmed by: **sputum culture** and sensitivities. No consolidation on **CXR**.
	Initial management: simple analgesia and antibiotics if continued purulent sputum.

Acute left ventricular failure due to ?cardiac event, valvular disease, electrolyte imbalance, arrhythmia	*Suggested by:* onset minutes to hours. Breathless, distressed and clammy, displaced tapping apex beat, 3rd heart sound, bilateral basal late fine inspiratory crackles. Often also signs of right ventricular failure (↑JVP, swollen legs).
	Confirmed by: **CXR**: fluffy opacification (greatest around the hila), horizontal linear opacities peripherally, bilateral effusions, large heart. Impaired left ventricular function on **echocardiogram**.
	Initial management: sit patient up, controlled O_2, diuretics IV. nitrates IV if very breathless and systolic BP >90. Identify and treat potential causes. Chronic: thiazide or loop diuretic, ACE inhibitor (or angiotensin receptor blocker). β-blocker and spironolactone (monitor K^+).
Anaphylaxis ?precipitant	*Suggested by:* dramatic onset over minutes, recent allergen exposure. Flushing, sweating facial oedema, urticaria, and warm but clammy extremities, tachypnoea, bronchospasm, and wheeze. Tachycardia and hypotension.
	Confirmed by: precipitant identification and response to adrenaline (epinephrine) IM.
	Initial management: remove antigen (e.g. bee sting, medication). Adrenaline IM 1 in 10,000. High flow O_2, fast fluids IV, steroids IV, and antihistamines IV. If stridor, secure airway early as laryngeal oedema may progress, and transfer to HDU/ITU.

Chronic breathlessness

Initial investigations (other tests in **bold** below): FBC, U&E, ECG, CXR, serial peak flow rates (PFRs)

Main differential diagnoses and typical outline evidence, etc.	
Obesity and muscle deconditioning	*Suggested by:* more breathlessness on exertion. No cough or other symptoms. High BMI, but no other abnormality on examination, and normal baseline tests.
	Confirmed by: normal or mild restrictive defect on s**pirometry, CXR, and ECG**. Improvement with weight loss and graduated aerobic exercise programme.
	Initial management: weight loss and reconditioning.
Asthma precipitated by allergens, e.g. pollen, house mites, etc.	*Suggested by:* wheeze, chronic cough worse at night/early morning, specific triggers. Family history or childhood history of asthma or atopy.
	Confirmed by: **spirometry:** reduced peak flow. FEV_1 that improves by >15% with treatment.
	Initial management: high flow O_2, prednisolone PO or hydrocortisone IV. Nebulized salbutamol and Atrovent® ± magnesium IV and aminophylline IV. Long-term care: identify precipitants. Stop smoking. Trial of bronchodilator prn and inhaled steroids, long-acting β-agonist/steroid combinations, leukotriene inhibitors/antihistamines.
COPD caused by smoking, smoke pollution, α1-antitrypsin deficiency	*Suggested by:* long history of cough ± sputum, many pack years of smoking, recurrent 'exacerbations'. **CXR:** radiolucent lungs.
	Confirmed by: **spirometry:** FEV_1<80% predicted and FEV/FVC ratio <0.7. <15% reversibility. Emphysema on **CT chest** ± ↓α1-antitrypsin levels.
	Initial management: stop smoking. Trials of bronchodilators prn, then regular long-acting bronchodilators. Regular inhaled steroids if FEV <50% predicted and three COPD exacerbations per year. If cough and breathless persists, prednisolone PO. If respiratory failure, home O_2.
Left ventricular dysfunction caused or made worse by atrial fibrillation, ischaemic heart disease, mitral stenosis, or regurgitation, hypertension. Anaemia, thyrotoxicosis, chest infections	*Suggested by:* fatigue, orthopnoea, and reduced exercise capability. Resting tachycardia with S3 and displaced apex, bibasal crackles. Evidence of causes.
	Confirmed by: reduced left ventricular function on **echocardiogram. CXR:** large cardiac shadow, upper lobe vein dilatation, loss of costophrenic angle, hilar shadows.
	Initial management: thiazide or loop diuretics, ACE inhibitors (or angiotensin receptor blockers). β-blockers, spironolactone to improve prognosis. Treat causes.

Pulmonary fibrosis/ interstitial lung disease	*Suggested by:* chronic dry cough, occupational exposure or evidence of underlying connective tissue disease. Clubbing, cyanosis, reduced chest expansion, coarse late inspiratory bibasal crackles.
NB. majority of cases have no cause identified	*Confirmed by:* ↓lung volumes and reticular nodular shadowing on **CXR**. Interstitial shadowing and/or subpleural fibrosis on **high resolution CT chest**.
	Initial management: home O_2 if saturations <93%. Refer for specialist opinion for detailed lung function, lung biopsy, immunosupression, antifibrotics, palliation.
Neuromuscular disease complicated by respiratory failure	*Suggested by:* muscle weakness, orthopnoea, daytime sleepiness and/or early morning headaches (due to nocturnal hypoventilation). Muscle wasting, fasciculation, calf hypertrophy, etc. Abnormal ABG.
	Confirmed by: clinical presentation and muscle biopsy. Restrictive defect on **spirometry + FVC**, and fall in FVC by ≥20% on lying flat. Small volume lungs on CXR.
	Initial management: non-invasive ventilation if ABGs show respiratory failure. Follow-up by neurologist and multidisciplinary team.
Pulmonary hypertension	*Suggested by:* features of underlying cause. Loud P2. Desaturation in pulse oximetry on walking and low transfer factor.
(1° pulmonary hypertension in 20%; in 80%, 2° to previous pulmonary emboli, vasculitis, chronic lung disease)	*Confirmed by:* ↑pulmonary pressures and/or right ventricular dysfunction on **echocardiogram**.
	Initial management: treat underlying cause (anticoagulate with heparin and warfarin if severe pulmonary hypertension—even if no proven pulmonary emboli). O_2 to maintain saturations >93%. Managed.
Psychogenic	*Suggested by:* no other associated features of pulmonary or cardiac disease. Underlying anxiety (e.g. high Nijmegan score), triggered by stressful situations.
	Confirmed by: no appearance of organic cause over time.
	Initial management: relaxation, control breathing exercises. Explanation and reassurance.
Chronic thrombo-emboli with or without pulmonary hypertension	*Suggested by:* underlying risk factors, borderline hypoxia (e.g. saturations of 92–95%), resting tachycardia. No loud P2.
	Confirmed by: **echocardiogram** showing no signs of pulmonary hypertension. **CT-PA** showing occluded vessels or **V/Q scans** (showing ventilation/perfusion mismatch (better at detecting peripheral smaller clots below 4th division of pulmonary arteries).
	Initial management: warfarin for at least 3mo, treat risk factors.

Frank haemoptysis (or sputum-streaked with blood)

Haemoptysis rarely causes hypovolaemia from blood loss, but if there is hypotension or tachycardia, consider their causes (see 📖pp.246 and 258). If tuberculosis (TB) is suspected, patient should be isolated whilst tests are carried out. Initial investigations (other tests in bold below): FBC, U&E, CXR.

Main differential diagnoses and typical outline evidence, etc.	
Acute viral or bacterial bronchitis	*Suggested by:* days of fever, mucopurulent sputum, dyspnoea. Typically only streaky haemoptysis and self-limiting.
	Confirmed by: **sputum culture** and sensitivities, response to appropriate antibiotics.
	Initial management: analgesia and consider antibiotics.
Pulmonary embolus/ infarction arising from deep veins	*Suggested by:* sudden breathlessness, pleural rub, cyanosis, tachycardia, loud P2, associated DVT, or predisposing risk factors such as recent surgery, immobility, malignancy, etc.
	Confirmed by: **CT pulmonary angiogram** showing clot in pulmonary artery.
	Initial management: LMW heparin (treatment dose), then warfarin. Thrombolysis if ↓BP, large bilateral clots, or acutely dilated right ventricle on echocardiogram.
Carcinoma of lung	*Suggested by:* weeks or months of weight loss, chest pain, typically smoking history, associated with new or worsening cough. Opacity on **CXR and/or CT**.
	Confirmed by: tumour cells on **sputum cytology** or on endobronchial/**CT guided biopsy**.
	Initial management: O$_2$ if dyspnoea or hypoxic. Analgesia, including diamorphine if distressed. Nebulized adrenaline and tranexamic acid PO before an urgent bronchoscopy.
Pulmonary TB	*Suggested by:* weeks or months of fever, malaise, weight loss, and a contact history/high-risk groups.
	Confirmed by: **CXR**: opacification, especially in apical segments but can be anywhere. Acid-fast bacilli (AFB) on **smear sputum, culture** and/or response to treatment (when cultures negative and no other explanation for symptoms).
	Initial management: isolate patient until smear test known. Isoniazid, pyrazinamide, rifampicin for 2mo, then isoniazid and rifampicin for 4mo. Ethambutol for 6mo if risk of resistance (if non-UK origin, immunosupression). If malnourished, add pyridoxine. Refer for contact tracing. Needs specialist management.

Upper respiratory tract infection (URTI), abnormalities, and bleeding e.g. nasal polyps, laryngeal carcinoma, pharyngeal tumours	*Suggested by:* days of purulent rhinorrhoea (blood from URTI swallowed or inhaled and coughed back up).
	Confirmed by: **nasendoscopy, CT/MRI, head and neck and surgery/biopsy.**
	Initial management: packing, cautery of (Little's) bleeding area, removal of lesion.

Lung abscess	*Suggested by:* days or weeks of copious and foul-smelling sputum, fevers, chest pain. Typically preceded by a prior significant respiratory infection (e.g. pneumonia).
	Confirmed by: **CXR**: circular opacity with fluid level, **sputum culture/culture of CT guided aspirate.**
	Initial management: analgesia, high dose broad-spectrum antibiotics IV for Gram +ve and Gram –ve bacteria, e.g. co-amoxiclav + flucloxacillin + metronidazole for 14d ± CT guided drainage (send for TB and fungal cultures) or surgical removal.

Bronchiectasis	*Suggested by:* progression over months or years. Cupful(s) of pus-like sputum per day. Clubbing, typically bilateral consolidation, and bilateral coarse late inspiratory crackles. Typically obstructive deficit on **spirometry**.
	Confirmed by: **CXR**: cystic shadowing; high resolution **CT chest**: honeycombing and thickened dilated bronchi.
	Initial management: chest physiotherapy (including postural drainage and cough clearance), sputum cultures. Mucolytics, bronchodilators, regular exercise, winter vaccinations. When unwell, treatment with 10–14d antibiotics IV according to last sputum cultures. NB. Anti-*pseudomonas* treatment (aminoglycoside cover). Monitor for weight loss.

Wegener's granulomatosis	*Suggested by:* months of cough, breathless ± microscopic haematuria (i.e. triad of upper/lower respiratory tract and renal abnormalities). Arthritis, myalgia, skin rashes, and nasal bridge collapse.
	Confirmed by: **CXR** showing cavitating shadows. **↑cANCA antibody titre**, and microscopic arteritis on **biopsy**.
	Initial management: immunosuppression with steroids, azathioprine, and cyclophosphamide jointly by renal, respiratory physicians, etc.

(Continued)

Frank haemoptysis (continued)

Main differential diagnoses and typical outline evidence, etc. *(continued)*	
Pneumonia	*Suggested by:* onset over hours or days. Rusty brown sputum (i.e. purulent sputum tinged with blood). Sharp chest pains worse on inspiration, fever, cough, signs of consolidation, etc.
	Confirmed by: patchy shadowing on **CXR** and **sputum/blood culture**.
	Initial management: 5-d course of oral amoxicillin/clarithromycin PO unless more features of CRB-65 (Confusion, Respiratory rate >30/min, Blood pressure <90/60 mmHg and age >65y). If so, amoxicillin/co-amoxiclav IV or cefuroxime with controlled O_2 and fluids. If reduced consciousness/aspiration, then cefuroxime/metronidazole IV. If hospital/nursing home acquired, cefuroxime or piperacillin with tazobactam IV.
Pulmonary arterio-venous malformation	*Suggested by:* haemoptysis alone. No other symptoms. CXR normal or showing coin-shaped lesion with feeding blood vessel.
	Confirmed by: vascular red-blue lesion on **bronchoscopy** (if endobronchial) or enhancing lesion on a **CT chest** with (delayed) contrast, **pulmonary arteriogram** shows feeding vessels.
	Initial management: embolization if bleeding is recurrent or a large quantity. Lobectomy if this fails.
Also	Opportunistic mycobacteria, Goodpasture's syndrome, aspergilloma, mitral valve stenosis (if on warfarin), other endobronchial tumours (including benign lesions), hereditary haemorrhagic telangiectasia, endobronchial amyloid, any cause of systemic clotting abnormality.

Cough with sputum

Initial investigations (other tests in **bold** below): FBC, U&E, CXR.

Main differential diagnoses and typical outline evidence, etc.	
Chronic bronchitis (overlaps with COPD)	*Suggested by:* long history of cough (productive grey/white sputum or dry). Typically >10 pack year smoking. Recurrent 'exacerbations' of cough lasting days, needing antibiotics. *Confirmed by:* **spirometry** shows FEV$_1$<80% predicted and FEV/FVC ratio <0.7, little reversibility (FEV$_1$ improves <15% with treatment). *Initial management:* stop smoking. Winter vaccinations.
Acute viral bronchitis	*Suggested by:* onset over hours or days. Fever, myalgia, fatigue, and white/yellow sputum. *Confirmed by:* no focal chest signs, no consolidation on **CXR**, resolution within 5d. *Initial management:* rest and simple analgesia such as paracetamol.
Acute bacterial bronchitis	*Suggested by:* onset over hours or days. Fever, mucopurulent sputum, dyspnoea. *Confirmed by:* no focal chest signs, **FBC**: ↑neutrophils, no consolidation on **CXR**, pathogens in sputum culture, and rapid response to appropriate antibiotics. *Initial management:* simple analgesia, amoxicillin/clarithromycin PO for 5–7d.
Pneumonia	*Suggested by:* onset over hours or days. Rusty brown sputum. Sharp chest pain (worse on inspiration), fever, cough, signs of consolidation. *Confirmed by:* patchy shadowing on **CXR** and sputum/blood culture. *Initial management:* 5-d course of amoxicillin/clarithromycin PO unless 2 or more features of CRB-65 (<u>C</u>onfusion, <u>R</u>espiratory rate >30min, <u>B</u>lood pressure <90/60mmHg and age >65y). If so, amoxicillin/co-amoxiclav IV or cefuroxime with controlled O$_2$ and fluids. If reduced consciousness/aspiration, then cefuroxime/metronidazole IV. If hospital/nursing home acquired, cefuroxime or piperacillin with tazobactam IV.

Lung abscess	*Suggested by:* days or weeks of copious and foul-smelling sputum, fever, chest pain. Typically preceded by a prior significant respiratory infection (e.g. pneumonia).
	Confirmed by: **CXR**: circular opacity with fluid level, **sputum culture/culture of CT guided aspirate**.
	Initial management: analgesia, high dose broad-spectrum antibiotics IV for Gram +ve and Gram −ve bacteria, e.g. co-amoxiclav + flucloxacillin + metronidazole for 14d ± CT guided drainage (send for TB and fungal cultures) or surgical removal.
Also	Broncho-alveolar cell carcinoma, pulmonary alveolar proteinosis, bronchiectasis associated with immunodeficiency states/primary ciliary dyskinesia, etc.

Persistent dry cough with no sputum

The duration of symptoms, severity, and progression will help determine the causes of a dry cough. No cause is found in up to 15% patient. As this symptom is non-life-threatening, initial management can be delayed until the exact cause is found. Initial investigations (other tests in **bold** below): FBC, U&E, CXR.

Main differential diagnoses and typical outline evidence, etc.	
Smoking	*Suggested by:* smoking history.
	Confirmed by: stopping smoking, cough often worsens initially as ciliary motility is restored, but improves within 3mo.
	Initial management: give generic advice and consider adjunct pharmacotherapy. Refer to smoking cessation specialist, if available, and patient is keen to stop.
Chronic asthma	*Suggested by:* chronic cough, worse at night and early morning. Seasonal variation and other specific triggers (e.g. aerosol sprays, cold air, perfumes, smoke, infections exercise, etc.). Family history or childhood history of asthma or atopy.
	Confirmed by: reduced or variable peak flow (classical dipping early morning/late evening) and **FEV$_1$** that improve by >15% with treatment.
	Initial management: identify precipitants, stop smoking, trial of bronchodilator prn, regular inhaled steroids, long-acting β-agonist/steroid combinations, leukotriene inhibitors/antihistamines. Managed in chest clinic.
Gastro-oesophageal reflux	*Suggested by:* cough worse lying flat and after heavy meals. Heart burn/indigestion. Absent stomach bubble on **CXR** (of hiatus hernia).
	Confirmed by: **24-h oesophageal pH monitoring** or improvement in cough on raising head of bed and with acid suppression (often need very high doses of more than one antacid, combined with promotility drugs).
	Initial management: proton pump inhibitor (PPI) bd combined with H$_2$ antagonist (e.g. ranitidine 150mg bd) and metoclopramide tds, domperidone 20mg tds, and even baclofen bd, in a stepwise fashion.
Post-nasal drip	*Suggested by:* feeling of catarrh and drip in back of throat, worse at night, nasal polyps.
	Confirmed by: improvement with nasal decongestion.
	Initial management: nasal steroids and or nasal ipratropium sprays. Antihistamines. Refer to ENT specialist if fails.
Viral infection with slow recovery	*Suggested by:* original onset over days, fever, sore throat, generalized aches.
	Confirmed by: spontaneous (slow) improvement.
	Initial management: observe.

ACE inhibitors	*Suggested by:* drug history (NB. symptoms can start after taking ACE inhibitors for a long time).
	Confirmed by: cough improves when ACE inhibitor stopped.
	Initial management: substitute with angiotensin receptor blocker for ACE inhibitor.
COPD caused by smoking, smoke pollution, $\alpha1$-antitrypsin deficiency	*Suggested by:* long history of cough ± sputum, many pack years of smoking, recurrent 'exacerbations'. **CXR**: radiolucent lungs.
	Confirmed by: **spirometry**: FEV_1 <80% predicted and FEV/FVC ratio <0.7. <15% reversibility. Emphysema on **CT chest ± ↓$\alpha1$-antitrypsin levels**.
	Initial management: stop smoking. Trials of bronchodilators prn, then regular long-acting bronchodilators. Inhaled steroids if FEV <50% predicted and three COPD exacerbations per year. If cough and breathless persists, prednisolone PO. If respiratory failure, home O_2.
Carcinoma of lung	*Suggested by:* weeks or months of weight loss, chest pain, typically smoking history, associated with new or worsening cough. Opacity on **CXR and/or CT**.
	Confirmed by: tumour cells on **sputum cytology** or on endobronchial/**CT guided biopsy**.
	Initial management: O_2 if dyspnoea or hypoxic. Analgesia, including diamorphine if distressed. Nebulized adrenaline and tranexamic acid PO before an urgent bronchoscopy.
Pulmonary TB	*Suggested by:* weeks or months of fever, malaise, weight loss, and a contact history/high-risk groups.
	Confirmed by: **CXR**: opacification, especially in apical segments, but can be anywhere. AFB on **smear sputum, culture** and/or response to treatment (when cultures negative and no other explanation for symptoms).
	Initial management: isolate patient until smear test known. Isoniazid, pyrazinamide, rifampicin for 2mo, then isoniazid and rifampicin for 4mo. Ethambutol for 6mo if risk of resistance (if non-UK origin, immunosuppression). If malnourished, add pyridoxine. Refer for contact tracing. Needs specialist management.
Interstitial lung disease	*Suggested by:* chronic dry cough, occupational exposure, or evidence of underlying connective tissue disease. NB. Majority of cases have no cause identified. Clubbing, cyanosis↑ yanosis, reduced chest expansion, coarse late inspiratory bibasal crackles.
	Confirmed by: reduced lung volumes and reticular nodular shadowing on **CXR**. Interstitial shadowing and/or subpleural fibrosis on **high resolution CT chest**.
	Initial management: O_2 if saturations <93%. Refer for specialist opinion for detailed lung function, lung biopsy, immunosuppression, antifibrotics, palliation.
Also	Inhaled foreign body, benign endobronchial lesions (e.g. hamartomas), psychogenic.

Hoarseness

Hoarseness of some weeks' or months' duration may have some sinister causes that need urgent attention. Initial investigations (other tests in **bold** below): FBC, U&E, CXR.

Main differential diagnoses and typical outline evidence, etc.	
Inhaled steroids	*Suggested by:* drug history.
	Confirmed by: improvement on stopping steroids.
	Initial management: improve inhaler technique (especially using spacer) and rinsing mouth after inhalers.
Chronic laryngitis	*Suggested by:* onset over months or years. History of recurrent acute laryngitis.
	Confirmed by: inflamed cords at **laryngoscopy** and no other pathology.
	Initial management: stop smoking and reduce alcohol.
Singer's nodes	*Suggested by:* onset over months. Long history, often occupational in teachers or singers due to voice strain, singing, alcohol, fumes, etc.
	Confirmed by: nodules on cord at **laryngoscopy**.
	Initial management: speech therapy, ENT referral for surgical removal.
Laryngeal carcinoma (glottic, supra-glottic, or subglottic tumour)	*Suggested by:* progressive hoarseness over weeks to months. Smoker, including cannabis. Dysphagia, haemoptysis, ear pain.
	Confirmed by: **laryngoscopy**, biopsy, staging.
	Initial management: ENT referral for possible surgical removal.
Vocal cord paresis due to vagal nerve trauma, cancer (thyroid, oesophagus, pharynx, bronchus) or tuberculosis, multiple sclerosis, polio, syringomyelia, (no cause identified in 15%)	*Suggested by:* onset after surgery or otherwise over weeks and months. Bovine cough. Symptoms of cause. Abnormal **CXR, barium swallow, MRI**.
	Confirmed by: paresis or abnormal movement of cords on **laryngoscopy**.
	Initial management: urgent ENT referral. May be considered for vocal cord prosthesis/implant after treatment of cause.

Functional hoarseness	*Suggested by:* recurrence at times of stress. Variable symptoms, able to cough normally.
	Confirmed by: no abnormality **laryngoscopy**.
	Initial management: counselling and behavioural therapy.
Myxoedema	*Suggested by:* onset over months or years. Fatigue, puffy face, obesity, cold intolerance, bradycardia, slow relaxing reflexes.
	Confirmed by: swollen vocal cords at **laryngoscopy**. **↑TSH, ↓FT4**.
	Initial management: thyroxine replacement.
Acromegaly	*Suggested by:* swollen vocal cords at **laryngoscopy**. Large wide face, embossed forehead, jutting jaw (prognathism), widely spaced teeth, and large tongue.
	Confirmed by: **↑IGF**, failure to suppress growth hormone to <2mU/L with **oral GTT**. **Skull X-ray** confirming bony abnormalities. **Hand X-ray** showing typical tufts on terminal phalanges. **MRI or CT scan** showing enlarged pituitary fossa.
	Initial management: hormone replacement and pituitary surgery/radiotherapy.
Sicca syndrome due to old age, Sjögren's syndrome, rheumatoid, sarcoid, etc.	*Suggested by:* onset over months to years. Dry mouth and eyes.
	Confirmed by: clinical presentation and inflamed cords at laryngoscopy and no other pathology.
	Initial management: lubricant lozenges ± artificial tears, address related conditions.
Granulomas due to syphilis, TB, sarcoid, Wegener's	*Suggested by:* onset over months with symptoms and signs in other systems. Abnormal CXR or other system involvement.
	Confirmed by: granulomata on cords at **laryngoscopy**. **Biopsy**. **Culture and sensitivity**.
	Initial management: if TB cultured, refer to a respiratory specialist for 6mo of triple/quadruple therapy. If Wegener's granulomatosis/sarcoid, immunosuppression with systemic steroids + azathioprine + cyclophosphamide. Surgical referral for possible vocal cord prosthesis.

Some thoughts when examining the respiratory system

The findings are described here in the sequence of inspection, palpation, percussion, and then auscultation. While inspecting, think of blood gas status, and when palpating, think of the mechanisms of ventilation. When percussing, think of the pleural surfaces, contents of the pleural cavity, and lung tissue. When auscultating, think of the state of the lung and overlying tissue as well as the airways.

Appearance suggestive of blood gas disturbance

Look at hands for cyanosis, feel for warmth, ask patient to hold arms out and extended at the wrists to see if there is a coarse tremor and/or muscle twitching in the arms. Look at the fingers for peripheral cyanosis and more importantly here, the tongue and lips for central cyanosis. Initial investigations (other tests in **bold** below): FBC, U&E, CXR, ABG.

Main differential diagnoses and typical outline evidence, etc.	
Hypoxic	*Suggested by:* blue fingernails (peripheral) and tongue (central cyanosis), restless, confused, drowsy, or unconscious.
	Confirmed by: P_aO_2 <8kPa on **blood gas analysis** (or **pulse oximetry** of <92% (mild) or <85% (severe)).
	Initial management: controlled O_2 via Venturi and continuous clinical/physiological monitoring whilst addressing underlying cause.
CO_2 retention	*Suggested by:* warm hands, bounding pulse, dilated veins on hands and face, twitching of facial muscles, headaches, confusion, and drowsy.
	Confirmed by: P_aCO_2 >6.5kPa on **blood gas analysis**. Typically >8.0 kPa to be symptomatic.
	Initial management: control O_2 delivery <28% (with Venturi mask to keep O_2 saturation 88–92%). Address underlying cause of respiratory depression if respiratory rate <10 breaths per min.
Hypocapnia	*Suggested by:* dizzy, anxious, paraesthesiae around lips or fingers, tachypnoea.
	Confirmed by: P_aCO_2 <4.5kPa on **blood gas analysis**.
	Initial management: address underlying illness; give supplemental O_2. If CO_2 low, then slow breathing by getting patient to relax; can try rebreathing with a paper bag.

Respiratory rate low (<10/min)

Count the number of respirations for a whole minute if rate appears low. Initial management is to check patient is conscious and secure airway as per Basic Life Support. Remove any obvious cause (e.g. high flow O_2 if saturations are >88%, needlesticks, etc). These patients typically have reduced consciousness and therefore, are at risk of losing their airway patency (e.g. aspiration) so they must be treated in a high dependency area. Initial investigations (other tests in **bold** below): FBC, U&E, CXR, ABG.

Main differential diagnoses and typical outline evidence, etc.	
CO_2 narcosis (very high blood CO_2) due to excess O_2 administration	*Suggested by:* warm hands, bounding pulse, dilated veins on hands and face, twitching of facial muscles, drowsy. High flow O_2 being given.
	Confirmed by: P_aCO_2 >6.5kPa on **blood gas analysis**.
	Initial management: reduce inhaled O_2 to keep saturation 88–92%. Address underlying cause of respiratory depression if respiratory rate is <10 breaths per min.
Drugs, e.g. opiates, alcohol, benzodiazepines, muscle relaxants	*Suggested by:* pinpoint pupils (needle track marks). History of ingestion, empty medication bottle.
	Confirmed by: response to drug withdrawal or antidotes, e.g. naloxone IV/IM, flumazenil IV. Drug levels on **toxicology screen**.
	Initial management: if saturations >90% and no other airway or cardiovascular compromise, observation only until the sedative wears off. Secure airway and trial of antidote; needs high dependency setting with anaesthetist support.
Raised intracranial pressure	*Suggested by:* papilloedema, focal neurology, severe headaches, and vomiting.
	Confirmed by: **CT brain** (loss of normal sulci, cerebral oedema).
	Initial management: secure airway, breathing, and circulation. Monitor neuro-observations. Nurse with head up at 45°. Consider dexamethasone IV, mannitol IV, and phenytoin IV if fits. Neurology referral.
Head injury (without raised intracranial pressure) or cervical cord trauma	*Suggested by:* history and signs of assault/trauma. Other abnormal neurology (upper or lower motor neurone signs).
	Confirmed by: **CT brain** (loss of normal sulci, cerebral oedema).
	Initial management: ATLS (Advanced Trauma Life Support) algorithm. NB. Care stabilizing cervical spine.

Acute (-on-chronic) neuromuscular disease, e.g. Guillain-Barré syndrome	*Suggested by:* known neurological disease, recent viral illness, autonomic dysfunction, ascending weakness, etc. ± other lower motor neurone signs.
	Confirmed by: muscle weakness and $\downarrow P_aO_2$, $\uparrow P_aCO_2$ **on blood gas analysis.**
	Initial management: ventilatory support (if appropriate), supplemental O_2. Specific measures depending on cause.
Severe hypothermia	*Suggested by:* exposure, immobility, reduced **CS**, bradycardia.
	Confirmed by: core temp <33°C.
	Initial management: gentle rewarming (space blankets, fluids IV, bladder irrigation, etc.)

Chest wall abnormalities

Inspect the chest shape and then its change on movement for asymmetry.
Initial investigations (other tests in **bold** below): FBC, U&E, CXR.

Main differential diagnoses and typical outline evidence, etc.	
Pectus carinatum (developmental or associated with emphysema)	*Suggested by:* prominent sternum, often associated with indrawing of the ribs (Harrison's sulci) above the costal margins. *Confirmed by:* **CXR**. *Initial management:* manage emphysema.
Pectus excavatum (developmental defect)	*Suggested by:* depression of the lower end or whole sternum. *Confirmed by:* **CXR**. *Initial management:* explanation.
Kyphosis (congenital or due to anterior collapse of spinal vertebrae, e.g. severe osteoporosis, spinal TB)	*Suggested by:* spine curved forward. *Confirmed by:* **CXR**, **spinal X-ray**. *Initial management:* assess partly using **blood gases**, need for (nocturnal) Non-Invasive Ventilatory support (NIV) if symptoms of ventilatory failure and/or P_aO_2 <8kPa with P_aCO_2 >6.5kPa.
Scoliosis (congenital, neuromuscular disease, surgery, spinal TB)	*Suggested by:* spine curved laterally. *Confirmed by:* CXR, spinal X-ray. *Initial management:* assess partly using blood gases, need for (nocturnal) Non-Invasive Ventilatory support (NIV) if symptoms of ventilatory failure and/or ↓PaO2 <8kPa with ↑PaCO2 >6.5kPa.
Absence of part of chest wall bone structure (congenital—Poland's syndrome—or post-surgery, e.g. thoracoplasty for TB, cancer)	*Suggested by:* absence of ribs, pectoralis muscle, clavicle, etc. *Confirmed by:* history, scars, **CXR**, **spinal X-ray**. *Initial management:* assess partly using **blood gases**, need for (nocturnal) NIV support if symptoms of ventilatory failure and/or P_aO_2 <8kPa with P_aCO_2 >6.5kPa

Bilateral poor chest expansion

Consider all the causes of a low respiratory rate (see 📖 p.308) and also the following that typically do not cause a low respiratory rate. Initial investigations (other tests in **bold** below): FBC, U&E, CXR, ABG.

Main differential diagnoses and typical outline evidence, etc.	
Obesity possibly causing obesity hypoventilation syndrome	*Suggested by:* insidious onset of breathlessness in obese individual. *Confirmed by:* examination (BMI often needs to be >40kg/m^2 to cause chest wall compromise). *Initial management:* weight loss, including dietitian referral and weight-lowering medications. Assess partly using **blood gases**, need for (nocturnal) NIV support if symptoms of ventilatory failure and P_aO_2 <8kPa with P_aCO_2 >6.5kPa (obesity hypoventilation syndrome).
Emphysema (overlaps with COPD) caused by smoking, smoke pollution, α1-antitrypsin deficiency	*Suggested by:* long history of cough ± sputum, many pack years of smoking, recurrent 'exacerbations', pursed lip, breathing (a chronic behavioural adaptation), hyperinflation, reduced chest expansion, reduced breath sounds and hyper-resonance. **CXR**: radiolucent lungs. *Confirmed by:* **spirometry**: FEV$_1$ <80% predicted and FEV/FVC ratio <0.7. <15% reversibility. Emphysema on **CT chest** ± ↓α1-antitrypsin levels. *Initial management:* stop smoking. Trials of bronchodilators prn, regular long-acting bronchodilators. Regular inhaled steroids if FEV <50% predicted and three COPD exacerbations per year. If cough and breathless persists, prednisolone PO. If respiratory failure, home O$_2$.
Pulmonary fibrosis/interstitial lung disease NB. majority of cases have no cause identified.	*Suggested by:* chronic dry cough, occupational exposure, or evidence of underlying connective tissue disease. Clubbing, cyanosis, reduced chest expansion, coarse late inspiratory bibasal crackles. *Confirmed by:* ↓lung volumes and reticular nodular shadowing on **CXR**. Interstitial shadowing and/or subpleural fibrosis on **high resolution CT chest**. *Initial management:* home O$_2$ if saturations <93%. Refer for specialist opinion about detailed lung function, lung biopsy, immunosuppression, antifibrotics, palliation.

Muscular dystrophy (other rarer myopathies, e.g. limb-girdle dystrophy, acid maltase deficiency, etc.)	*Suggested by:* early age onset, family history, calf hypertrophy, lower motor neurone signs. *Confirmed by:* restrictive deficit on **spirometry** (especially when lying flat). Sparing of transfer factor, globally low volumes, especially reduced residual volumes and mouth (inspiratory) pressures on **detailed lung function; muscle biopsy**. *Initial management:* assess need for (nocturnal) NIV support if symptoms of ventilatory failure and/or **blood gases** show P_aO_2 <8kPa with P_aCO_2 >6.5kPa. Refer to neurologist for long-term care.
Motor neurone disease	*Suggested by:* late-onset mixed upper and lower motor neurone signs, tongue fasciculation, bulbar palsy. *Confirmed by:* clinical and **electromyography** (EMG). Restrictive deficit (globally low volumes) on **spirometry** (especially when lying flat). Sparing of transfer factor, reduced residual volumes and mouth (inspiratory) pressures on **detailed lung function**. *Initial management:* medications to reduce upper airway secretions. Assess need for (nocturnal) NIV support if symptoms of ventilatory failure and/or **blood gases** show P_aO_2 <8kPa with P_aCO_2 >6.5kPa. Urgent referral to neurologist.
Multiple sclerosis	*Suggested by:* restrictive deficit (globally low volumes) on spirometry (especially when lying flat). *Confirmed by:* **MRI brain**, **visual evoked responses**. Sparing of transfer factor, reduced residual volumes and mouth (inspiratory) pressures on **detailed lung function**. *Initial management:* assess need for (nocturnal) NIV support if symptoms of ventilatory failure and/or **blood gases** show P_aO_2 <8kPa with P_aCO_2 >6.5kPa. Refer to neurologist for long-term care.
Guillain–Barré syndrome	*Suggested by:* ascending weakness, autonomic disturbances, and recent infection. Restrictive deficit on **lung function** (especially when lying flat). *Confirmed by:* rapid deterioration on lung function (FVC). Sparing of corrected transfer factor. Progress of illness worsening over days to weeks, then improvement. *Initial management:* ventilatory support if P_aO_2 falling and/or P_aCO_2 rising, steroids, and plasmapheresis/globulin infusions.
Also	Myasthenia gravis, Eaton-Lambert syndrome, muscle relaxant drugs, e.g. suxamethonium, neurotoxins (including organophosphates), severe electrolyte abnormalities ($\downarrow\uparrow K^+$, $\downarrow Ca^{2+}$).

Unilateral poor chest expansion

If the patient has become ill rapidly, then this sign has a short differential diagnosis: tension pneumothorax, (which needs to be treated without doing 'initial tests'), flail segment, or severe pneumonia, and need rapid diagnosis and urgent treatment. Less urgent causes are more common; the more dangerous are given precedent here. Initial investigations (other tests in **bold** below): FBC, U&E, CXR, ABG.

Main differential diagnoses and typical outline evidence, etc.	
Pneumothorax ('tension', moderate, or mild)	*Suggested by:* pain in centre or side of chest with abrupt breathlessness, diminished breath sounds, and hyper-resonance to percussion.
	Confirmed by: tracheal deviation and distress suggesting tension pneumothorax, or **expiration CXR** showing loss of lung markings outside sharp line ('moderate' if >5cm gap from lung edge to chest wall, 'mild' if <5cm.)
	Initial management: if tension pneumothorax, insert large Venflon into 2nd intercostal (IC) space, mid-clavicular line. Give O_2 if breathless. Analgesia. Aspirate if moderate; if this is unsatisfactory or prior lung disease, insert IC drain into 'triangle of safety'. If 'mild' (<5cm gap) and not breathless, observe.
Flail segment following trauma	*Suggested by:* paradoxical movement of part of chest wall.
	Confirmed by: **CXR**.
	Initial management: apply direct pressure and 'splint' the segment. Apply ATLS algorithm.
Extensive consolidation due to bacterial infection, but possibly autoimmune disease, malignancy, or drugs.	*Suggested by:* reduced breath sounds, bronchial breathing, increased tactile vocal fremitus, reduced percussion note.
	Confirmed by: CXR.
	Initial management: if not very ill, but fever and ↑neutrophil count, analgesia, and an empiric 5-d course of amoxicillin/clarithromycin PO. If ≥2 features of CRB-65, then amoxicillin/co-amoxiclav IV or cefuroxime with controlled O_2 and fluids. If history of reduced consciousness/aspiration, then cefuroxime/metronidazole IV. If hospital/nursing home acquired infection, cefuroxime or piperacillin with tazobactam IV. If no fever or WCC normal, investigate non-infective possibilities.

Fractured ribs possibly complicated by pneumothorax, haemothorax	*Suggested by:* history of trauma, focal tenderness.
	Confirmed by: **CXR**.
	Initial management: analgesia and rest. Admit to hospital for observation if breathless or worsening pain.

Pleural effusion	*Suggested by:* reduced breath sounds, reduced tactile vocal fremitus, stony dull percussion note.
	Confirmed by: homogeneous opacification with meniscus level on **CXR** and fluid on **US scan/CT chest**.
	Initial management: if breathless at rest, aspirate 500mL (therapeutic) and send fluid for tests, not draining to dryness if cause unknown as thoracoscopy/pleural biopsy required. If known malignancy, also insert IC drain directly and refer for pleurodesis.

Musculoskeletal e.g. previous thoracoplasty	*Suggested by:* history, scar.
	Confirmed by: **CXR**.
	Initial management: assess need for (nocturnal) NIV support if symptoms of ventilatory failure and/or **blood gases** show P_aO_2 <8kPa with P_aCO_2 >6.5kPa. Refer to neurologist for long-term care.

Trachea displaced

First assess the patient—if clinically compromised, suspect tension pneumothorax. Although this is a rare cause of displaced trachea, it must be managed immediately both in primary and secondary care. Palpate with middle finger and with the index and ring finger on either side of trachea. Localize apex beat to see if lower mediastinum is also displaced. Initial investigations (after treating any tension pneumothorax based on clinical diagnosis—other tests in **bold** below): FBC, U&E, CXR, ABG.

Main differential diagnoses and typical outline evidence, etc.	
Pushed by contralateral tension pneumothorax	*Suggested by:* in *extremis* with high pulse rate and hypotension, reduced/absent breath sounds, reduced tactile vocal fremitus, hyper-resonant percussion note.
	Confirmed by: escape of air after insertion of a Venflon into 2nd IC space, opposite side of tracheal deviation.
	Initial management: insertion of Venflon as above; expertly secured emergency IC drain insertion. O_2 and analgesia.
Pulled by ipsilateral pneumothorax ('tension', moderate, or mild)	*Suggested by:* pain in centre or side of chest with abrupt breathlessness, diminished breath sounds, and hyper-resonance to percussion.
	Confirmed by: tracheal deviation and distress suggesting tension pneumothorax, or **expiration CXR** showing loss of lung markings outside sharp line ('moderate' if >5cm gap from lung edge to chest wall, 'mild' if <5cm.)
	Initial management: if tension pneumothorax, insert large Venflon into 2nd IC space, mid-clavicular line. Give O_2 if breathless. Analgesia. Aspirate if moderate; if this is unsatisfactory or prior lung disease, insert IC drain into 'triangle of safety'. If 'mild' (<5cm gap) and not breathless, observe.
Pulled by ipsilateral upper lobe fibrosis, collapse, or removal	*Suggested by:* TB (chronic), radiation fibrosis (skin changes, tattoo marks), surgery (scar), ankylosing spondylitis, chronic sarcoidosis. If smoker and focal lobar collapse, consider endobronchial tumour. Reduced upper chest wall expansion.
	Confirmed by: **CXR** showing diminished abnormal chest anatomy 'pulling' on mediastinum with trachea deviated towards the same side.
	Initial management: review old CXR; for **CT chest and bronchoscopy** if new upper lobe collapse. Assess need for (nocturnal) NIV support if symptoms of ventilatory failure and/or **blood gases** show P_aO_2 <8kPa with P_aCO_2 >6.5kPa.

Pushed by contralateral pleural effusion	*Suggested by:* reduced breath sounds, reduced tactile vocal fremitus, stony dull percussion note.
	Confirmed by: **CXR** showing large homogeneous white opacification 'pushing' on mediastinum.
	Initial management: if breathless at rest, aspirate 500mL (therapeutic) and send fluid for tests. Do not drain to dryness if cause unknown, thoracoscopy/pleural biopsy is required. If known cause (e.g. malignancy), aspirate 500mL or insert IC drain directly and refer for pleurodesis.
Scoliosis	*Suggested by:* chest wall deformity and curved spine.
	Confirmed by: **spinal X-ray, CXR**.
	Initial management: analgesia, physiotherapy, calcium supplements. Assess need for (nocturnal) NIV support if symptoms of ventilatory failure and/or **blood gases** show P_aO_2 <8kPa with P_aCO_2 >6.5kPa.

Reduced tactile vocal fremitus

If *in extremis*, treat as tension pneumothorax. If not, Initial investigations (other tests in **bold** below): FBC, U&E, CXR.

	Main differential diagnoses and typical outline evidence, etc.
Pleural effusion	*Suggested by:* reduced breath sounds, reduced tactile vocal fremitus, stony dullness to percussion.
	Confirmed by: homogeneous opacification with meniscus level on **CXR** and fluid on **US scan/CT chest**.\
	Initial management: if breathless at rest, aspirate 500mL (therapeutic) and send fluid for tests. Do not drain to dryness if cause unknown, thoracoscopy/pleural biopsy is required. If known cause (e.g. malignancy), aspirate 500 mL or insert IC drain directly and refer for pleurodesis.
Pneumothorax ('tension', moderate or mild)	*Suggested by:* pain in centre or side of chest with abrupt breathlessness, diminished breath sounds, and hyper-resonance to percussion.
	Confirmed by: above findings, tracheal deviation, and distress suggesting tension pneumothorax, or **expiration CXR** showing loss of lung markings outside sharp line ('moderate' if >5cm gap from lung edge to chest wall, 'mild' if <5cm.)
	Initial management: If tension pneumothorax, insert large Venflon into 2nd IC space, mid-clavicular line. Give O_2 if breathless. Analgesia. Aspirate if moderate; if this unsatisfactory or prior lung disease, insert IC drain into 'triangle of safety'. If 'mild' (<5cm gap) + not breathless, observe.
Collapsed lobe with no consolidation	*Suggested by:* reduced breath sounds, reduced expansion, normal percussion note.
	Confirmed by: **CXR** (collapse of different lobes will have different patterns radiologically, e.g. showing fan-shaped shadow arising from mediastinum, mediastinal shift, raised hemidiaphragm, displaced horizontal fissure or 'sail sign'). **CT thorax** confirms lobar collapse.
	Initial management: bronchoscopy to remove any foreign body or debris, or to biopsy obstructive growth.

Increased tactile vocal fremitus

Initial investigations (other tests in **bold** below): FBC, U&E, CXR.

Main differential diagnoses and typical outline evidence, etc.	
Extensive consolidation due to bacterial infection, but possibly autoimmune disease, malignancy, or drugs.	*Suggested by:* reduced breath sounds, bronchial breathing, increased tactile vocal fremitus, reduced percussion note.
	Confirmed by: **CXR**.
	Initial management: if not very ill, but fever and ↑neutrophil count on **FBC**, analgesia and an empiric 5-d course of amoxicillin/clarithromycin PO. If ≥2 features of CRB-65, then amoxicillin/co-amoxiclav IV or cefuroxime with controlled O_2 and fluids. If history of reduced consciousness/aspiration, then cefuroxime/metronidazole IV. If hospital/nursing home acquired infection, cefuroxime or piperacillin with tazobactam IV. If no fever or WCC normal, investigate non-infective possibilities.

Stony dull percussion

This implies pleural effusion. The causes of pleural effusion are traditionally divided into transudates and exudates. Initial investigations (other tests in **bold** below): FBC, U&E, CXR diagnostic pleural aspiration.

Main differential diagnoses and typical outline evidence, etc.	
Transudates	*Suggested by:* bilateral effusions, underlying clinical cause.
	Confirmed by: **protein in pleural effusion** <30g/L or <0.5 ratio to serum protein (except can be higher in treated heart failure).
Left heart failure (LVF), superior vena cava (SVC) obstruction, pericarditis, peritoneal dialysis	*Suggested by:* peripheral oedema, ↑JVP, basal crackles, 3rd heart sound, if LVF. Headache, swollen/plethoric face, and dilated superficial venules across anterior chest if SVC obstruction.
	Confirmed by: **CXR, echocardiogram, CT thorax** (if considering SVC obstruction).
	Initial treatment: diuretics and ACE inhibitors if LVF. Steroids and anticoagulation if SVC obstruction. NSAIDs and treat cause if pericardial effusion.
Low albumin states, e.g. liver cirrhosis, nephrotic syndrome	*Suggested by:* malnutrition, generalized oedema. Evidence of other disease.
	Confirmed by: ↓**serum albumin**.
	Initial treatment: try to correct serum albumin with appropriate diet.
Rare causes	Hypothyroidism, Meig's syndrome.
Exudates	*Suggested by:* typically unilateral effusion (but may be bilateral). Signs and symptoms of underlying disease.
	Confirmed by: protein in effusion >30g/dL or >0.5 ratio to serum protein.
Infective: bacterial/ empyema, TB, viral, etc.	*Suggested by:* history, fever, ↓pH, ↓glucose in pleural fluid.
	Confirmed by: **pleural aspiration** of pus with organisms on **Gram stain or culture** in bacterial pneumonia. ↑lymphocytes suggest TB (confirmed by +ve cultures or **Ziehl-Neelsen (ZN)** stain on fluid or pleural biopsy or of caseating granuloma).
	Initial management: appropriate antibiotic treatment and IC drain to remove fluid or pus.
Neoplastic: lung 1° or 2°, breast, ovarian, reticuloses, Kaposi's, local chest wall tumours, mesothelioma	*Suggested by:* history, especially weight loss. Signs of local or distal spread.
	Confirmed by: **pleural aspiration** (cytology), **pleural biopsy** or other tissue histology.
	Initial management: once cancer confirmed, typically needs IC drain, and drain to dryness followed by pleurodesis. Referral to oncology for active treatment or palliative care.

Rheumatoid, systemic lupus erythematosus, etc.	*Suggested by:* history, other organ specific involvement, e.g. joints, +ve rheumatoid factor in fluid, very low fluid glucose.
	Confirmed by: +ve **autoantibodies** and clinical criteria, response to immunosuppression.
	Initial management: steroids/azathioprine/ cyclophosphamide.
Pulmonary infarction/ embolus	*Suggested by:* sudden/acute worsening of breathlessness, pleural rub, cyanosis, tachycardia, loud P2, associated DVT, or risk factors such as recent surgery, immobility, previous emboli, malignancy, etc. Other tests typically show raised D-dimers, tachycardia or right heart strain, and rarely S1Q3T3 on ECG.
	Confirmed by: **CT pulmonary angiogram** showing clot in pulmonary artery. Echocardiogram (right heart strain) is useful for risk stratification if pulmonary embolus confirmed.
	Initial management: LMW heparin (treatment dose not prophylactic dose) and 3mo anticoagulation with warfarin (longer if ongoing risk factors). Consider thrombolysis if ↓BP, large and bilateral clots, no response to anticoagulation or acutely dilated right ventricle on echocardiogram.

Dull to percussion but not stony dull

Initial investigations (other tests in **bold** below): FBC, U&E, CXR.

Main differential diagnoses and typical outline evidence, etc.	
Consolidation due to bacterial infection, but possibly autoimmune disease, malignancy, or drugs.	*Suggested by:* reduced breath sounds, bronchial breathing, increased tactile vocal fremitus, reduced percussion note.
	Confirmed by: **CXR**.
	Initial management: if not very ill, but fever and ↑neutrophil count on **FBC**, analgesia and an empiric 5-d course of amoxicillin/clarithromycin PO. If ≥2 features of CRB-65, then amoxicillin/co-amoxiclav IV or cefuroxime with controlled O_2 and fluids. If history of reduced consciousness/aspiration, then cefuroxime/metronidazole IV. If hospital/nursing home acquired infection, cefuroxime or piperacillin with tazobactam IV. If no fever or WCC normal, investigate non-infective possibilities.
Pulmonary oedema due to acute left ventricular failure or chronic (congestive) cardiac failure due to ischaemic heart disease, mitral stenosis	*Suggested by:* background fatigue and exertional breathlessness, cardiac risk factors. Displaced apex beat, 3rd heart sound, bilateral basal fine crackles. ↑JVP and leg swelling.
	Confirmed by: **CXR**: fluffy opacification, especially near hila. Loss of costophrenic angle. Impaired left ventricular function on **echocardiogram**.
	Initial management: sit patient up, controlled O_2, diuretics IV. nitrates IV if very breathless and systolic BP> 90.
	Chronic: thiazide or loop diuretic, ACE inhibitor (or angiotensin receptor blocker). β-blocker and spironolactone (monitor K^+).
Elevated hemidiaphragm	*Suggested by:* typically asymptomatic, reduced/absent breath sounds, no other abnormalities unless from underlying cause, e.g. pulmonary embolus, tumour, phrenic nerve scar, etc. (often no cause found).
	Confirmed by: **CXR**.
	Initial management: anticoagulate if pulmonary embolus, seek old CXR to see if longstanding.
Severe fibrosis/ collapse	*Suggested by:* clubbing and signs of underlying cause, reduced chest expansion, tracheal deviation. Reduced breath sounds, course crackles.
	Confirmed by: **CXR, high resolution CT thorax**.
	Initial management: bronchoscopy if new lobar collapse.
Severe pleural thickening, e.g. due to pleural secondaries or mesothelioma	*Suggested by:* chest pain, weight loss, history of asbestos exposure, clubbing, reduced breath sounds.
	Confirmed by: **CT thorax and pleural biopsy**.
	Initial management: analgesia (e.g. opiates) and controlled O_2. Refer to oncologist/chest physician for specialist treatment.

Hyper-resonant percussion

If *in extremis*, consider the rare, but immediately life-threatening, cause of tension pneumothorax. Initial investigations (other tests in **bold** below): FBC, U&E, CXR, ABG.

Main differential diagnoses and typical outline evidence, etc.	
Emphysema (overlaps with COPD) caused by smoking, smoke pollution, α-1 antitrypsin deficiency	*Suggested by:* long history of cough ± sputum, many pack years of smoking, recurrent 'exacerbations', pursed lip, breathing (a chronic behavioural adaptation), hyperinflation, reduced chest expansion, reduced breath sounds, and hyper-resonance. CXR: radiolucent lungs.
	Confirmed by: **spirometry**: FEV$_1$ <80% predicted and FEV/FVC ratio <0.7. <15% reversibility. Emphysema on **CT chest ± ↓α1-antitrypsin levels**.
	Initial management: stop smoking. Trials of bronchodilators prn, regular long-acting bronchodilators. Regular inhaled steroids if FEV <50% predicted and three COPD exacerbations per year. If cough and breathless persists, prednisolone PO. If respiratory failure, home O$_2$.
Large bullae	*Suggested by:* other signs of emphysema but can be isolated finding, and often congenital in otherwise normal lungs.
	Confirmed by: **CT thorax**.
	Initial management: observe. Can mimic partial pneumothorax (do not insert intercostal drain). Cardiothoracic surgical referral for bullectomy if symptomatic and no widespread emphysema.
Pneumothorax ('tension', moderate, or mild)	*Suggested by:* pain in centre or side of chest with abrupt breathlessness, diminished breath sounds, and hyper-resonance to percussion.
	Confirmed by: above findings, tracheal deviation, and distress suggesting tension pneumothorax, or **expiration CXR** showing loss of lung markings outside sharp line ('moderate' if >5cm gap from lung edge to chest wall, 'mild' if <5cm.)
	Initial management: if tension pneumothorax, insert large Venflon into 2nd IC space, mid-clavicular line. Give O$_2$ if breathless. Analgesia. Aspirate if moderate; if this is unsatisfactory or prior lung disease, insert IC drain into 'triangle of safety'. If 'mild' (<5cm gap) and not breathless, observe.

Reduced breath sounds

When auscultating the lungs, think of the underlying lung parenchyma and overlying tissues. Ensure patient breathes with mouth open, regularly and deeply, and does not vocalize (e.g. groaning). Reduced breath sounds may be because:

- air is not entering/leaving the lung(s);
- excess air, fat, or fluid between lung and your stethoscope;
- good air entry but abnormal lung parenchyma.

Initial investigations (other tests in **bold** below): FBC, U&E, CXR, ABG.

Air is not entering/leaving the lung(s): Main differential diagnoses and typical outline evidence, etc.	
Poor respiratory effort	*Suggested by:* reduced consciousness/cooperation, any cause of poor chest wall expansion (see 📖pp.312). *Confirmed by:* **ABG** (type 2 failure). *Initial management:* treat cause (e.g. remove high flow O_2, respiratory sedative) and consider non-invasive ventilation.
Endobronchial obstruction, e.g. tumour, retained secretions, inhaled foreign body	*Suggested by:* cough, stridor, unilateral signs of dullness to percussion, crackles, and unilateral reduced breath sounds (unless pathology is above the carina). *Confirmed by:* **CT thorax, bronchoscopy.** *Initial management:* bronchoscopy and removal obstruction, if possible.
Severe asthma or anaphylaxis (bronchoconstriction)	*Suggested by:* history, sudden onset, often precipitating factor. Patient *in extremis*, reduced consciousness. *Confirmed by:* **peak flow rate** undetectable. **ABG** shows type 2 respiratory failure. *Initial management:* high flow O_2, high dose bronchodilators (β2-agonists and anticholinergics) via nebulizer, Hydrocortisone IV 200mg. magnesium IV, antihistamines IV, and aminophylline IV can be considered. NB. Keep hydrated and monitor ABG and serum K^+. Refer to HDU if drowsy, ↑CO_2.

Excess air, fat, or fluid between lung and your stethoscope:
Main differential diagnoses and typical outline evidence, etc.

Obesity (leading to ventilatory failure = obesity hypoventilation syndrome)	*Suggested by:* insidious onset of breathlessness with rising weight. *Confirmed by:* examination (BMI typically >40kg/m² to cause chest wall compromise). *Initial management:* weight loss, including dietitian referral and weight-lowering medications. Assess need for (nocturnal) NIV support (i.e. if symptoms of ventilatory failure and P_aO_2 <8kPa with P_aCO_2 >6.5kPa).
Pneumothorax ('tension', moderate, or mild)	*Suggested by:* pain in centre or side of chest with abrupt breathlessness, diminished breath sounds, and hyper-resonance to percussion. *Confirmed by:* above findings, tracheal deviation, and distress suggesting tension pneumothorax, or **expiration CXR** showing loss of lung markings outside sharp line ('moderate' if >5cm gap from lung edge to chest wall, 'mild' if <5cm.) *Initial management:* if tension pneumothorax, insert large Venflon into 2nd IC space, mid-clavicular line. Give O_2 if breathless. Analgesia. Aspirate if moderate; if this is unsatisfactory or prior lung disease, insert IC drain into 'triangle of safety'. If 'mild' (<5cm gap) and not breathless, observe.
Pleural effusion	*Suggested by:* reduced breath sounds, reduced tactile vocal fremitus, stony dull percussion note. *Confirmed by:* homogeneous opacification with meniscus level on **CXR** and fluid on **US scan/CT chest**. *Initial management:* if breathless at rest, aspirate 500mL (therapeutic) and send fluid for tests, not draining to dryness if cause unknown, as thoracoscopy/pleural biopsy required. If known malignancy, also insert IC drain directly and refer for pleurodesis.
Severe pleural thickening, e.g. due to pleural secondaries or mesothelioma	*Suggested by:* chest pain, weight loss, history of asbestos exposure, clubbing, reduced breath sounds. *Confirmed by:* **CT thorax and pleural biopsy**. *Initial management:* analgesia (e.g. opiates) and controlled O_2. Refer to oncologist/chest physician for specialist treatment.

(Continued)

Reduced breath sounds (continued)

Good air entry but abnormal lung parenchyma:
Main differential diagnoses and typical outline evidence, etc.

Emphysema (overlaps with COPD) caused by smoking, smoke pollution, α1-antitrypsin deficiency	*Suggested by:* long history of cough $\pm$ sputum, many pack years of smoking, recurrent 'exacerbations', pursed lip, breathing (a chronic behavioural adaptation), hyperinflation, reduced chest expansion, reduced breath sounds, and hyper-resonance. CXR: radiolucent lungs.
	Confirmed by: **spirometry**: FEV_1 <80% predicted and FEV/FVC ratio <0.7. <15% reversibility. Emphysema on **CT chest $\pm$ $\downarrow\alpha$1-antitrypsin levels**.
	Initial management: stop smoking. Trials of bronchodilators prn, regular long-acting bronchodilators. Regular inhaled steroids if FEV <50% predicted and three COPD exacerbations per year. If cough and breathless persists, prednisolone PO. If respiratory failure, home O_2.
Large bullae	*Suggested by:* other signs of emphysema but can be isolated finding, and often congenital in otherwise normal lungs.
	Confirmed by: **CT thorax**.
	Initial treatment: observe. Can mimic partial pneumothorax, but do NOT insert IC drain. Refer to cardiothoracics for bullectomy if symptomatic and not widespread emphysema.
Consolidation due to bacterial infection, but possibly autoimmune disease, malignancy, or drugs.	*Suggested by:* reduced breath sounds, bronchial breathing, increased tactile vocal fremitus, reduced percussion note.
	Confirmed by: **CXR**.
	Initial management: if not very ill, but fever and $\uparrow$neutrophil count, analgesia, and an empiric 5-d course of amoxicillin/clarithromycin PO. If $\geq$2 features of CRB-65, then amoxicillin/co-amoxiclav IV or cefuroxime with controlled O_2 and fluids. If history of reduced consciousness/aspiration, then cefuroxime/metronidazole IV. If hospital/nursing home acquired infection, cefuroxime or piperacillin with tazobactam IV. If no fever or WCC normal, investigate non-infective possibilities.

Bronchial breathing

Prolonged expiration phase with a definite silence between inspiration and expiration (same as sound heard with stethoscope bell over trachea). Initial investigations (other tests in **bold** below): FBC, U&E, CXR.

Main differential diagnoses and typical outline evidence, etc.	
Consolidation due to bacterial infection, but possibly autoimmune disease, malignancy, or drugs.	*Suggested by:* reduced breath sounds, bronchial breathing, increased tactile vocal fremitus, reduced percussion note.
	Confirmed by: **CXR**.
	Initial management: if not very ill, but fever and ↑neutrophil count on FBC, analgesia, and an empiric 5-d course of amoxicillin/clarithromycin PO. If ≥2 features of CRB-65, then amoxicillin/co-amoxiclav IV or cefuroxime with controlled O₂ and fluids. If history of reduced consciousness/aspiration, then cefuroxime/metronidazole IV. If hospital/nursing home acquired infection, cefuroxime or piperacillin with tazobactam IV. If no fever or WCC normal, investigate non-infective possibilities.
Lung cavity	*Suggested by:* localized bronchial breathing, otherwise normal examination.
	Confirmed by: **CXR**, **CT thorax** (should have greater than 2mm wall thickness to differentiate from a lung cyst).
	Initial management: compare with old CXR. Consider TB and lung cancer. Refer to chest physician.
Pulmonary fibrosis/ interstitial lung disease NB. Majority of cases have no cause identified.	*Suggested by:* chronic dry cough, occupational exposure or evidence of underlying connective tissue disease. Clubbing, cyanosis, reduced chest expansion, coarse late inspiratory bibasal crackles.
	Confirmed by: ↓lung volumes and reticular nodular shadowing on **CXR**. Interstitial shadowing and/or subpleural fibrosis on **high resolution CT chest**.
	Initial management: home O₂ if saturations <93%. Refer for specialist opinion about detailed lung function, lung biopsy, immunosuppression, antifibrotics, palliation.

Fine inspiratory crackles

Very fine crackles are like the sound made when hair next to the ear is rolled between finger and thumb, or opening a velcro pad! Initial investigations (other tests in **bold** below): FBC, U&E, CXR, ABG.

Main differential diagnoses and typical outline evidence, etc.	
Incidental due to normal secretions	*Suggested by:* late in inspiration, disappear on coughing. *Confirmed by:* **CXR** showing normal lung fields.
Pulmonary oedema due to acute left ventricular failure or chronic (congestive) cardiac failure due to ischaemic heart disease, mitral stenosis	*Suggested by:* background fatigue and exertional breathless, cardiac risk factors. Displaced apex beat, 3rd heart sound, bilateral basal fine crackles. ↑JVP and leg swelling. *Confirmed by:* **CXR**: fluffy opacification, especially near hila. Loss of costophrenic angle. Impaired left ventricular function on **echocardiogram**. *Initial management:* sit patient up, controlled O_2, diuretics IV. nitrates IV if very breathless and systolic BP >90. Chronic: thiazide or loop diuretic, ACE inhibitor (or angiotensin receptor blocker). β-blocker and spironolactone (monitor K^+).
Pulmonary oedema due to acute lung injury	*Suggested by:* late in inspiration, dullness to percussion at lung bases (in associated effusion), no S3. Severe hypoxia, patient critically ill. Evidence of cause cause, e.g. infection. *Confirmed by:* **CXR** showing bilateral hilar fluffy shadows, normal-sized heart, and linear opacities in upper lobes. **Echocardiogram** showing normal left ventricular contraction. *Initial management:* treat underlying cause. Supplemental O_2, specialist ventilatory support.
Pulmonary fibrosis/ interstitial lung disease NB. Majority of cases have no cause identified.	*Suggested by:* chronic dry cough, occupational exposure or evidence of underlying connective tissue disease. Clubbing, cyanosis, reduced chest expansion, coarse late inspiratory bibasal crackles. *Confirmed by:* ↓lung volumes and reticular nodular shadowing on **CXR**. Interstitial shadowing and/or subpleural fibrosis on **high resolution CT chest**. *Initial management:* home O_2 if saturations <93%. Refer for specialist opinion about detailed lung function, lung biopsy, immunosuppression, antifibrotics, palliation.
Chronic bronchitis (overlaps with COPD)	*Suggested by:* long history of cough (productive grey/ white sputum or dry). Typically >10 pack year smoking. Recurrent 'exacerbations' of cough lasting days, needing antibiotics. *Confirmed by:* spirometry shows FEV_1 <80% predicted and FEV/FVC ratio <0.7, little reversibility (FEV_1 improves <15% with treatment). *Initial management:* stop smoking. Winter vaccinations.

Emphysema (overlaps with COPD) caused by smoking, smoke pollution, α1-antitrypsin deficiency	*Suggested by:* long history of cough ± sputum, many pack years of smoking, recurrent 'exacerbations', pursed lip, breathing (a chronic behavioural adaptation), hyperinflation, reduced chest expansion, reduced breath sounds, and hyper-resonance. **CXR**: radiolucent lungs.
	Confirmed by: **spirometry**: FEV$_1$ <80% predicted and FEV/FVC ratio <0.7. <15% reversibility. Emphysema on **CT chest ± ↓α1-antitrypsin levels**.
	Initial management: stop smoking. Trials of bronchodilators prn, regular long-acting bronchodilators. Regular inhaled steroids if FEV <50% predicted and three COPD exacerbations per year. If cough and breathless persists, prednisolone PO. If respiratory failure, home O$_2$.
Consolidation due to bacterial infection,	*Suggested by:* reduced breath sounds, bronchial breathing, increased tactile vocal fremitus, reduced percussion note.
	Confirmed by: **CXR**.
but possibly autoimmune disease, malignancy, or drugs.	*Initial management:* if not very ill, but fever and ↑neutrophil count on **FBC**, analgesia, and an empiric 5-d course of oral amoxicillin/clarithromycin. If ≥2 features of CRB-65, then amoxicillin/co-amoxiclav IV or cefuroxime with controlled O$_2$ and fluids. If history of reduced consciousness/aspiration, then cefuroxime/metronidazole IV. If hospital/nursing home acquired infection, cefuroxime or piperacillin with tazobactam IV. If no fever or WCC normal, investigate non-infective possibilities.

Coarse crackles

Bubbly crackles, often heard in both inspiration and expiration. Initial investigations (other tests in **bold** below): FBC, U&E, CXR.

Main differential diagnoses and typical outline evidence, etc.	
Bronchiectasis	*Suggested by:* progression over months or years. Cupful(s) of pus-like sputum per day. Clubbing, typically bilateral consolidation, and bilateral coarse late inspiratory crackles. Typically obstructive deficit on **spirometry**.
	Confirmed by: **CXR**: cystic shadowing; high resolution **CT chest**: honeycombing and thickened dilated bronchi.
	Initial management: chest physiotherapy (including postural drainage and cough clearance), sputum cultures. Mucolytics, bronchodilators, regular exercise, winter vaccinations. When unwell, treatment with 10–14d antibiotics IV according to last sputum cultures. NB. Anti-*pseudomonas* treatment (aminoglycoside cover). Monitor for weight loss.
Pulmonary fibrosis/ interstitial lung disease NB. Majority of cases have no cause identified.	*Suggested by:* chronic dry cough, occupational exposure or evidence of underlying connective tissue disease. Clubbing, cyanosis, reduced chest expansion, coarse late inspiratory bibasal crackles.
	Confirmed by: ↓lung volumes and reticular nodular shadowing on **CXR**. Interstitial shadowing and/or subpleural fibrosis on **high resolution CT chest**.
	Initial management: home O_2 if saturations <93%. Refer for specialist opinion about detailed lung function, lung biopsy, immunosuppression, antifibrotics, palliation.

Pleural rub

This sound can be reproduced by placing one finger over your ear and scratching the nail bed with your opposite index finger (or crunching through snow). Pleural rub is caused by inflammation of the pleura. Initial investigations (other tests in **bold** below): FBC, U&E, CXR.

Main differential diagnoses and typical outline evidence, etc.	
Pneumonia with pleurisy	*Suggested by:* onset over hours or days, rusty brown sputum ± blood. Sharp pains worse on inspiration, fever, cough, crackles, dullness to percussion, bronchial breathing, **WCC**: ↑neutrophils, ↑**CRP**.
	Confirmed by: patchy shadowing on **CXR** and sputum/blood culture
	Initial management: analgesia and provisional antibiotic e.g. amoxicillin/clarithromycin PO for 5d. If >2 features of <u>C</u>onfusion, <u>R</u>esp rate >30/min, <u>B</u>P <90/60, age >65y), then antibiotic IV, e.g. amoxicillin/co-amoxiclav or cefuroxime, and controlled O₂ and fluids. If suspected aspiration, then anti-anaerobics, e.g. cefuroxime/metronidazole IV. If hospital/nursing home acquired, cefuroxime or piperacillin with tazobactam IV.
Pulmonary embolus/ infarction arising from deep veins or in left atrium	*Suggested by:* sudden breathlessness, pleural rub, cyanosis, tachycardia, loud P2, associated DVT, or risk factors such as recent surgery, immobility, previous emboli, malignancy, etc.
	Confirmed by: **CT pulmonary angiogram** showing clot in pulmonary artery.
	Initial management: LMW heparin (treatment dose), then warfarin. Thrombolysis if ↓BP, large bilateral clots or acutely dilated right ventricle on echocardiogram.
Severe pleural thickening, e.g. due to pleural secondaries or mesothelioma	*Suggested by:* chest pain, weight loss, history of asbestos exposure, clubbing, reduced breath sounds.
	Confirmed by: **CT thorax** and **pleural biopsy**.
	Initial management: analgesia (e.g. opiates) and controlled O₂. Refer to oncologist/chest physician for specialist treatment.

Stridor ± inspiratory wheeze

This suggests obstruction in or near the larynx. This represents a <u>medical emergency</u>. Attempts to examine the upper airway outside of a specialist setting may make matters worse. Initial investigations (other tests in **bold** below): FBC, U&E, CXR.

Main differential diagnoses and typical outline evidence, etc.	
Epiglottitis	*Suggested by:* fever, URTI coryzal symptoms (the 4 Ds = drooling, drawn facies, dysphonia, dysphagia).
	Confirmed by: **indirect laryngoscopy** under controlled (anaesthetic) conditions.
	Initial management: penicillin IV, and refer for emergency treatment with ENT and anaesthetic opinion.
Croup	*Suggested by:* high-pitched cough in infants.
	Confirmed by: above presentation and findings.
	Initial management: refer for paediatric support if respiratory compromise.
Inhaled foreign body	*Suggested by:* history of inhaled peanut, bead, etc. typically right-sided chest signs.
	Confirmed by: **CXR, CT thorax, bronchoscopy**.
	Initial management: slap between shoulder blades/Heimlich manoeuvre if acutely ill. CT and bronchoscopy if not acutely ill.
Rapidly progressive laryngomalacia	*Suggested by:* change in voice over months to years.
	Confirmed by: **indirect laryngoscopy**, **CT thorax**.
	Initial management: ENT surgical referral.
Laryngeal papillomas	*Suggested by:* change in voice over weeks to months.
	Confirmed by: **indirect laryngoscopy**.
	Initial management: ENT surgical referral.
Anaphylaxis causing laryngeal oedema	*Suggested by:* onset over minutes, history of recent allergen exposure, feeling of dread, flushing, sweating, facial oedema, urticaria, warm clammy extremities, dyspnoea and tachypnoea, wheeze. Tachycardia and ↓BP.
	Confirmed by: clinical presentation and response to adrenaline (epinephrine) IM. Results of controlled allergen exposure.
	Initial management: remove antigen (e.g. bee sting, medication). Adrenaline IM 1 in 10,000. Secure airway early if stridor. High flow O_2, fast fluids IV, steroids IV, and antihistamines IV. Transfer to HDU/ITU.

Inspiratory monophonic wheeze

This suggests large airway obstruction, often very proximal. A lesion just above the carina can be immediately life-threatening as neither lung can be ventilated, and tracheostomy will also not get below the obstruction. Initial investigations (other tests in **bold** below): FBC, U&E, CXR.

Main differential diagnoses and typical outline evidence, etc.	
Acute bilateral vocal cord paralysis	*Suggested by:* change in voice, bilateral reduced breath sounds, and wheeze. *Confirmed by:* **laryngoscopy**. *Initial management:* ENT surgical referral.
Inhalation of foreign body	*Suggested by:* history of putting an object in mouth, e.g. peanut. Sudden stridor, severe cough, low-pitched, monophonic wheeze, and reduced breath sounds, typically on the right. *Confirmed by:* if not *in extremis*, **CXR/CT thorax** or **bronchoscopy** to show foreign body. *Initial management:* if *in extremis*, slap back between the shoulder blades with patient leaning forward; if fails, perform Heimlich manoeuvre.
Tracheal tumours or stenosis after ventilation	*Suggested by:* stridor, over weeks to months, bilateral reduced breath sounds, and bilateral wheeze. *Confirmed by:* **CXR, CT thorax and neck, bronchoscopy**. Initial treatment: controlled O_2, and/or steroids IV.
Extrinsic compression of large airways by mediastinal masses	*Suggested by:* neck/chest discomfort ± swelling over weeks to months. Look for signs of SVC obstruction. Can be focal (unilateral) or bilateral wheeze, depending on site of obstruction. *Confirmed by:* **CT thorax and neck**. *Initial management:* steroids and referral to oncology for palliative chemo-radiotherapy.
Extrinsic compression by oesophageal tumours	*Suggested by:* dysphagia, weight loss over weeks to months. *Confirmed by:* **CT thorax and neck**. *Initial management:* soft pureed diet. Barium swallow if high dysphagia or oesophago-gastroduodenoscopy (OGD) if low dysphagia.
Tracheal blunt trauma	*Suggested by:* history, pain and swelling, change in voice over minutes or hours after trauma. *Confirmed by:* **laryngoscopy, bronchoscopy**. *Initial management:* early intubation and steroids.

Expiratory monophonic wheeze

This suggests obstruction of a large airway. Initial investigations (other tests in **bold** below): FBC, U&E, CXR.

Main differential diagnoses and typical outline evidence, etc.	
Endobronchial carcinoma (benign lesions very rare)	*Suggested by:* smoker, weight loss, cough, chest pain, and haemoptysis, clubbed. Unilateral wheeze (typically occur below the carina) and unilateral reduced breath sounds. Often signs of consolidation distal to obstruction. CXR can be normal.
	Confirmed by: **sputum cytology, CT chest, bronchoscopy and biopsy.**
	Initial management: referral for possible radiotherapy, tracheal stenting, cryotherapy, laser therapy, brachytherapy (radioactive source put close to tumour).
Acute bilateral vocal cord paralysis	*Suggested by:* change in voice, bilateral reduced breath sounds, and wheeze.
	Confirmed by: **laryngoscopy.**
	Initial management: ENT surgical referral for possible intubation and tracheostomy.
Inhalation of foreign body	*Suggested by:* history of putting an object in mouth, e.g. peanut. Sudden stridor, severe cough, low-pitched, monophonic wheeze, and reduced breath sounds, typically on the right.
	Confirmed by: If not *in extremis*, **CXR/CT thorax or bronchoscopy** to show foreign body.
	Initial management: if *in extremis*, slap back between the shoulder blades with patient leaning forward; if fails, perform Heimlich manoeuvre.
Tracheal tumours	*Suggested by:* stridor over weeks to months, bilateral reduced breath sounds, and bilateral wheeze.
	Confirmed by: **CXR, CT thorax and neck, bronchoscopy.**
	Initial treatment: controlled O_2, and/or steroids IV.
Extrinsic compression by mediastinal masses	*Suggested by:* neck/chest discomfort ± swelling over weeks to months. Look for signs of SVC obstruction. Can be focal (unilateral) or bilateral wheeze, depending on site of obstruction.
	Confirmed by: **CT thorax and neck.**
	Initial management: steroids and oncology referral for palliative chemo-radiotherapy.
Extrinsic compression by oesophageal tumours	*Suggested by:* dysphagia, weight loss over weeks to months.
	Confirmed by: **CT thorax and neck.**
	Initial management: soft pureed diet. Barium swallow if high dysphagia or OGD if low dysphagia.
Tracheal blunt trauma	*Suggested by:* history, pain and swelling, change in voice over minutes or hours after trauma.
	Confirmed by: **laryngoscopy, bronchoscopy.**
	Initial management: steroids and ENT referral for possible intubation and tracheostomy.

Expiratory polyphonic, high-pitched wheeze

This suggest small airways obstruction. Initial investigations (other tests in **bold** below): FBC, U&E, CXR.

Main differential diagnoses and typical outline evidence, etc.	
Exacerbati on of asthma	*Suggested by:* widespread polyphonic wheeze with exacerbations over hours. Silent chest if severe. Anxiety, tachypnoea, tachycardia, and use of accessory muscles.
	Confirmed by: reduced peak flows. **FEV₁** that improves by >15% with treatment.
	Initial management: high flow O_2, prednisolone PO or Hydrocortisone IV. Nebulized salbutamol and ipratropium ± magnesium IV and aminophylline IV. NB. Keep hydrated, and monitor ABG and serum K^+. Refer to HDU if drowsy, ↑CO_2.
'Wheezy bronchitis'	*Suggested by:* wheeze association with infective episodes of bronchitis alone.
	Confirmed by: **FEV₁** response to bronchodilators and antibiotics.
	Initial management: consider antibiotics if high fever, mucopurulent sputum.
Viral wheeze	*Suggested by:* wheeze associated URTI viral illness, poor response to bronchodilators.
	Confirmed by: resolving spontaneously.
	Initial management: analgesic and antipyretic, e.g. paracetamol.
Anaphylaxis	*Suggested by:* onset over minutes, history of recent allergen exposure, feeling of dread, flushing, sweating, facial oedema, urticaria, warm clammy extremities, dyspnoea and tachypnoea, wheeze. Tachycardia and ↓BP.
	Confirmed by: clinical presentation and response to adrenaline (epinephrine) IM. Results of controlled allergen exposure.
	Initial management: remove antigen (e.g. bee sting, medication). Adrenaline IM 1 in 10,000. Secure airway early if stridor. High flow O_2, fast fluids IV, steroids IV, and antihistamines IV. Transfer to HDU/ITU.
Pulmonary oedema due to acute left ventricular failure or chronic (congestive) cardiac failure due to ischaemic heart disease, mitral stenosis	*Suggested by:* background fatigue and exertional breathless, cardiac risk factors. Displaced apex beat, 3rd heart sound, bilateral basal fine crackles. ↑JVP and leg swelling.
	Confirmed by: **CXR:** fluffy opacification, especially near hila. Loss of costophrenic angle. Impaired left ventricular function on **echocardiogram**.
	Initial management: sit patient up, controlled O_2, diuretics IV, nitrates IV if very breathless and systolic BP >90.
	Chronic: thiazide or loop diuretic, ACE inhibitor (or angiotensin receptor blocker). β-blocker and spironolactone (monitor K^+).

Gastrointestinal symptoms and physical signs

Unintentional weight loss over weeks or months

The more rapid and severe the weight loss, the more probable it is to be due to a serious cause. Initial investigations (other tests in **bold** below): test urine for sugar and protein, FBC, ESR or CRP, fasting blood glucose, U&E, calcium and bone profile, LFT, PSA, TSH, and FT4, CXR, US scan abdomen.

Main differential diagnoses and typical outline evidence, etc.	
Any advanced malignancy (e.g. gastrointestinal (GI), lung, lymphoma)	*Suggested by:* progressive onset over weeks or months of specific symptoms, e.g. change of bowel habit, rectal bleeding, haemoptysis, neurological deficit, etc.
	Confirmed by: tumour on GI endoscopy or **bronchoscopy**, lymph node biopsy, metastases on CXR or CT thorax, metastases on **US scan of liver or CT abdomen**, or leukaemic changes on FBC, etc.
	Initial management: assess diet, give food supplements, counselling, analgesia if pain, plan treatment of any underlying diagnosis.
Psychiatric illness (mainly severe depression)	*Suggested by:* sleep disorder, poor concentration, social withdrawal, lack of interest in usual activities, etc.
	Confirmed by: response to antidepressants and/or psychotherapy.
	Initial management: after excluding physical cause, consider selective serotonin reuptake inhibitors (SSRI), psychiatric advice.
Non-malignant GI diseases (e.g. peptic ulcer disease, inflammatory bowel disease, malabsorption, etc.)	*Suggested by:* dysphagia, vomiting, diarrhoea, abdominal pain, melaena, alcohol intake, etc.
	Confirmed by: **GI endoscopy, US scan of abdomen**, anaemia on FBC, etc.
	Initial management: assess diet, give food supplements, counselling, analgesia if pain, plan treatment of underlying condtion.
Alcoholism (complicated by liver disease, gastritis, peptic ulceration, seizures, or delirium tremens on withdrawal)	*Suggested by:* depression, anxiety, visual hallucination, social withdrawal, lack of interest in non-drinking activities, anorexia, etc.
	Confirmed by: history of alcohol abuse, presence of signs of chronic liver disease, etc.
	Initial management: withdrawal of alcohol, short course of sedative—initially to prevent withdrawal symptoms, benzodiazepine if seizure occurs.

Undiagnosed or uncontrolled diabetes mellitus	*Suggested by:* thirst, polydipsia, polyuria, pruritis.
	Confirmed by: **fasting blood glucose** 7.0 mmol/L (on two occasions) OR random or **GTT** glucose 11.1mmol/L once only in the presence of symptoms.
	Initial management: lifestyle modification—diet, exercise ± metformin. Insulin if type 1 diabetes or ketotic.
Thyrotoxicosis	*Suggested by:* heat intolerance, tremor, nervousness, palpitation, frequency of bowel movements, goitre, fine tremor, warm and moist palm.
	Confirmed by: ↓TSH, ↑FT4 ± ↑FT3.
	Initial management: propranolol to control symptoms. Carbimazole or propylthiouracil to reduce T4.
Pulmonary tuberculosis (TB)	*Suggested by:* night sweats, fever, malaise, chronic cough.
	Confirmed by: CXR showing opacification of pneumonia and presence of **acid-fast bacilli (AFB) in sputum** on microscopy and culture.
	Initial management: broad-spectrum antibiotics provisionally; if TB confirmed, antituberculous regimen, e.g. isoniazid, rifampicin, pyrazinamide, and ethambutol for 2mo, then isoniazid and rifampicin for 4mo with pyridoxine supplement.
Addison's disease	*Suggested by:* lethargy, weakness, dizziness, pigmentation (buccal, scar), hypotension.
	Confirmed by: ↓9 a.m plasma cortisol and impaired response to **short Synacthen test**.
	Initial management: if ↓BP, fluids IV or colloids; if ↓glucose, 10% dextrose IV. If ill, hydrocortisone IV, otherwise PO ± fludrocortisone.
Also	Acute infections: HIV, subacute bacterial endocarditis, parasites. Drugs: digoxin, metformin, levodopa. Neurological disease: stroke, Parkinson's disease, dementia. Connective tissue disease: SLE, scleroderma. Idiopathic or unknown.

Weight gain

In addition to usual details (speed of onset, etc.), assess the distribution of body fat. Is it mainly truncal or general (trunk and limbs)? Differentiate between increased oedema (pitting) and adiposity (non-pitting). Initial investigations (other tests in **bold** below): test urine for protein and glucose, do FBC, fasting glucose, U&E, TSH, and FT4.

Main differential diagnoses and typical outline evidence, etc.	
Excessive caloric intake (by far the main cause: >95%), often with mild depression	*Suggested by:* gradual and progressive weight increase over months to years, no other associated symptoms. *Confirmed by:* history of overeating, all other investigations normal. *Initial management:* ↓calorie intake, ↑physical activity.
Drugs, e.g. steroids, NSAIDs, sulphonylureas, insulin, oestrogen, etc.	*Suggested by:* history of medication. *Confirmed by:* weight decreasing following reduction or withdrawal of causative drug. *Initial management:* stop or reduce causative drugs.
Congestive cardiac failure	*Suggested by:* weight gain over days to months, dyspnoea, orthopnoea, paroxysmal nocturnal dyspnoea (PND), liver enlargement and tenderness, gallop rhythm, leg oedema. *Confirmed by:* **CXR** and **echocardiogram**. *Initial management:* furosemide, ACE inhibitor.
Hypothyroidism	*Suggested by:* weight gain over weeks to months, cold intolerance, constipation, lethargy, coarse and dry skin, puffy eyelids. *Confirmed by:* ↑TSH, ↓FT4, **↑thyroid antibodies.** *Initial management:* thyroxine.
Premenstrual fluid retention	*Suggested by:* premenstrual weight gain over days, breast swelling and tenderness, finger swelling. *Confirmed by:* oedema and weight decrease after menstruation. *Initial management:* weight reduction, salt reduction, spironolactone.
Polycystic ovary syndrome (associated with insulin resistance or sometimes type 2 diabetes mellitus)	*Suggested by:* weight gain over years, truncal obesity, hirsutism, abdominal striae, acne, head hair thinning. *Confirmed by:* ↑**testosterone**, ↓**SHBG**, ↑**LH, FSH** normal, **24h urinary free cortisol** normal, ovarian cysts on **US scan.** *Initial management:* metformin, oestrogens ± cyproterone for hirsutism, acne, or head hair thinning.

Pregnancy (common condition but unusual to present as weight gain)	*Suggested by:* weight gain over weeks, amenorrhoea, and mass in pelvis (cannot get below it). *Confirmed by:* +ve **urine pregnancy test** or **plasma-hCG**. Also **abdominal US scan**. *Initial management:* antenatal clinic referral.
Liver cirrhosis with ascites	*Suggested by:* weight gain over weeks to months, bilateral bulging flanks, shifting dullness, fluid thrill, sudden and rapid weight gain. *Confirmed by:* **US scan liver and abdomen**. *Initial management:* bed rest, salt restriction, fluid restriction if Na^+ <120mmol/L, spironolactone ± furosemide, monitor daily weight. Ascitic tap—paracentesis if gross ascites and symptomatic.
Nephrotic syndrome	*Suggested by:* weight gain over weeks to months, generalized oedema, puffy eyelids, abdominal distension, weight gain may be sudden and rapid. *Confirmed by:* ↓serum albumin, 24h urine protein >3g. *Initial management:* salt restriction, furosemide ± metolazone, statins, ACE inhibitors, treat cause.
Cushing's syndrome due to ACTH-secreting pituitary tumour (Cushing's disease); adrenal adenoma; steroid therapy	*Suggested by:* weight gain over months to years, 'moon face', truncal obesity, hirsutism, 'buffalo hump', abdominal striae, proximal weakness, thin skin, bruising, purple striae. *Confirmed by:* **24h urinary free cortisol, ↑midnight cortisol** and/or failure to suppress cortisol after **dexamethasone test** 0.5mg 6-hourly for 48h. *Initial management:* reduce any glucocorticoid if drug-induced, consider metyrapone to control cortisol prior to surgery.
Also	Smoking cessation, alcohol excess, menopause, Klinefelter syndrome, Other endocrine disorders: hypopituitarism, acromegaly, insulinoma, hypogonadism. Hypothalamic disorder: craniopharyngioma, Congenital disorders: Prader–Willi syndrome, Laurence–Moon–Biedl syndrome.

Vomiting

Vomiting is not only a feature of GI disorders, but is also associated with a wide variety of local and systemic disorders. Therefore, look for better diagnostic leads. Ask about the amount, frequency, and nature of vomitus—red blood, 'coffee-ground', timing of vomit, i.e. in relation to meals, AND ask about weight loss, fever, headache, and abdominal pain. Initial investigations (other tests in **bold** below): test urine for protein and glucose, do FBC, fasting glucose, U&E, TSH, and FT4.

Try subdividing into:
- Vomiting *with* weight loss
- Vomiting *without* weight loss
- Vomiting *(within hours)* of food
- Vomiting unrelated to food but *with abdominal pain AND fever*
- Vomiting unrelated to food *with abdominal pain but NO fever* (non-metabolic)
- Vomiting unrelated to food *with abdominal pain but NO fever* (metabolic)
- Vomiting unrelated to food *without* abdominal pain *but with headaches*
- Vomiting *unrelated* to food and *without* abdominal pain or headaches

Vomiting with weight loss

Vomiting with weight loss

Many causes are shared with weight loss alone. Initial investigations (other tests in **bold** below): test urine for sugar, request FBC, ESR or CRP, fasting blood glucose, U&E, calcium and bone profile, LFT, PSA, TSH, and FT4 before specific tests below.

Main differential diagnoses and typical outline evidence, etc.	
Oesophageal stricture	*Suggested by:* undigested solid food and fluid in vomitus.
	Confirmed by: **barium swallow, oesophagogastroscopy** showing food residue and fixed narrowing.
	Initial management: small meals, avoiding fat, Proton pump inhibitor (PPI). Severe: nasogastric (NG) tube + nil by mouth ± fluids IV, proton pump inhibitor (PPI). All: surgical referral (e.g for endoscopic balloon dilatation, surgery).
Oesophageal carcinoma	*Suggested by:* dysphagia to solid food first, then semisolid, and finally fluid.
	Confirmed by: **barium swallow** showing filling defect, **fibreoptic gastroscopy** with biopsy of tumour.
	Initial management: NG tube, fluids IV ± antibiotic prophylaxis, referral for dilatation or stent insertion
Gastric carcinoma	*Suggested by:* satiety after small meal.
	Confirmed by: **oesophagogastroscopy** showing and allowing biopsy of visible tumour, **barium meal** showing filling defect.
	Initial management: if hypovolaemia and poor nutrition, NG tube ± fluids IV, surgical referral.
Small intestinal tumour, e.g. lymphoma	*Suggested by:* abdominal pain, anorexia, bilious vomitus.
	Confirmed by: **small bowel follow-through, CT abdomen, flexible enteroscopy with biopsy**.
	Initial management: if hypovolaemia and poor nutrition, NG tube ± fluids IV, surgical referral.
Achalasia	*Suggested by:* vomiting after large meals, undigested solid food and fluid, nocturnal regurgitation.
	Confirmed by: **barium swallow** demonstrating the absence of peristaltic contractions, **oesophagogastroscopy** showing dilatation.
	Initial management: smooth muscle dilator—nifedipine, verapamil, or isosorbide mononitrate. Refer for endoscopic balloon dilatation or injection of botulinum toxin.

Vomiting without weight loss

Initial investigations (other tests in **bold** below): FBC, ESR or CRP, fasting blood glucose, U&E, calcium and bone profile, LFT, US scan abdomen before specific tests below.

Main differential diagnoses and typical outline evidence, etc.	
Oesophagitis and ulceration	*Suggested by:* retrosternal pain, heartburn, dyspepsia, 'waterbrash'.
	Confirmed by: **oesophagogastroscopy** showing inflammation and/or ulceration.
	Initial management: mild: small frequent meals long before bedtime, elevate head of bed, PPI. Severe: nil by mouth, fluids IV, PPI, antibiotics for any *Helicobacter* (*H.*) *pylori*.
Pharyngeal pouch	*Suggested by:* no pain, regurgitation of undigested food, aspiration ± pneumonia.
	Confirmed by: **barium swallow** showing saccular opacification outside pharynx.
	Initial management: fluids IV and NG tube + nil by mouth, if severe and/or aspiration, enteral feeding. Surgical referral (e.g. stapling, diverticulotomy, crico-pharyngeal myotomy, or diverticulectomy if large).
Achalasia	*Suggested by:* vomiting after large meals, undigested solid food and fluid, dysphagia to fluid, nocturnal regurgitation.
	Confirmed by: **barium swallow** demonstrating the absence of peristaltic contractions, **oesophagogastroscopy** showing dilatation.
	Initial management: smooth muscle dilator, e.g. nifedipine, verapamil, or isosorbide mononitrate. Refer for endoscopic balloon dilatation or injection of botulinum toxin.

Vomiting shortly after food

Initial investigations (other tests in **bold** below): test urine and request FBC, fasting blood glucose, U&E, calcium, etc., LFT, serum amylase, CXR, ECG, abdominal X-ray (AXR); specific tests depending on suspected diagnoses.

Main differential diagnoses and typical outline evidence, etc.	
Gastritis/peptic ulcer disease: duodenal ulcer (DU) or gastric ulcer (GU)	*Suggested by:* vomiting during or soon after a meal, epigastric pain/discomfort (worse after food suggests GU, relieved by food suggests DU. *Confirmed by:* **oesophagogastroscopy, barium meal,** *and* **pH study.** *Initial management:* stop smoking, avoid NSAIDs and aspirin. Antacids. PPI for 4wk for DU, 8wk for GU + antibiotic regimen for any *H pylori.*
Gastric outlet obstruction e.g. carcinoma, lymphoma, chronic scarring, congenital pyloric stenosis in newborn	*Suggested by:* intermittent vomiting ≥1h after eating, abdominal fullness or bloating, distended upper abdomen, succussion splash. *Confirmed by:* **oesophagogastroscopy** *and* **biopsy, double contrast barium meal** shows structural abnormality. *Initial management:* if hypovolaemia and poor nutrition: fluids IV, NG tube + nil by mouth. Surgical referral.
Small intestinal tumour e.g. lymphoma	*Suggested by:* abdominal pain, anorexia, bilious vomitus, weight loss. *Confirmed by:* **small bowel barium meal** *and* **follow-through** showing filling defect, **CT abdomen** showing abnormal tumour in wall, **flexible enteroscopy** with biopsy showing abnormal histology. *Initial management:* if hypovolaemia and poor nutrition: fluids IV, NG tube + nil by mouth. Surgical referral.
Gastroparesis due to diabetes mellitus	*Suggested by:* intermittent vomiting, occurs ≥1h after eating, abdominal fullness or bloating, distended upper abdomen, succussion splash, history of diabetes. *Confirmed by:* **oesophagogastroscopy, double contrast barium meal** showing normal mucosa but dilatation. *Initial management:* low-fat diet, frequent small meals; if severe, liquid meals + vitamins.
Acute cholecystitis due to cholelithiasis	*Suggested by:* nausea and vomiting after fatty food with colicky abdominal pain. Tenderness in the right upper quadrant (RUQ) or Murphy's sign +ve or jaundice. *Confirmed by:* **US scan** of biliary tree and gallbladder showing stones. *Initial management:* nil by mouth, fluids IV, pain relief with opioid analgesia, antibiotics IV, e.g. metronidazole + cephalosporin.

Acute pancreatitis	*Suggested by:* severe epigastric/central abdominal pain, jaundice, tachycardia, Cullen's sign (periumbilical discoloration) or Grey Turner's sign (discoloration at the flank).
	Confirmed by: ↑↑**serum amylase**, ↓**Ca²⁺**.
	Initial management: pain relief, e.g. pethidine, if abdominal distension due to paralytic ileus, NG tube + nil by mouth, fluids IV ± plasma expander/blood.

Vomiting with abdominal pain and fever

The vomiting is usually unrelated to eating. Also assess for consequences such as hypovolaemia. Initial investigations (other tests in **bold** below): test urine, examine stools (and send for culture, etc). Also request FBC, U&E, LFT, calcium, etc., serum amylase, CXR, AXR; specific tests depending on suspected diagnoses.

Main differential diagnoses and typical outline evidence, etc.	
Gastroenteritis (from live microbes, e.g. salmonella)	*Suggested by:* diarrhoea, ↑bowel sounds. *Confirmed by:* **stools for culture**. *Initial management:* oral rehydration solution (containing glucose and salt); if severe vomiting, fluids IV etc.
Food poisoning (from toxins of dead microbes, e.g. *staphylococci*)	*Suggested by:* within hours of ingestion, associated with diarrhoea ± eating companions affected. *Confirmed by:* **stools for WBC and culture, cultures of vomitus, food and blood** *(–ve)*. *Initial management:* oral rehydration solution (containing glucose and salt); if severe vomiting, fluids IV etc.
Urinary tract infection ± pyelonephritis	*Suggested by:* dysuria, frequency, 'dipstick' indicating blood, protein, and nitrites (if Gram –ve infection). *Confirmed by:* **MSU microscopy and culture** (± US scan showing anatomical abnormality). *Initial management:* hydration, provisional antibiotic (e.g trimethoprim) then based on culture and sensitivity; antibiotic IV, e.g. cephalosporin if severe infection.
Acute appendicitis	*Suggested by:* right lower quadrant (RLQ) pain, anorexia, fever. *Confirmed by:* tenderness at McBurney's point, guarding ± rebound or right-sided rectal tenderness. *Initial management:* nil by mouth, fluids IV, NG tube if vomiting, broad-spectrum antibiotic, e.g. cephalosporin, surgical referral for appendicectomy.
Mesenteric adenitis or non-specific abdominal pain (NSAP)	*Suggested by:* RLQ pain, anorexia, fever. *Confirmed by:* diffuse RLQ tenderness, no guarding, no rebound, no right-sided rectal tenderness, self-limiting outcome. *Initial management:* analgesia.
Hepatitis A or B	*Suggested by:* RUQ pain, jaundice. *Confirmed by:* ↑ALT ↑bilirubin, **hepatitis serology**. *Initial management:* antipyretics, fluids IV, anti-emetics prn, colestyramine for pruritus.

Toxic shock syndrome	*Suggested by:* history of tampon use, nasal packing, high fever, vomiting, profuse watery diarrhoea, confusion, skin rash, hypotension, myalgia. FBC: ↑WCC, ↓platelets. ↑CPK.
	Confirmed by: **cultures of blood, stool, vaginal swab,** for *staphylococcus* and toxin.
	Initial management: ICU care, removal of tampon or nasal packings; fluids IV, dopamine IV if ↓↓BP; antibiotics IV, e.g oxacillin or nafcillin.
Pneumonia (lower lobe)	*Suggested by:* cough, dyspnoea, fever, ↑WCC.
	Confirmed by: CXR shows consolidation. **Sputum and blood cultures. Serology** if atypical.
	Initial management: give O_2, monitor SpO_2, BP, pulse, fluids IV if dehydrated, paracetamol for fever. Provisional antibiotics, e.g. erythromycin, azithromycin, etc. pending sensitivities. Metronidazole if aspiration.
Pelvic inflammatory disease	*Suggested by:* lower abdominal pain, fever, vaginal discharge.
	Confirmed by: high vaginal swab, ↑ESR and CRP. FBC: leucocytosis, **pelvic US scan ± laparoscopy.**
	Initial management: analgesia, fluids IV if dehydrated, empirical antibiotics, e.g. cefoxitin or other 2nd generation cephalosporin + doxycycline 100mg bd, etc.
Haemolytic uraemic syndrome	*Suggested by:* haematuria, fever, confusion.
	Confirmed by: FBC: thrombocytopaenia, fragmented RBC on **blood film**, renal failure on **U&E**.
	Initial management: fluids IV, U&E, BP control, prophylaxis for seizures, dialysis.
Malaria (*Plasmodium* (*P.*). *vivax, P. ovale, P. malariae, P. falciparum*)	*Suggested by:* recent travel to malaria zone, periodic paroxysms of rigors, fever, sweating, nausea.
	Confirmed by: plasmodium in **blood smear**.
	Initial management: paracetamol for fever, blood transfusion if anaemic ++. Chloroquine for *P. vivax, P. ovale, P. malariae,* and primaquine for *P. vivax* and *P. ovale* hepatic phase; mefloquine or pyrimethamine/ sulfadoxine (Fansidar®) if chloroquine-resistant; quinine for *P. falciparum,* quinine IV if very ill. Please refer to WHO guidelines for the up to date treatment regimens at http:// www.who.int/topics/malaria/en/

Vomiting with abdominal pain alone (unrelated to food and no fever)— non-metabolic causes

Look for better leads with the history and examination. Initial investigations (other tests in **bold** below): FBC, U&E, LFT, calcium, etc., serum amylase, CXR, ECG, AXR.

Main differential diagnoses and typical outline evidence, etc.	
Large bowel obstruction, e.g. malignancy, strangulated hernia	*Suggested by:* faecal vomiting, abdominal distension. *Confirmed by:* **AXR** showing bowel dilation, **barium enema, colonoscopy.** *Initial management:* NG tube + nil by mouth, fluids IV, fluid balance, antibiotics, surgical referral.
Hepatic carcinoma, 1° or 2°	*Suggested by:* RUQ pain and mass, jaundice. *Confirmed by:* **weight loss over weeks to months, US scan/CT of liver** showing hepatic mass. *Initial management:* analgesia, surgical referral.
Mesenteric artery occlusion	*Suggested by:* periumbilical pain, diarrhoea, melaena, absent bowel sounds. *Confirmed by:* **mesenteric angiography** showing filling defect. *Initial management:* fluids IV, analgesia, antibiotics, surgical referral
Renal calculi	*Suggested by:* colicky loin pain, haematuria. *Confirmed by:* **plain AXR, US scan, intravenous urography (IVU).** *Initial management:* opioid analgesics + anti-emetics, urology referral.
Ectopic pregnancy, miscarriage	*Suggested by:* cramping pain, spotting, PV bleeding. *Confirmed by:* +ve **pregnancy test, US scan of pelvis.** *Initial management:* analgesia, fluids IV, gynaecology referral.
Acute inferior myocardial infarction	*Suggested by:* central chest pain, sweating, nausea. *Confirmed by:* ↑ST or ↓T wave on ECG *with* ↑**cardiac enzymes,** e.g. CK-MB **or** troponin. *Initial management:* ECG monitor (best in CCU), O_2, GTN (IV if pain persists), morphine, aspirin 300mg, and clopidogrel 300mg stat, thrombolysis (if ST↑ and <12h from the onset), LMW heparin for unstable angina or NSTEMI.
Congestive cardiac failure (and liver congestion)	*Suggested by:* dyspnoea, orthopnoea, PND, liver enlargement and tenderness, leg oedema. *Confirmed by:* **CXR** *and* **echocardiogram.** *Initial management:* ECG monitor, O_2, slow furosemide IV, morphine or diamorphine, GTN (?IV), dobutamine if hypotensive.

Vomiting with abdominal pain alone (unrelated to food and no fever)—metabolic causes

Look for better leads in the history and examination. Initial investigations (other tests in **bold** below): FBC, U&E, LFT, calcium, etc., serum amylase, CXR, ECG, AXR.

Main differential diagnoses and typical outline evidence, etc.	
Drugs overdose, e.g. digoxin	*Suggested by:* drug history.
	Confirmed by: ↑**serum digoxin levels**.
	Initial management: O₂, ECG monitoring, IV access, stop digoxin, check U&E, digoxin. Fab antibody if severe, arrhythmias, or hyperkalaemia.
Diabetic ketoacidosis	*Suggested by:* polyuria, dehydration ± Kussmaul respiration.
	Confirmed by: ↑**blood glucose, ↓pH, ketonuria** or ↓**plasma bicarbonate** <15mmol/L.
	Initial management: large volumes 0.9% saline IV with K⁺, insulin sliding scale, hourly blood glucose, NG tube, bicarbonate if pH<7.0, treat any infection.
Hypercalcaemia	*Suggested by:* lethargy, confusion, constipation, muscle weakness, polydipsia and polyuria.
	Confirmed by: ↑↑**serum Ca²⁺**.
	Initial management: large volumes 0.9% saline IV with K⁺, furosemide IV, central venous pressure (CVP) monitoring.
Addison's disease	*Suggested by:* lethargy, weakness, dizziness, pigmentation (buccal, scar), hypotension.
	Confirmed by: ↓9 **a.m. plasma cortisol** and impaired response to **short Synacthen test**.
	Initial management: if ↓BP, fluids IV or colloids, if ↓glucose, 10% dextrose IV. If ill, hydrocortisone IV, otherwise PO ± fludrocortisone.
Acute intermittent porphyria	*Suggested by:* LFT, peripheral neuropathy, hypertension, psychosis, urine dark after standing.
	Confirmed by: ↑**urinary aminolevulinic acid** *and* **porphobilinogen, plasma porphyrins**.
	Initial management: fluids IV, haematin IV, analgesics, prorpranolol for tachycardia and hypertension, diazepam for seizures, high carbohydrate intake.

Phaeochromocytoma	*Suggested by:* headache, sweating, palpitations, pallor, nausea, hypertension (intermittent or persistent), tachycardia.
	Confirmed by: ↑**24h urinary metanephrines**, ↑**serum catecholamines (adrenaline, noradrenaline), CT abdomen, MRI scan**.
	Initial management: fluids IV with CVP monitoring before α- and then β-blockade, e.g. phenoxybenzamine ± phentolamine, then β-blockade, e.g. propranolol. Endocrine surgical referral.
Lead poisoning	*Suggested by:* anorexia, personality changes, headaches, metallic taste, loss of sensation.
	Confirmed by: ↑**whole blood lead concentration** >2.4micromol/L.
	Initial management: stop exposure, analgesia, anti-emetic. If severe, 0.9% saline IV, NG tube + nil by mouth, intestinal irrigation with polyethylene glycol, diazepam IV for convulsion; if lead >2.16micromol/L (45 mcg/dL), chelation + supplements, including iron.
Vitamin A intoxication	*Suggested by:* ↑intracranial pressure, drowsiness, headache, irritability, muscle pain and weakness.
	Confirmed by: symptoms and signs go within 1–4wk after stopping vitamin A ingestion.
	Initial management: stop vitamin A, fluids IV if vomiting, diarrhoea or hypercalcaemia, O_2.

Vomiting with headache alone (unrelated to food and no abdominal pain)

Look for better leads with the history and examination. Initial investigations (other tests in **bold** below): FBC, U&E, LFT, CXR, ECG, CT scan.

Main differential diagnoses and typical outline evidence, etc.	
Migraine	*Suggested by:* throbbing headache with preceding visual auras or other transient sensory symptoms and 'trigger' factors, e.g. premenstrual, stress, foods.
	Confirmed by: history, but if in doubt, **MRI scan** to exclude anatomical abnormalities.
	Initial management: rest in dark and quiet; if mild, paracetamol, NSAIDs, dextropropoxyphene, or combinations; if worse, 5HT agonist, e.g. sumatriptan or ergot, e.g. ergotamine. Prevention: avoid 'trigger' factors, prescribe β-blocker, tricyclics, serotonergics.
Raised intracranial pressure	*Suggested by:* being worse in morning, on coughing and leaning forward, papilloedema, pupillary dilatation, bradycardia, increased pulse pressure.
	Confirmed by: **CT scan head** showing flattening of sulci and darkening of brain tissue.
	Initial management: ICU care, neuro obs, treat cause, hyperventilation to keep P_aCO_2 down, mannitol IV.
Meningitis (viral or bacterial)	*Suggested by:* photophobia, fever, neck stiffness.
	Confirmed by: **CT scan**—no signs of ↑intracranial pressure and **lumbar puncture** (LP): ↑lymphocytes and normal glucose in viral, ↑neutrophils and ↓glucose in bacterial + organisms on staining and culture.
	Initial management: paracetamol, nurse in dark and quiet room. Fluids IV. Antivirals if varicella or herpes. Bacterial—after LP: 3rd gen. cephalosporin, e.g. cefotaxime (+ vancomycin if high local prevalence of penicillin-resistant *pneumococci*); dexamethasone IV if Glasgow Coma Score 8–11.
Haemorrhagic stroke	*Suggested by:* sudden onset of headache, then hemiparesis, (but not upper face) dysarthia ± dysphasia, extensor plantar response.
	Confirmed by: **CT brain scan**—high attenuation area representing haemorrhage.
	Initial management: IV access, nil by mouth + NG tube, control BP neurosurgical referral.

Severe hyper-tension	*Suggested by:* continuous throbbing headache (non-severe hypertension is usually asymptomatic), but headache ± visual disturbance in malignant hypertension.
	Confirmed by: **serial BP measurement**: usually >140mmHg diastolic and/or >240mmHg systolic.
	Initial management: labetalol IV or nitroprusside to lower diastolic BP to 100–105 in 2–6h.
Acute glaucoma	*Suggested by:* blurred vision, painful red eye, coloured haloes.
	Confirmed by: ↑**intraocular pressure** on measurement.
	Initial management: nurse supine, no eye covering ± analgesics ± anti-emetics. Pilocarpine 2–4% eyedrops ± oral acetazolamide. Ophthalmology referral.
Epilepsy Idiopathic or 2° to brain tumour or cerebrovascular disease or acute hypotension or metabolic disturbance	*Suggested by:* aura, altered consciousness, abnormal movements.
	Confirmed by: **EEG** result—spikes and waves over focus.
	Initial management: BP and ECG monitoring, pulse oximetry ± intubation, fluids IV ± U&E, diazepam IV stat ± infusion for status ± phenytoin IV. CT brain to exclude intracranial pathology if first presentation.

Vomiting alone (unrelated to food and without abdominal pain or headaches)

Look for better leads with the history and examination Initial investigations (other tests in **bold** below): FBC, U&E, LFT, CXR, ECG.

Main differential diagnoses and typical outline evidence, etc.	
Gastroenteritis	*Suggested by:* diarrhoea, ↑bowel sounds.
	Confirmed by: **stools for WBC and culture**.
	Initial management: glucose PO + salt solution; fluids IV if severe vomiting; antibiotic if agent identified.
Acute viral labyrinthitis	*Suggested by:* vertigo, tinnitus, hearing loss, nystagmus.
	Confirmed by: being dehydrated over days.
	Initial management: bed rest. fluids IV and anti-emetics (e.g. metoclopramide, prochlorperazine) if severe nausea and vomiting.
Drugs e.g. antibiotics, cytotoxics, metformin, any overdose, excessive alcohol ingestion, etc.	*Suggested by:* history of drug ingestion, vomiting soon after taking medication.
	Confirmed by: response of symptoms to avoidance of causative drug.
	Initial management: stop offending drug, no alcohol.
Sliding hiatus hernia	*Suggested by:* occasional chest pain precipitated by heavy meals, lying flat.
	Confirmed by: **barium meal** showing reflux.
	Initial management: reduce weight if overweight, avoid stooping, semi-sitting position for sleep, correct constipation, antacids or H_2 blockers for pain.
Chronic renal failure (**CRF**)	*Suggested by:* fatigue, pruritus, anorexia, nausea, 'lemon-tinged' skin.
	Confirmed by: **↑↑serum creatinine, ↓↓creatinine clearance**. ↓**Hb** (if chronic), and small kidneys on **renal US scan**.
	Initial management: treat cause if possible. Low phosphate, low K^+ diet, fluid restriction. BP control, erythropoietin ± transfusion if ↓Hb, calcium carbonate to lower serum phosphate, calcium ± calcitriol if ↓serum Ca^{2+}; loop diuretics if overload. Plan renal replacement therapy.
Pregnancy—hyperemesis gravidarum	*Suggested by:* being worse soon after waking better later, amenorrhoea <3mo.
	Confirmed by: pregnancy test +ve.
	Initial management: fluids IV, anti-emetic, e.g. metoclopramide, obstetric referral.

Ménière's disease	*Suggested by:* vertigo, tinnitus, deafness.
	Confirmed by: **audiometry**—sensory hearing loss.
	Initial management: acute—anticholinergics, antihistamine, and benzodiazepine; then salt restriction, diuretics ± betahistine.
Acute otitis media (in children)	*Suggested by:* fever, earache, decreased hearing, otorrhoea if eardrum is perforated, accompanying upper respiratory infection symptoms.
	Confirmed by: **otoscopy** or **tympanometry**.
	Initial management: analgesics ± amoxicillin, ENT referral—?myringotomy.
Anaphylaxis	*Suggested by:* bronchospasm, laryngeal oedema, flushing, urticaria, angioedema.
	Confirmed by: relief with antihistamines or steroids.
	Initial management: adrenaline 1 in 1000 (1mg/mL) IM or SC, repeat every 5–10min until pulse and BP normal; fluids IV if ↓BP, O_2, corticosteroids + nebulized salbutamol if bronchospasm ± intubation.
Addison's disease	*Suggested by:* lethargy, weakness, dizziness, pigmentation (buccal, scar), hypotension.
	Confirmed by: ↓9 a.m. plasma cortisol and impaired response to **short Synacthen® test**.
	Initial management: if ↓BP, fluids IV or colloids, if ↓glucose, 10% dextrose IV. If ill, hydrocortisone IV, otherwise PO ± fludrocortisone
Functional	*Suggested by:* vomiting during or soon after a meal ± other psychological disturbance, and no symptoms and physical signs of organic disease.
	Confirmed by: response to psychotherapy.
	Initial management: psychotherapy referral.
Also	Diabetic gastroparesis, ↑intracranial pressure, oesophageal or pyloric obstruction, any viral or bacterial infection, etc.

Jaundice

This can be a symptom reported by the patient or a physical sign. It is confirmed by high bilirubin in the plasma. Yellow sclerae and skin usually becomes visible when serum bilirubin level is >35micromol/L, so urine tests may provide the first clue. First subdivide into the five leads below. Remember that haemolysis causes ↑urinary urobilinogen and decreased serum haptoglobin. Hepatic failure causes increased serum unconjugated bilirubin, but intrahepatic or extrahepatic biliary obstruction results in increased serum conjugated bilirubin. Initial investigations (other tests in **bold** below): FBC + reticulocyte count, U&E, LFT, clotting screen, viral antibodies.

Main differential diagnoses and typical outline evidence, etc.	
Carotinaemia	*Suggested by:* onset over months. Skin yellow with white sclerae, normal stools and normal urine. Diet rich in yellow vegetables/fruits).
	Confirmed by: no bilirubin, no **urobilinogen** in the urine, and normal **serum bilirubin**. Normal **LFT**. Response to diet change.
	Initial management: diet change.
'Pre-hepatic' jaundice due to haemolysis	*Suggested by:* jaundice and anaemia (the combination seen as 'lemon' or pale yellow). Normal dark stools and normal-looking urine.
	Confirmed by: ↑(unconjugated and thus insoluble) **serum bilirubin**, but normal (conjugated and soluble) bilirubin, and thus no ↑bilirubin in urine. ↑**urine urobilinogen** and ↓**serum haptoglobin**. Normal LFT. ↑**reticulocyte count, ↓Hb**.
	Initial management: stop drugs that can cause haemolysis, give folic acid, fluids IV if dehydrated.
'Hepatic' jaundice due to congenital enzyme defect	*Suggested by:* normal-looking stools and normal-looking urine.
	Confirmed by: ↑**serum bilirubin** (unconjugated), but no (conjugated) bilirubin in urine. No **urobilinogen in urine** and *normal* **haptoglobin**. Normal **LFT**.
	Initial management: symptomatic treatment.
'Hepatocellular' jaundice ('hepatic' with element of 'obstructive' jaundice)	*Suggested by:* onset of jaundice over days or weeks, stools pale or normal, but dark urine.
	Confirmed by: ↑**serum** (conjugated) **bilirubin** and thus ↑**urine bilirubin**. Normal urine urobilinogen. LFT all abnormal especially ↑**ALT**.
	Initial management: fluids IV if dehydrated, treat underlying cause.

'Obstructive' jaundice	*Suggested by:* onset of jaundice over days or weeks with pale stools and dark urine. bilirubin (i.e. conjugated and thus soluble) in urine.
	Confirmed by: ↑**serum conjugated bilirubin** and thus ↑**urine bilirubin** but no ↑urobilinogen in urine. ↑↑**alkaline phosphatase**, but less abnormal LFT and ↑γGT.
	Initial management: if dehydrated, fluids IV, give O_2, ECG monitor, NG suction, antibiotics IV; treat underlying cause.

Pre-hepatic jaundice due to haemolysis

Suggested by: jaundice and anaemia (the combination often seen as 'lemon' or pale yellow). Normal dark stools and normal-looking urine.

Confirmed by: ↑**serum bilirubin** (unconjugated and thus insoluble), but normal conjugated and thus soluble bilirubin, and in turn no bilirubin in urine. Evidence of haemolysis as: ↑**urinary urobilinogen** and ↓**serum haptoglobin**. ↑**reticulocyte count**. Normal **LFT**, ↓**Hb**.

Main differential diagnoses and typical outline evidence, etc.

Hereditary haemolytic anaemia	*Suggested by:* LFT, anaemia, splenomegaly, leg ulcers.
	Confirmed by: above evidence of haemolysis, ↑osmotic fragility; enzyme deficiency, e.g. G6PD, **pyruvate kinase**.
	Initial management: no fava beans in G6PD deficiency, Transfusion, referral for splenectomy if required (+ prior immunization for *H. influenza* and *S. pneumoniae*).
Acquired haemolytic anaemia	*Suggested by:* sudden onset, in later life, and on medication.
	Confirmed by: above evidence of haemolysis, **blood film**, +ve **Coombs' test** in autoimmune type.
	Initial management: stop drugs that cause immune haemolysis, prescribe folic acid ± blood transfusion.
Septicaemic haemolysis due to pneumonia, urinary tract infection (UTI), etc.	*Suggested by:* fever ± shock symptoms and signs of infection.
	Confirmed by: evidence of haemolysis, **blood culture** +ve.
	Initial management: fluids ± blood transfusion if ↓BP + active haemolysis; paracetamol if fever; antibiotics.
Malaria	*Suggested by:* recent travel to malaria zone, periodic paroxysms of rigors, fever, sweating, nausea.
	Confirmed by: plasmodium in **blood smear**.
	Initial management: paracetamol if fever, blood transfusion if severe anaemia; chloroquine for *P. vivax, P. ovale, P. malariae*, add primaquine for *P. vivax* and *P. ovale* hepatic phase; mefloquine or pyrimethamine/ sulfadoxine (Fansidar®) if chloroquine resistant; quinine for *P. falciparum*, quinine IV if very ill.

Hepatic jaundice due to congenital enzyme defect

Suggested by: jaundice. Normal-looking stools and normal-looking urine.

Confirmed by: ↑**serum bilirubin** (unconjugated), but no (conjugated) bilirubin in urine. No **urobilinogen in urine** and *normal* **haptoglobin**. Normal **LFT**.

Main differential diagnoses and typical outline evidence, etc.

Gilbert's syndrome (normal lifespan)	*Suggested by:* above evidence of impaired conjugation, asymptomatic. *Confirmed by:* demonstration of unconjugated hyperbilirubinaemia with normal LFT, no haemolysis. Rise in **bilirubin when fasting and after nicotinic acid**. *Initial management:* no treatment necessary. Reassure.
Crigler–Najjar syndrome (type I: severe, neonatal and often fatal; type II: normal lifespan)	*Suggested by:* above evidence of impaired conjugation. *Confirmed by:* unconjugated hyperbilirubinaemia with otherwise normal LFT, no haemolysis. No rise in **bilirubin when fasting or after nicotinic acid.** *Initial management:* type 1: refer for phototherapy and plasmapheresis to lower serum bilirubin, liver transplant is definitive treatment; type 2: supportive therapy, no specific treatment for the hyperbilirubinaemia,

Hepatocellular jaundice (due to hepatitis or very severe liver failure)

> *Suggested by:* onset of jaundice over days or weeks, stools pale or normal but dark urine.
>
> *Confirmed by:* ↑**serum** (conjugated) **bilirubin** and thus ↑**urine bilirubin**. Normal urine urobilinogen. LFT all increasingly abnormal especially ↑**ALT**.

Main differential diagnoses and typical outline evidence, etc.

Drug-induced hepatitis e.g. paraceta-mol, halothane	*Suggested by:* drug history, recent surgery.
	Confirmed by: drug levels and improvement after stopping the offending drug.
	Initial management: withdrawal of the drug which causes hepatitis, supportive therapy—fluids, etc.
Acute (viral) hepatitis A	*Suggested by:* tender hepatomegaly.
	Confirmed by: presence of **hepatitis A IgM antibody** suggests acute infection.
	Initial management: antipyretics, fluids IV and anti-emetics if nausea and vomiting, colestyramine for pruritus.
Acute hepatitis B	*Suggested by:* history of IV drug user, blood transfusion, needle punctures, tattoos, tender hepatomegaly.
	Confirmed by: presence of **HBsAg in serum**.
	Initial management: antipyretics, colestyramine for pruritus; if acute hepatic failure, monitor blood glucose, U&E, LFT, coagulation profile. 5% dextrose IV (10% if ↓blood glucose), NG tube + nil by mouth, neomycin PO, lactulose, vitamin K IV.
Acute hepatitis C	*Suggested by:* history of IV drug user, mild illness, blood transfusion, tender hepatomegaly.
	Confirmed by: presence of **anti-HCV antibody**, **HCV-PCR**.
	Initial management: antipyretics, colestyramine for pruritus, interferon may be effective at reducing the rate of chronicity; if acute hepatic failure, monitor blood glucose, U&E, LFT, coagulation profile. 5% dextrose IV (10% if ↓blood glucose), NG tube + nil by mouth, neomycin PO, lactulose, vitamin K IV.
Alcoholic hepatitis	*Suggested by:* history of drinking, presence of spider naevi and other signs of chronic liver disease. **AST:ALT ratio** >2.
	Confirmed by: resolution with abstinence.
	Initial management: stop alcohol, give folate, thiamine, vitamin K IV if coagulopathy; if acute hepatic failure, monitor blood glucose, U&E, LFT, coagulation profile. 5% dextrose IV (10% if ↓blood glucose), NG tube + nil by mouth, neomycin PO, lactulose, vitamin K IV.

1° hepatoma	*Suggested by:* weight loss, abdominal pain, RUQ mass.
	Confirmed by: **US scan/CT liver, liver biopsy,** ↑alpha-fetoprotein.
	Initial management: surgical referral for resection and adjunct chemotherapy.
Right heart failure	*Suggested by:* ↑JVP, hepatomegaly, ankle oedema.
	Confirmed by: **CXR:** large heart. **Echocardiogram:** dilated right ventricle.
	Initial management: stop smoking, salt and fluid restriction, O_2, furosemide IV or PO ± K^+ supplement.
Glandular fever (infectious mononucleosis)	*Suggested by:* cervical lymphadenopathy, sharp edge ± splenomegaly ± jaundice.
	Confirmed by: **Paul–Bunnell,** +ve **heterophil antibody test**.
	Initial management: gargles/lozenges, analgesics, paracetamol. No aspirin (associated with Reye syndrome).

Obstructive jaundice

	Suggested by: jaundice with pale stools and dark urine. Bilirubin in urine (i.e. conjugated and thus soluble).
	Confirmed by: ↑conjugated bilirubin and thus **urine bilirubin** but no ↑urobilinogen in urine. ↑↑**alkaline phosphatase**, but less abnormal LFT and ↑γGT.

Main differential diagnoses and typical outline evidence, etc.

Common bile duct stones	*Suggested by:* pain or tenderness in RUQ ± Murphy's sign.
	Confirmed by: **US scan liver**—dilatation of biliary ducts.
	Initial management: acute—analgesic, anti-emetics, nil by mouth, fluids IV, (no specific treatment for biliary colic, usually dehydration); antibiotic IV, e.g. cephalosporin if acute (infective) cholecystitis.
Cancer of head of pancreas	*Suggested by:* progressive painless jaundice, palpable gallbladder (Courvoisier's law), weight loss.
	Confirmed by: **US scan liver**—dilatation of biliary ducts. **CT pancreas; ERCP** or **MRCP**: obstruction within head of pancreas.
	Initial management: low fat, high-protein diet, pain control, pancreatic enzyme supplement, phenothiazine or colestyramine for pruritis, gastro referral for stenting, surgical referral for resection.
Sclerosing cholangitis	*Suggested by:* progressive fatigue, pruritus.
	Confirmed by: ↑**ALP. US scan liver**: no gallstones. ERCP (beading of the intra- and extrahepatic biliary ducts).
	Initial management: nil by mouth during acute phase, control sepsis—antibiotics for Gram −ve aerobes, enterococci and anaerobes, treat underlying cause.
1° biliary cirrhosis	*Suggested by:* scratch marks, non-tender hepatomegaly ± splenomegaly, xanthelasmata and xanthomas, arthralgia.
	Confirmed by: +ve **anti-mitochondrial antibody,** ↑**serum IgM**, infiltrate around hepatic bile ducts, and cirrhosis on **liver biopsy**.
	Initial management: no alcohol, colestyramine or ursodeoxycholic acid for pruritus.
Drug-induced	*Suggested by:* drug history of oral contraceptive pill, phenothiazines, anabolic steroids, erythromycin, etc.
	Confirmed by: symptoms receding when drug discontinued.
	Initial management: stop offending drug(s).
Pregnancy (last trimester)	*Suggested by:* jaundice during pregnancy.
	Confirmed by: resolution following delivery.
	Initial management: antipruritics.

Alcoholic hepatitis or cirrhosis	*Suggested by:* history of excess alcohol intake, presence of spider naevi and other signs of chronic liver disease.
	Confirmed by: **US scan** or **CT liver, liver biopsy,** improvement if abstinence.
	Initial management: stop alcohol, no specific folate and thiamine, vitamin K IV if coagulopathy; if acute hepatic failure, monitor blood glucose, U&E, LFT, coagulation profile. 5% dextrose IV (10% if ↓blood glucose), NG tube + nil by mouth, neomycin PO, lactulose, vitamin K IV.
Dubin–Johnson syndrome (decreased excretion of conjugated bilirubin)	*Suggested by:* intermittent jaundice and associated pain in the right hypochondrium. No hepatomegaly.
	Confirmed by: normal **ALP**, normal LFT, ↑**urinary bilirubin**. Pigment granules on **liver biopsy**.
	Initial management: analgesia as necessary.

Dysphagia for solids which stick

It is important to distinguish between oropharyngeal and oesophageal dysphagia. The patient is often able to point to a specific point where the food sticks. Dysphagia to solids alone is more likely to be due to a mechanical obstruction. Initial investigations (other tests in **bold** below): FBC, CRP or ESR, U&E, ECG, CXR.

Main differential diagnoses and typical outline evidence, etc.	
Oesophageal stricture	*Suggested by:* history of gastro-oesophageal reflux, ingestion of corrosives, radiation or trauma.
	Confirmed by: **barium swallow and meal, fibreoptic endoscopy** show necrotic mucosa ± ulceration.
	Initial management: no fatty food, small slow meals, H₂-blocker or PPI. Severe: nil by mouth, fluids IV, PPI, referral for endoscopic balloon dilatation or surgery.
Carcinoma of oesophagus	*Suggested by:* progressive dysphagia, weight loss.
	Confirmed by: **barium swallow** shows filling defect, **fibreoptic endoscopy** with biopsy of mass.
	Initial management: fluids IV ± antibiotic prophylaxis, surgical referral for oesophageal dilatation or stent insertion by endoscopy.
Carcinoma of cardia of stomach	*Suggested by:* weight loss, epigastric pain, vomiting.
	Confirmed by: **barium swallow** shows filling defect, **fibreoptic endoscopy** with biopsy of mass.
	Initial management: NG tube + nil by mouth, fluids IV, analgesics, surgical referral.
External oesophageal compression	*Suggested by:* few other GI symptoms.
	Confirmed by: **barium swallow** shows filling defect, **endoscopy** shows normal mucosa, **CT thorax** shows extrinsic mass from retrosternal goitre, neoplasms (lung or mediastinal tumours, lymphoma), aortic aneurysm.
	Initial management: treat underlying cause.
Also	Pharyngeal carcinoma, foreign bodies, mediastinal lymphadenopathy, left atrial enlargement, substernal thyroid, etc.

Dysphagia for solids (which do not stick) > fluids

It is important to distinguish from odynophagia—painful swallowing. Initial investigations (other tests in **bold** below): FBC, CRP or ESR, U&E, ECG, CXR.

Main differential diagnoses and typical outline evidence, etc.	
Globus pharyngeus	*Suggested by:* feeling of a lump in the throat which needs to be swallowed, may be associated with anxiety.
	Confirmed by: normal **barium swallow/endoscopy**, **resolution** with reassurance and/or **psychotheraphy**.
	Initial management: reassurance, treat underlying psychological disorder. Referral for psychotherapy.
Xerostomia e.g. drugs, elderly, Sjögren's syndrome, post-parotidectomy	*Suggested by:* dryness of mouth, elderly, especially females.
	Confirmed by: clinical appearance of atrophic, dry oral mucosa.
	Initial management: stop drugs that cause xerostomia, sips of water or sugar-free chewing gum, hypromellose or methylcellulose; pilocarpine or cevimeline.
Pharyngeal pouch (pharyngo-oesophageal diverticulum)	*Suggested by:* regurgitation of undigested food, a sensation of a lump in the throat, halitosis, neck bulge on drinking, aspiration into lungs.
	Confirmed by: **barium swallow** shows extra luminal collection (oesophagoscopy avoided).
	Initial management: fluids IV. NG tube + nil by mouth if vomiting or dysphagia to prevent aspiration and for enteral feeding. Surgical referral, e.g. for endoscopic stapling, diverticulotomy, cricopharyngeal myotomy or diverticulectomy.
Post-cricoid web congenital or Plummer–Vincent or Paterson–Kelly syndrome	*Suggested by:* untreated, severe iron deficiency anaemia.
	Confirmed by: **barium swallow** shows a thin, horizontal shelf; **endoscopy** to exclude malignancy.
	Initial management: iron supplements, transfusion if severe anaemia, referral for dilatation or resection.

Sore throat

Sore throat—pain in the throat that worsens with swallowing. Odynophagia—pain that occurs only with swallowing. Initial investigations (other tests in **bold** below): FBC, CRP or ESR, U&E, throat swab.

Main differential diagnoses and typical outline evidence. etc.	
Viral pharyngitis	*Suggested by:* sore throat, pain on swallowing, fever, cervical lymphadenopathy and injected fauces. ↑lymphocytes, normal or ↓leucocytes.
	Confirmed by: –ve **throat swab** for bacterial culture, dehydration: resolution within days.
	Initial management: gargles/lozenges, paracetamol, etc.
Acute follicular tonsillitis (streptococcal)	*Suggested by:* severe sore throat, pain on swallowing, fever, enlarged tonsils with white patches (like strawberries and cream). Cervical lymphadenopathy, especially in angle of jaw. Fever, ↑leucocytes in WCC.
	Confirmed by: **throat swab** for culture and sensitivities of organisms.
	Initial management: analgesic, antibiotics, e.g. penicillin V or cephalosporin or clavulanic acid + amoxicillin.
Infectious mononucleosis (glandular fever) due to Epstein–Barr virus	*Suggested by:* very severe throat pain with enlarged tonsils covered with grey mucoid film. Petechiae on palate. Profound malaise. Generalized lymphadenopathy, splenomegaly.
	Confirmed by: ↑atypical lymphocytes in WBC. **Paul–Bunnell** or **Monospot®** test +ve. **Viral titres**.
	Initial management: gargles/lozenges, analgesics, e.g. paracetamol (amoxycilin causes rash, aspirin may cause Reye syndrome).
Candidiasis of buccal or oesophageal mucosa	*Suggested by:* painful dysphagia, white plaque, history of immunosuppression/diabetes/recent antibiotics.
	Confirmed by: **oesophagoscopy** showing erythema and plaques, **brush cytology ± biopsy** showing spores and hyphae.
	Initial management: analgesics, antifungal lozenges or solutions, e.g. nystatin suspension or oral fluconazole.
Agranulocytosis e.g. antithyroid drugs	*Suggested by:* sore throat, history of taking a drug (e.g carbimazole) or contact with noxious substance.
	Confirmed by: low or absent neutrophil count.
	Initial management: stop offending drug, broad-spectrum antibiotics IV or PO, if febrile.
Also with oropharyngeal ulceration;	Herpes zoster infection, Herpes simplex infection, local herpangina, aphthous ulceration, etc.
without oropharyngeal ulceration	Reflux oesophagitis, epiglottitis, blood dyscrasia, etc.

Dysphagia for fluids > solids

This implies that there is a neuromuscular as opposed to an obstructive cause. Initial investigations (other tests in **bold** below): FBC, CRP or ESR, U&E, CXR.

Main differential diagnoses and typical outline evidence, etc.	
Pseudobulbar palsy due to brain-stem stroke, multiple sclerosis, motor neurone disease, etc.	*Suggested by:* nasal, 'Donald Duck'-like speech, small spastic tongue. *Confirmed by:* inhalation of **Gastrografin®** clinical features of brainstem stroke, multiple sclerosis, motor neurone disease, etc. *Initial management:* NG tube + nil by mouth initially, thickened fluids if swallowing mechanism adequate, if not refer for percutaneous gastrostomy (PEG).
Scleroderma	*Suggested by:* reflux symptoms: cough and inhalation of fluids, tight skin, hooked nose, mouth rugae. *Confirmed by:* **barium swallow**—diminished or absent peristalsis, **oesophageal manometry**—subnormal or absent lower oesophageal sphincter tone. *Initial management:* raise head of bed, small meals; physiotherapy, nifedipine for Raynaud's; antibiotics if bacterial overgrowth, fat-soluble vitamins for malabsorption.
Bulbar palsy	*Suggested by:* nasal, quiet, or hoarse speech; flaccid, fasciculating tongue. *Confirmed by:* clinical features of motor neurone disease/Guillain–Barré syndrome/brainstem tumour/syringobulbia/pontine demyelination. *Initial management:* Initial management: NG tube + nil by mouth initially, thickened fluids if swallowing mechanism adequate; if not, refer for PEG.
Myasthenia gravis	*Suggested by:* difficult start to swallowing movement, cough (inhalation) precipitated by swallowing. *Confirmed by:* inhalation on **Gastrografin®** *swallow.* Response to **Tensilon® test, ↑anti-acetylcholine receptor antibody.** *Initial management:* stop drugs which exacerbate; e.g. β-aminoglycosides; pyridostigmine ± corticosteroids if severe. Monitor FVC; intubation if FVC <1L
Motor neurone disease	*Suggested by:* combination of upper and lower motor neurone signs. *Confirmed by:* **EMG and nerve conduction studies.** *Initial management:* NG tube + nil by mouth initially, thickened fluids if swallowing mechanism adequate; if not, refer for PEG.

Diffuse oesophageal spasm (intermittent)	*Suggested by:* intermittent crushing retrosternal pain.
	Confirmed by: **barium swallow**—sometimes 'corkscrew oesophagus', **oesophageal manometry** show abnormal pressure profiles.
	Initial management: calcium channel blocker, e.g diltiazem, antidepressant, e.g imipramine, or isosorbide dinitrate.
Achalasia (progressive)	*Suggested by:* dysphagia with almost every meal, regurgitation (postural and effortless, contains undigested food).
	Confirmed by: **barium swallow, oesophageal manometry, oesophagoscopy** demonstrate absence of progressive peristalsis.
	Initial management: symptomatic treatment with smooth muscle dilator, e.g. nifedipine, diltiazem or isosorbide mononitrate may be helpful. Referral for endoscopic balloon dilatation of lower oesophageal sphincter or injection of botulinum toxin.

Acute pain in the upper abdomen

Trying to localize the pain to the right, left, or middle may be difficult for the patient. More information such as the site of tenderness will become available from examining the abdomen. Initial investigations (other tests in bold below): FBC, U&E, CXR, AXR.

Main differential diagnoses and typical outline evidence, etc.	
Gallstone colic (with no acute inflammation or infection)	*Suggested by:* jaundice, biliary colic, pain in epigastrium or RUQ radiating to right lower scapula. No fever. Tenderness in the RUQ. WCC normal.
	Confirmed by: **US scan of gallbladder and biliary ducts**.
	Initial management: pain relief, e.g. pethidine, nil by mouth, fluids IV, anti-emetic.
Acute cholecystitis	*Suggested by:* fever, guarding, and +ve Murphy's sign. WCC: leucocytosis.
	Confirmed by: **US scan gallbladder and biliary ducts**.
	Initial management: fluids IV, opioid analgesia, antibiotics IV, e.g. metronidazole + cephalosporin.
Acute pancreatitis	*Suggested by:* pain radiating straight through to the back, better on sitting up or leaning forward. General abdominal tendeness, reduced bowel sounds.
	Confirmed by: ↑↑**serum amylase, CT pancreas**.
	Initial management: pethidine, fluids IV, NG tube + nil by mouth if ileus + colloid ± blood; monitor serum Ca^{2+} and glucose.
Acute cholangitis	*Suggested by:* fever, RUQ abdominal pain, and jaundice (Charcot's triad), hypotension. WCC: leucocytosis.
	Confirmed by: **US scan gallbladder and biliary ducts, blood cultures**.
	Initial management: fluids IV, opioid analgesia, antibiotics IV, e.g. metronidazole + cephalosporin, gastro or surgical referral.
Gastric carcinoma	*Suggested by:* marked anorexia, fullness, pain, Troisier's sign (a 'Virchow's' node, i.e. large lymph node in the left supraclavicular fossa).
	Confirmed by: **upper GI endoscopy with biopsy**.
	Initial management: NG tube + nil by mouth, fluids IV, analgesics, surgical referral.
Gastritis	*Suggested by:* epigastric pain, dull or burning discomfort, nocturnal pain
	Confirmed by: **oesophagogastroscopy, barium meal** *and* **pH study**.
	Initial management: antacids, H_2 blocker or PPI if symptoms persist.

Oesophagitis	*Suggested by:* retrosternal pain, heartburn.
	Confirmed by: **oesophagogastroscopy**.
	Initial management: small meal often, no food before bed, elevate head of bed, antacids; if severe: nil by mouth, fluids IV, H_2 blocker or PPI; if *H. pylori*, antibiotics to eradicate.
Hiatus hernia	*Suggested by:* heartburn, worsens with stooping or lying, relieved by antacids.
	Confirmed by: **oesophagogastroscopy, barium meal**.
	Initial management: lose weight, no stooping, semi-sitting for sleep, correct constipation, antacids or H_2 blockers if pain.
Acute coronary syndrome (unstable angina or infarction)	*Suggested by:* chest tightness or pain on exertion.
	Confirmed by: **ECG ± coronary angiography** if troponin normal, or later if ↑troponin.
	Initial management: ECG monitor (best in CCU), O_2, GTN (IV if pain persists), morphine, aspirin 300mg and clopidogrel 300mg stat, if ↑ST thrombolysis (and <12h from the onset), LMW heparin for unstable angina or NSTEMI.
Also	Pericarditis, pneumonia, empyema, herpes zoster, etc.

Acute central abdominal pain

Examination of the abdomen may provide better leads. Initial investigations (other tests in **bold** below): FBC, U&E, CXR, AXR.

Main differential diagnoses and typical outline evidence, etc.	
Small bowel obstruction	*Suggested by:* vomiting, constipation with complete obstruction.
	Confirmed by: **AXR** shows small bowel loops and fluid levels.
	Initial management: NG tube + nil by mouth, fluids IV, surgical referral.
Abdominal aortic dissection	*Suggested by:* tearing pain, hypertension, (hypotension and shock indicate grave prognosis).
	Confirmed by: **US scan** *or* **CT abdomen**.
	Initial management: pain control with morphine, group and crossmatch, IV access, reduce systolic BP to 100–120mmHg with labetalol IV or propranolol ± nitroprusside. Surgical referral.
Crohn's disease	*Suggested by:* chronic diarrhoea with abdominal pain, weight loss, palpable RLQ mass or fullness, mouth ulcers.
	Confirmed by: **colonoscopy with biopsy, barium studies** showing 'skip lesions', string sign in advanced cases.
	Initial management: antimotility or antidiarrhoeal drugs; acute: fluids IV, corticosteroids IV or PO, high dose 5-ASA analogues (e.g. mesalazine, sulfasalazine), analgesics, elemental diet ± parenteral nutrition.
Mesenteric artery occlusion	*Suggested by:* vomiting, bowel urgency, melaena, diarrhoea.
	Confirmed by: **mesenteric angiography, exploratory laparotomy**.
	Initial management: fluids IV ++ if ↓BP, analgesics, broad-spectrum antibiotics, surgical referral.

Acute lateral abdominal pain

Examination of the abdomen may provide better leads. Initial investigations (other tests in **bold** below): FBC, U&E, CXR, AXR.

Main differential diagnoses and typical outline evidence, etc.	
Appendicitis	*Suggested by:* pain initially central, then radiating to RLQ, anorexia, low-grade fever, constipation. RLQ tenderness and guarding.
	Confirmed by: inflamed appendix at **laparotomy**
	Initial management: nil by mouth, fluids IV, NG tube + nil by mouth if vomiting, broad-spectrum antibiotic, surgical referral.
Pyelonephritis	*Suggested by:* pain in loin (upper lateral), rigors, fever, vomiting, frequency of micturition, renal angle tenderness.
	Confirmed by: FBC: leucocytosis. **MSU:** pyuria, urine and blood culture and sensitivities.
	Initial management: fluids IV, analgesics, anti-emetic; provisional antibiotics pending sensitivities, e.g. ampicillin + gentamicin or 3rd generation cephalosporin.
Renal calculus	*Suggested by:* renal colic, mainly in loin (upper lateral), haematuria.
	Confirmed by: **urinalysis, renal US scan, IVU, CT/MRI.**
	Initial management: fluids IV, analgesic, anti-emetics, e.g. prochlorperazine.
Ureteric calculus	*Suggested by:* renal colic, moving from loin (upper lateral) down to RLQ, haematuria.
	Confirmed by: *urinalysis, renal US scan,* **IVU, CT/MRI.**
	Initial management: fluids IV, analgesic, anti-emetics, e.g. prochlorperazine.
Salpingitis	*Suggested by:* fever, nausea, vomiting, mucopurulent cervical discharge, irregular menses. Bilateral lower abdominal tenderness and guarding.
	Confirmed by: FBC: leucocytosis. **High vaginal swab, laparoscopy.**
	Initial management: analgesics, anti-emetics, antibiotics, e.g. cephalosporin, cefoxitin + doxycycline.
Also	Ruptured ovarian cyst or torsion, endometriosis, etc.

Acute lower central (hypogastric) abdominal pain

Examination of the abdomen may provide better leads. Initial investigations (other tests in **bold** below): FBC, U&E, CXR, AXR.

Main differential diagnoses and typical outline evidence, etc.	
Cystitis due to bacterial infection	*Suggested by:* frequency, urgency, dysuria ± haematuria. *Confirmed by:* **MSU** for microscopy and culture. *Initial management:* fluids IV if dehydrated, antibiotics.
Pelvic inflammatory disease	*Suggested by:* vaginal discharge, dysuria, dyspareunia, pelvic tenderness on moving cervix, ↑ESR and CRP. WCC: leucocytosis. *Confirmed by:* **high vaginal swab** *for* culture and sensitivity, **pelvic US scan** ± **laparoscopy**. *Initial management:* analgesia, fluids IV if dehydrated, provisional antibiotic, e.g. cefoxitin pending sensitivities
Pelvic endometriosis	*Suggested by:* dysmenorrhoea, ovulation pain, dyspareunia, infertility, pelvic mass. *Confirmed by:* **laparoscopy**. *Initial management:* analgesics, fluids IV for hypovolaemia, blood transfusion for severe bleeding, gynae referaal for large or ruptured endometriosis.
Ectopic pregnancy	*Suggested by:* constant unilateral pain ± referred shoulder pain, amenorrhoea, vaginal bleeding (usually less than normal period), faintness with an acute rupture. *Confirmed by:* **pregnancy test** +ve, bimanual examination finding enlarged uterus, **pelvic US scan** showing empty uterus with thickened decidua. *Initial management:* analgesics, fluids ++ if hypotension or shock, urgent gynae/surgical referral.
Large bowel obstruction	*Suggested by:* severe distension, late vomiting, visible peristalsis, resonant percussion, increased bowel sounds. Supine AXR showing peripheral abdominal large bowel shadow (with haustra partly crossing the lumen). Fluid levels on erect film. *Confirmed by:* **US scan** *and* **laparotomy** *findings*. *Initial management:* NG tube, 'drip and suck', fluids IV, monitor intake/output, antibiotics, surgical referral.
Infective or ulcerative colitis	*Suggested by:* abdominal pain, diarrhoea with blood and mucus. *Confirmed by:* **stool microscopy and culture, colonoscopy**. *Initial management:* nil by mouth, fluids IV with K supplement, corticosteroids IV, antibiotic prophylaxis, may need parenteral nutrition, consult surgeon if toxic megacolon.

Acute abdominal pain in children

Examination of the abdomen may provide better leads. Initial investigations (other tests in **bold** below): FBC, U&E, CXR, AXR.

Main differential diagnoses and typical outline evidence, etc.	
Gastroenteritis (all ages)	*Suggested by:* crampy pain, low grade fever, diarrhoea, vomiting, symptoms resolve in 2wk. *Confirmed by:* virus in the **stool specimen**. *Initial management:* paracetamol for fever, oral rehydration solutions, fluids IV if severe dehydration.
Infantile colic (commonly between 2–16wk old)	*Suggested by:* prolonged crying lasting >3h occurs during late afternoon and early evening >3d per week. *Confirmed by:* history and normal physical findings. *Initial management:* reassurance.
Mesenteric adenitis	*Suggested by:* symptoms and signs similar to early appendicitis, but without guarding or rectal tenderness. *Confirmed by:* spontaneous resolution (or findings at **laparotomy** or **laparoscopy**). *Initial management:* analgesia, monitor for resolution.
UTI	*Suggested by:* vomiting, irritability, fever, poor feeding in baby; urgency, dysuria, suprapubic discomfort, fever in older children; (chills, nausea, loin pain in upper tract infection). *Confirmed by:* urine microscopy and culture. *Initial management:* antibiotics, e.g. oral amoxicillin or trimethoprim/sulfamethoxazole (>2mo old); 3rd generation cephalosporin IV if upper tract infection.
Intussusception (common between 6–9mo old)	*Suggested by:* child, usually between 6–9mo of life, acute onset of colicky intermittent abdominal pain, redcurrant 'jelly' PR bleed ± a sausage-shaped mass in upper abdomen. *Confirmed by:* US scan, **barium or air enema**, may reduce the intussusceptions with appropriate hydrostatic pressure. *Initial management:* fluids IV, NG tube + nil by mouth, analgesics, surgical referral for enema/hydrostatic reduction.
Acute appendicitis (mainly 5–15y)	*Suggested by:* vomiting, diarrhoea, pain initially central, then radiating to RLQ, anorexia, low-grade fever, constipation. RLQ tenderness and guarding. *Confirmed by:* inflamed appendix at **laparotomy**. *Initial management:* nil by mouth, fluids IV, NG tube + nil by mouth if vomiting, broad-spectrum antibiotic, surgical referral.
Also	Diabetic ketoacidosis, infections—mumps, Epstein–Barr mononucleosis, pneumonia (especially right lower lobe), torsion of testes, Henoch–Schönlein purpura, sickle crisis, Meckel's diverticulitis.

Recurrent abdominal pain in children

Majority of cases of recurrent abdominal pain in children will not have organic pathology. However, organic disease is more likely if the pain is associated with vomiting, weight loss or failure to thrive, and may wake the child from sleep. Examination of the abdomen may provide better leads. Initial investigations (other tests in **bold** below): FBC, U&E.

Main differential diagnoses and typical outline evidence, etc.	
Recurrent viral illness	*Suggested by:* recurrent fever, malaise, diarrhoea and vomiting, blocked nose, etc.
	Confirmed by: WCC shows lymphocytosis, viral serology.
	Initial management: explanation, reassurance.
Psychosomatic cause, e.g, stress, anxiety, depression, etc.	*Suggested by:* social withdrawal, irritability, poor attention, decreased activity, **school/home stress**, school avoidance.
	Confirmed by: **history**.
	Initial management: explanation, reassurance, referral to child psychologist/psychiatrist.
Constipation	*Suggested by:* infrequent and/or painful bowel movements, hard stools,
	Confirmed by: history, **AXR** may show faeces and evidence of bowel obstruction ± barium enema.
	Initial management: high-fibre diet, increased fluid intake, regular toilet sitting, disimpaction, e.g. with phosphate enema, polyethylene glycol solution PO, or stool softener.
Recurrent UTI	*Suggested by:* vomiting, irritability, fever, poor feeding in baby; urgency, dysuria, suprapubic discomfort, fever in older children; (chills, nausea, loin pain in upper tract infection).
	Confirmed by: **urine microscopy and culture, US scan** to detect any abnormal urinary tract anatomy.
	Initial management: antibiotics, e.g. amoxicillin PO or trimethoprim/sulfamethoxazole (>2mo old); 3rd generation cephalosporin IV if upper tract infection.
Inflammatory bowel disease (in adolescents)	*Suggested by:* chronic diarrhoea with abdominal pain, weight loss, RLQ mass or fullness, mouth ulcers.
	Confirmed by: **colonoscopy with biopsy, barium studies** showing 'skip lesions', string sign (in advanced cases) in Crohn's; or loss of haustration, mucosal oedema, ulceration in ulcerative colitis.
	Initial management: antimotility drugs (e.g loperamide) or antidiarrhoeal drugs; acute attack: fluids IV, corticosteroids PO or IV, high dose 5-ASA analogues (e.g. mesalazine, sulfasalazine), analgesics, elemental diet ± parenteral nutrition.
Also	Parasitic infestation of bowel, lactose intolerance, Hirschsprung's disease, ureteric reflux, lead poisoning, pica, etc.

Sudden diarrhoea, fever, and vomiting

Initial investigations (other tests in **bold** below): FBC, U&E, stool for culture and sensitivity. NB. Measures to prevent cross infection.

Main differential diagnoses and typical outline evidence, etc.	
Viral gastroenteritis (usually Norwalk virus)	*Suggested by:* diarrhoea in older children and adults, symptoms resolve in 2wk. *Confirmed by:* **detection of virus in the stool**. *Initial management:* paracetamol, oral rehydration solutions or fluids IV, anti-emetic; antidiarrhoeals, e.g. loperamide for patient without 'dysentery'.
Rotavirus	*Suggested by:* diarrhoea in children <5y, symptoms resolving in a week. *Confirmed by:* detection of virus in the stool by immmunoassays or PCR. *Initial management:* paracetamol, oral rehydration solutions or fluids IV, anti-emetic; antidiarrhoeals, e.g. loperamide for patient without 'dysentery'.
Antibiotic-induced bacterial opportunists, e.g. *Clostridium* (C.) *difficile*	*Suggested by:* diarrhoea with a history of recent antibiotic therapy, ↑WCC. *Confirmed by:* C. difficile toxin in **stool culture**. *Initial management:* stop offending antibiotic, paracetamol for fever, fluids IV if dehydrated, oral metronidazole or vancomycin for 10–14d .
Food poisoning/toxins *Salmonella typhimurium*	*Suggested by:* eating 'doubtful' meat, egg, poultry. Fever (with relative bradycardia), headache, dry cough. *Confirmed by:* **stool microscopy and culture**. *Initial management:* paracetamol for fever, oral rehydration solutions or fluids IV if dehydrated, ciprofloxacin or trimethoprim/sulfamethoxazole.
Clostridium perfringens	*Suggested by:* eating 'doubtful' meat, incubation period 8–16h, abdominal cramps, little vomiting, lasting 1–2d. *Confirmed by:* organism **isolation from faeces or suspected food**. *Initial management:* paracetamol for fever, oral rehydration solutions or fluids IV if dehydrated,
Staphylococcus (S.) *aureus*	*Suggested by:* eating 'doubtful' meat, incubation period <6h, marked vomiting. *Confirmed by:* isolation of S. aureus from **examination of suspected food**. nitial management: paracetamol for fever, oral rehydration solutions or fluids IV if dehydrated,

Bacillus cereus	*Suggested by:* eating 'doubtful' rice, incubation period <6h, marked vomiting.
	Confirmed by: **stool microscopy and culture**.
	Initial management: paracetamol for fever, oral rehydration solutions or fluids IV if dehydrated,
Vibrio para haemolyticus	*Suggested by:* 'doubtful' seafood, incubation period 16–72h.
	Confirmed by: **stool microscopy and culture**.
	Initial management: paracetamol for fever, oral rehydration solutions or fluids IV if dehydrated, tetracycline or doxycycline.
Botulism	*Suggested by:* eating 'doubtful' canned food, incubation period 18–36h (may vary from 4h to 8d), abdominal cramps, dry mouth, diplopia, progressive paralysis.
	Confirmed by: *C. botulinum* **toxin in serum or faeces;** *C. botulinum* **toxin isolation from suspected food**.
	Initial management: manage in ICU, monitor pulse, oximetry and spirometry, early intubation with ventilatory, botulinum antitoxin IV.

Recurrent diarrhoea with blood ± mucus—bloody flux

Initial investigations (other tests in **bold** below): FBC, U&E, stool for culture and sensitivity. NB. Measures to prevent cross infection.

Main differential diagnoses and typical outline evidence, etc.	
Crohn's disease	*Suggested by:* chronic diarrhoea with abdominal pain, weight loss, RLQ mass or fullness, mouth ulcers.
	Confirmed by: **colonoscopy with biopsy, barium studies** showing 'skip lesions', string sign (in advanced cases).
	Initial management: antimotility drugs (e.g loperamide) or antidiarrhoeal drugs; acute attack: fluids IV, corticosteroids PO or IV, high dose 5-ASA analogues (e.g. mesalazine, sulfasalazine), analgesics, elemental diet ± parenteral nutrition.
Ulcerative colitis	*Suggested by:* lower abdominal cramps, ↑urgency to defaecate, severe diarrhoea, ↑fever in acute attack. **FBC** showing ↑WCC, U&E; ↑urea and creatinine in dehydration.
	Confirmed by: **colonoscopy with biopsy, barium studies** show loss of haustration, mucosal oedema, ulceration.
	Initial management: nil by mouth, fluids IV with K⁺, corticosteroids IV, antibiotic prophylaxis ± parenteral nutrition; if toxic megacolon, surgical referral.
Colonic carcinoma	*Suggested by:* alternate diarrhoea and constipation.
	Confirmed by: **barium enema** showing filling defect, **colonoscopy with biopsy** shows mass and malignant histology.
	Initial management: surgical referral.
Colorectal carcinoma	*Suggested by:* sensation of incomplete evacuation.
	Confirmed by: **sigmoidoscopy with biopsy** showing mass and malignant histology, **barium enema** shows filling defect.
	Initial management: surgical referral.
Diverticular disease/diverticulitis	*Suggested by:* middle-aged or elderly, diarrhoea, LIF (LIF) pain and tenderness, abdominal and rectal mass.
	Confirmed by: **barium enema** showing opaque filling diverticula, **colonoscopy** showing inflammatory foci.
	Initial management: clear liquids only, ciprofloxacin + metronidazole PO for 7–10d, high-fibre diet when acute phase is over; severe: hospitalization, fluids IV, nil by mouth, paracetamol for fever, metronidazole IV + a 3ʳᵈ generation cephalosporin or a fluoroquinolone.

Acute bloody diarrhoea ± mucus— 'dysentery'

Initial investigations (other tests in **bold** below): FBC, U&E, stool for culture and sensitiviry. NB. Measures to prevent cross infection.

Main differential diagnoses and typical outline evidence, etc.	
Campylobacter enteritis	*Suggested by:* associated severe abdominal pain. *Confirmed by:* **stool microscopy and culture** of organism. *Initial management:* oral rehydration solution; fluids IV if severe vomiting, antidiarrhoeal, e.g. codeine, ciprofloxacin, or erythromycin.
Shigella (bacillary) dysentery	*Suggested by:* blood and mucus, fever, abdominal pain. *Confirmed by:* **stool microscopy** revealing red cells, pus cells, and appearance of organism. *Initial management:* oral rehydration solution; fluids IV if severe vomiting, antidiarrhoeal, ciprofloxacin or trimethoprim/sulfamethoxazole.
Enteroinvasive Escherichia (E.) coli	*Suggested by:* fever, watery diarrhea, later ± bloody diarrhoea. *Confirmed by:* **stool microscopy** and **culture** of organism. *Initial management:* paracetamol for fever, oral rehydration solutions or fluids IV if severe dehydration, antibiotic if frail or progressive.
Enterohaemorrhagic type 0157 E. coli	*Suggested by:* no fever, bloody diarrhoea ± haemolytic-uraemic syndrome. *Confirmed by:* **stool microscopy** *and* **culture** of organism. *Initial management:* oral rehydration solution or fluids IV if severe dehydration, correct electrolytes, watch for haemolytic-uraemic syndrome.
Entamoeba histolytica (amoebic) dysentery	*Suggested by:* abdominal discomfort, flatulence, frequent watery, bloody diarrhoea. *Confirmed by:* **stool microscopy** and **culture** of organism. *Initial manageme nt:* oral rehydration solution; fluids IV if severe vomiting, metronidazole PO for 10d.

Watery diarrhoea

Note that diarrhoea can result in severe dehydration. Initial investigations (other tests in **bold** below): FBC, U&E, stool for culture and sensitiviry. NB. Measures to prevent cross infection.

Main differential diagnoses and typical outline evidence, etc.	
Traveller's diarrhoea	*Suggested by:* recent travel, no obvious ingestion of contaminated water or food. *Confirmed by:* rapid resolution or response to ciprofloxacin. *Initial management:* reassure that most cases are self-limited; oral rehydration solutions if serve diarrhhoea; ciprofloxacin for 2d, or single dose of azithromycin; bismuth prep until diarrhoea resolves (up to x8); antimotility agents, e.g. loperamide or diphenoxylate.
Enterotoxigenic *E. coli* (commonest)	*Suggested by:* incubation period 12–72h in relation to contact to others with similar features. *Confirmed by:* **stool microscopy** and **culture**. *Initial management:* reassure that majority of cases are dehydration; oral rehydration solutions or fluids IV if severe dehydration.
Vibrio cholera	*Suggested by:* incubation period from a few hours to 5 days, profuse watery diarrhoea, fever, vomiting. *Confirmed by:* **stool microscopy and culture**. *Initial management:* oral rehydration solutions, fluids IV if >10% bodyweight loss from dehydration, tetracycline for 3d or one dose of doxycycline.
Rotavirus	*Suggested by:* diarrhoea in children <5y and symptoms resolve in a week. *Confirmed by:* **detection virus in the stool by immunoassays or PCR**. *Initial management:* paracetamol for fever, oral rehydration solutions or fluids IV if severe, no antimotility nor antispasmodics in children.
Norwalk virus	*Suggested by:* diarrhoea in older children and adults and symptoms resolve in 2wk. *Confirmed by:* detection of virus in **stool specimen**. *Initial management:* paracetamol to reduce fever, oral rehydration solutions or fluids IV if severe dehydration.

Recurrent diarrhoea with no blood in the stools, no fever

Initial investigations (other tests in **bold** below): FBC, U&E, LFT, random glucose, T4, TSH.

Main differential diagnoses and typical outline evidence, etc.	
Irritable bowel syndrome	*Suggested by:* no weight loss, intermittent daytime diarrhoea, pain relieved by defaecation, abdominal distension, mucus but no blood in the stool.
	Confirmed by: normal **colonoscopy and barium studies,** and no appearance of other cause of symptoms.
	Initial management: high-fibre diet; try metoclopramide, mebeverine, loperamide, lactulose; low dose tricyclic antidepressant and psychological therapy.
Faecal impaction with overflow	*Suggested by:* elderly patient and hard faeces on rectal examination.
	Confirmed by: **AXR** may show faecal impaction. Response to suppositories/removal of faeces.
	Initial management: laxatives and enemas ± gentle digital disimpaction.
Malabsorption due to coeliac disease, lactose intolerance, pancreatic disease, Whipple's disease	*Suggested by:* pale, bulky offensive stools, weight loss, signs of nutritional deficiencies.
	Confirmed by: **coeliac screen, small bowel biopsy or lactose tolerance test; intestinal biopsy** shows foamy macrophages containing PAS +ve glycoprotein in Whipple's.
	Initial management: nutritional support (treat cause).
Drug-induced	*Suggested by:* history of laxative abuse, magnesium alkalis, antibiotics, hypotensive agents, alcohol.
	Confirmed by: resolution on withdrawing drug.
	Initial management: stop offending drug.
HIV infection	*Suggested by:* weight loss, other opportunistic infection, lymphadenopathy, Kaposi's sarcoma.
	Confirmed by: **HIV serology, stool microscopy and cultures** showing *Cryptosporidium*, microsporidia, *Isospora belli*, enteropathy, etc.
	Initial management: try loperamide, empirical antibiotics, e.g ciprofloxacin + metronidazole (except if 0157 *E. coli* suspected).

Diabetic autonomic neuropathy	*Suggested by:* known diabetic, intermittent watery painless diarrhhoea, postural hypotension, impotence, urinary retention.
	Confirmed by: lying and standing BP, loss of **beat-to-beat variation** during slow deep breathing.
	Initial management: loperamide or codeine for diarrhhoea, co-amoxiclav + metronidazole for bacterial overgrowth, fludrocortisone for severe postural hypotension.
Thyrotoxicosis	*Suggested by:* heat intolerance, tremor, nervousness, palpitation, frequent bowel movements, goitre.
	Confirmed by: ↓**TSH**, ↑**FT4** or ↑**FT3**.
	Initial management: propranolol 40–80 mg 8-hourly to control symptoms, carbimazole, or propylthiouracil to treat thyroid overactivity.
Carcinoid syndrome	*Suggested by:* facial flushing ± wheeze, abdominal pain
	Confirmed by: ↑24h **urinary 5-HIAA**.
	Initial management: avoid precipitating factors, e.g. alcohol, physical activity. Codeine phosphate for diarrhoea, H_2 agonist or theophylline for asthma; surgical referral for resection of tumour.

Chronic diarrhoea in children

Note that certain conditions that cause chronic diarrhoea in children require special attention. Initial investigations (other tests in **bold** below): FBC, U&E, LFT.

Main differential diagnoses and typical outline evidence, etc.	
Lactose intolerance	*Suggested by:* bloatedness, colicky abdominal pain, diarrhoea after digestion of lactose-containing food.
	Confirmed by: stool analysis shows presence of reducing substances in the liquid portion of stool, and pH of stool <5.5.
	Initial management: no lactose-containing products.
Cow's milk protein intolerance	*Suggested by:* crampy abdominal pain, diarrhoea after ingestion of cow's milk formula, onset of symptoms may be delayed.
	Confirmed by: response to withdrawal of cow's milk formula.
	Initial management: no cow's milk protein.
Chronic infection of bowel (e.g. *Salmonella* sp., *Campylobacter*, *Giardia lambia*, etc.)	*Suggested by:* abdominal discomfort, flatulence, frequent watery ± bloody diarrhoea.
	Confirmed by: **stool microscopy** and **culture** of organism.
	Initial management: oral rehydration solution; fluids IV if severe vomiting, no antidiarrhoeal drugs, treat underlying infection.
Coeliac disease (usually present at 9–18mo)	*Suggested by:* anorexia, irritability, frequent bulky offensive stools, failure to thrive, abdominal distension.
	Confirmed by: **coeliac screen, duodenal biopsy.**
	Initial management: no gluten in diet, give nutritional supplements.
Cystic fibrosis (present in infancy)	*Suggested by:* LFT, meconium ileus in the neonate, fatty diarrhoea, malabsorption, recurrent chest infection, failure to thrive.
	Confirmed by: **sweat test**: Cl⁻ >60mmol/L and genetic testing: (1 mutation = mild disease, 2 mutations = severe), response to pancreatic enzyme replacement.
	Initial management: pancreatic enzyme replacement, treatment of any chest infections, postural drainage.
Inflammatory bowel disease (adolescents)	*Suggested by:* chronic diarrhoea with abdominal pain, weight loss, RLQ mass or fullness, mouth ulcers.
	Confirmed by: **colonoscopy with biopsy, barium studies** showing 'skip lesions', string sign (in advanced cases) in Crohn's; or loss of haustration, mucosal oedema, ulceration in ulcerative colitis.
	Initial management: antimotility drugs (loperamide 2–4mg tds) or antidiarrhoeal drugs; acute attack: fluids IV, corticosteroids IV or PO, high dose 5-ASA analogues (e.g. mesalazine, sulfasalazine), analgesics, elemental diet ± parenteral nutrition.

Constipation

Constipation is defined as a change in a person's normal bowel habit to infrequent or more difficult defaecation. It is important to establish what the patient means by the term 'constipation', what his or her normal bowel habit is, and how the presenting problem differ from 'normal'. Initial investigations (other tests in **bold** below): FBC, U&E, LFT, serum calcium, T4, TSH, AXR, sigmoidoscopy.

Main differential diagnoses and typical outline evidence, etc.	
Change in diet, e.g. low-fibre diet.	*Suggested by:* history of ↓diet fibre, ↓fluid intake.
	Confirmed by: normal **endoscopy** and response to diet change.
	Initial management: ↑dietary fibre and ↑fluid intake.
Change in the lifestyle or environment.	*Suggested by:* history.
	Confirmed by: normal **sigmoidoscopy or colonoscopy** and constipation resolves when resuming prior lifestyle or environment.
	Initial management: resume lifestyle, ↑dietary fibre.
Immobility	*Suggested by:* history.
	Confirmed by: normal **sigmoidoscopy or colonoscopy** and history.
	Initial management: mobilization, ↑dietary fibre.
Drug-induced	*Suggested by:* constipating drugs (opioids, hypotensive agents, aluminium alkalis, etc.), purgative dependence.
	Confirmed by: normal **sigmoidoscopy or colonoscopy** and response to withdrawal of suspected agent.
	Initial management: stop offending drug.
Anal fissure	*Suggested by:* skin tag, pain on defaecation, staining of toilet paper following defaecation.
	Confirmed by: physical examination of anal region.
	Initial management: high-fibre diet, stool softeners, warm sitz baths, analgesic cream, glyceryl trinitrate ointment, oral or topical diltiazem, botulinum toxin injection near to the fissures, surgical referral for sphincterotomy if medical therapy fails.
Haemorrhoids	*Suggested by:* rectal bleeding follows defaecation, perianal protrusion with pain.
	Confirmed by: anal inspection and **proctoscopy** (haemorrhoids drop over edge of proctoscope as it is withdrawn).
	Initial management: high-fibre diet, hydrocortisone suppositories to relieve irritation and pruritus ± surgical referral.

Poor fluid intake	*Suggested by:* history of ↓fluid intake.
	Confirmed by: normal **sigmoidoscopy or colonoscopy** and response to increased fluid intake.
	Initial management: ↑fluid intake.
Hypothyroidism	*Suggested by:* cold intolerance, lethargy, weight gain, coarse and dry skin, puffy eyelids.
	Confirmed by: ↑*TSH,* ↓*FT4* ± ↓*FT3.*
	Initial management: levothyroxine.
Rectal tumour	*Suggested by:* rectal bleeding with defaecation, blood limited to surface of stool.
	Confirmed by: **sigmoidoscopy with rectal biopsy.**
	Initial management: surgical referral.
Colonic carcinoma	*Suggested by:* alternate diarrhoea and constipation, anaemia or weight loss.
	Confirmed by: **colonoscopy with biopsy, barium enema.**
	Initial management: surgical referral.
Also	Hypercalcaemia, behavioural—'stool-holding' in children, external pelvic mass compression, etc.

Change in bowel habit

This may be an increase in constipation or diarrhoea or both alternating. Initial investigations (other tests in bold below): FBC, U&E, LFT, serum calcium, T4, TSH, AXR, sigmoidoscopy.

Main differential diagnoses and typical outline evidence, etc.	
Change in diet	*Suggested by:* history of ↓diet fibre, ↓fluid intake.
	Confirmed by: normal **sigmoidoscopy or colonoscopy** and response to diet change.
	Initial management: diet change—↑fibre and fluid intake.
Colonic carcinoma	*Suggested by:* alternate diarrhoea and constipation, anaemia or weight loss.
	Confirmed by: **colonoscopy with biopsy, CT abdomen, barium enema**.
	Initial management: surgical referral.
Drug-induced	*Suggested by:* constipating drugs (opioids, hypotensive agents, aluminium alkalis, etc.), purgative dependence.
	Confirmed by: normal **sigmoidoscopy or colonoscopy** and response to stopping causal agent.
	Initial management: stop offending drug.
Depression	*Suggested by:* sleep disorders, social withdrawal, lack of interest in usual activities, etc.
	Confirmed by: normal **sigmoidoscopy or colonoscopy**, and response to lifting of depression.
	Initial management: psychiatric referral
Immobility	*Suggested by:* history.
	Confirmed by: normal **sigmoidoscopy or colonoscopy** and history.
	Initial management: mobilization, ↑fibre.
Cerebral or spinal cord lesion	*Suggested by:* neurological symptoms and signs ± abnormal sphincter tone and anal sensation.
	Confirmed by: **CT or MRI**.
	Initial management: rehabilitation programmes, ↑fibre.
Metabolic disturbances: hypothyroidism, hyperthyroidism, hypercalcaemia, hypokalaemia	*Suggested by:* symptoms of metabolic disturbance or absence of anatomical abnormality.
	Confirmed by: **TFT, serum calcium, potassium**, etc.
	Initial management: correct electrolytes and metabolic disturbance, treat underlying cause.

Haematemesis ± melaena

Vomiting of bright red blood and/or passage of black tarry motions. This implies bleeding from the upper GI tract: oesophagus, stomach, and duodenum. Initial investigations (other tests in **bold** below): FBC, U&E, LFT, clotting screen, group and save, monitor Hb.

Main differential diagnoses and typical outline evidence, etc.	
Bleeding DU	*Suggested by:* epigastric pain and tenderness, nausea.
	Confirmed by: **oesophagogastroscopy** showing bleeding ulcer.
	Initial management: large bore IV or central line, fluids IV—colloid initially ± transfusion, CVP monitoring, NG tube + irrigation, urinary catheter to monitor output, surgical referral. H_2 blocker or PPI for 4wk; *H. pylori* eradication therapy if *H. pylori* +ve.
Bleeding GU	*Suggested by:* epigastric pain, dull or burning discomfort, nocturnal pain.
	Confirmed by: appearance of ulcer on **oesophagogastroscopy** and **pH study** showing hyperacidity.
	Initial management: treat acute severe bleed as DU; antacid; H_2 blocker or PPI for 8wk; *H. pylori* eradication therapy if *H. pylori* +ve.
Gastric erosion	*Suggested by:* history of NSAIDs or alcohol ingestion, epigastric pain, dull or burning discomfort, nocturnal pain.
	Confirmed by: appearance of erosion on **oesophagogastroscopy** and **pH study** showing hyperacidity.
	Initial management: treat acute bleed as DU; stop aspirin, NSAIDs, alcohol; antacids, H_2 blocker or PPI.
Oesophageal varices	*Suggested by:* liver cirrhosis, splenomegaly, prominent upper abdominal veins.
	Confirmed by: **oesophagogastroscopy** showing varicose mucosa and blood distally and in stomach.
	Initial management: if bleeding stopped, propranolol or long-acting nitrate. Still bleeding: large bore IV or central line, fluids IV (colloid initially) ± transfusion, CVP monitoring, NG tube + irrigation, urinary catheter to monitor output, correct coagulopathy with FFP and vitamin K IV. Surgical or gastro referral for banding or sclerotherapy.
Mallory–Weiss tear	*Suggested by:* preceding marked vomiting, later bright red blood.
	Confirmed by: **oesophagogastroscopy** showing tear.
	Initial management: monitor vital signs, Hb, fluids IV, nil by mouth, surgical referral if persistent bleeding requiring blood transfusion, treat underlying cause.

Oesophageal carcinoma	*Suggested by:* progressive dysphagia with solids which sticks, weight loss.
	Confirmed by: **barium swallow, fibreoptic gastroscopy with mucosal biopsy** showing malignant tissue.
	Initial management: treat severe bleed as DU. Nil by mouth, fluids IV, analgesics ± blood transfusion if bleeding continues ± antibiotic prophylaxis, surgical referral for oesophageal dilatation or stent insertion by endoscopy.
Gastric carcinoma	*Suggested by:* marked anorexia, fullness, pain, Troisier's sign (enlarged left supraclavicular lymph (Virchow's) node).
	Confirmed by: **oesophagogastroscopy with biopsy** showing malignant tissue.
	Initial management: NG tube + nil by mouth, fluids IV, analgesics ± transfusion, treat severe bleed as DU, surgical referral.
Gastro-oesophageal reflux	*Suggested by:* heartburn worse when lying flat, anorexia, nausea ± regurgitation of gastric content.
	Confirmed by: appearance of erosion on **oesophagoscopy, barium meal,** and **pH study** showing ↑acidity.
	Initial management: treat severe bleed as DU. Small meals, no food before bed, raise head of bed, antacids; Moderate to severe: nil by mouth, fluids IV, H₂ blocker or PPI, antibiotics to eradicate *H. pylori* if ulceration.
Hiatus hernia	*Suggested by:* heartburn, worse with stooping, relieved by antacids.
	Confirmed by: herniation of stomach into chest on plain X-ray or barium meal, appearance of erosion on **oesophagoscopy** and **pH study** showing hyperacidity.
	Initial management: treat severe bleed as DU. reduce weight avoid stooping, semi-sitting position for sleep, correct constipation, antacids, or H₂ blockers for pain.
Ingestion of corrosives	*Suggested by:* history of ingestion etc.
	Confirmed by: **oesophagogastroscopy** showing severe erosions.
	Initial management: removal of offending agent, fluids IV ± blood transfusion if hypotension or bleeding, laryngoscopy ± tracheostomy if respiratory distress; broad-spectrum antibiotics infection, steroids to reduce stricture formation.
Meckel's diverticulum	*Suggested by:* no haematemesis, usually asymptomatic, anaemia, rectal bleeding.
	Confirmed by: **technetium-labelled red blood cell scan** showing isotopes in gut lumen and laparotomy.
	Initial management: fluids IV, nil by mouth ± NG tube, transfusion if significant bleeding, surgical referral.

(Continued)

Haematemesis ± melaena (continued)

Main differential diagnoses and typical outline evidence, etc. *(continued)*	
False haematemesis	*Suggested by:* swallowed nose bleed or haemoptysis.
	Confirmed by: normal **oesophagogastroscopy** and **bleeding source** identified in nose.
	Initial management: treat underlying cause.
Also	Angiodysplasia, bleeding disorders.

Passage of blood per rectum

May not be noticed by the patient but only be discovered on rectal examination. Initial investigations (other tests in **bold** below): FBC, CRP or ESR, LFT, sigmoidoscopy or proctoscopy, AXR.

Main differential diagnoses and typical outline evidence, etc.	
Bleeding haemorrhoids	*Suggested by:* pain, discharge, pruritus, staining of toilet paper following defaecation.
	Confirmed by: physical and digital rectal examination, proctoscopy.
	Initial management: high-fibre diet, hydrocortisone suppositories for pruritus ± surgical referral.
Anal fissure	*Suggested by:* skin tag, pain on defaecation, staining of toilet paper following defaecation, exquisite anal tenderness.
	Confirmed by: history and clinical examination.
	Initial management: high-fibre diet, stool softeners, warm sitz baths, analgesic cream, glyceryl trinitrate ointment, oral or topical diltiazem, botulinum toxin injection, referral for sphincterotomy if above fails.
Diverticulitis	*Suggested by:* bloody 'splash in the pan', abdominal pain, usually LIF, diarrhoea and constipation.
	Confirmed by: **colonoscopy, barium enema**.
	Initial management: mild: clear liquids only, antibiotics, e.g. ciprofloxacin and metronidazole or co-amoxiclav for >7d, then high-fibre-diet. Severe: fluids IV, nil by mouth, metronidazole IV + a 3rd generation cephalosporin or a fluoroquinolone.
Carcinoma rectum	*Suggested by:* rectal bleeding with defaecation, unsatisfactory defaecation.
	Confirmed by: **sigmoidoscopy with biopsy**.
	Initial management: surgical referral.
Colonic carcinoma	*Suggested by:* red blood mixed with stool and alternate diarrhoea and constipation.
	Confirmed by: **flexible colonoscopy with biopsy**.
	Initial management: surgical referral.
Ulcerative colitis	*Suggested by:* lower abdominal pain, urgency to defaecate, severe bloody diarrhoea, fever in acute attack.
	Confirmed by: **colonoscopy with biopsy, barium studies** show loss of haustration, mucosal oedema, ulceration.
	Initial management: nil by mouth, fluids IV with K^{+} supplements, corticosteroids IV, antibiotics ± parenteral nutrition, surgical referral if toxic megacolon.

Massive upper GI bleed	*Suggested by:* bright or dark red 'maroon'-coloured stool.
	Confirmed by: **upper GI endoscopy**.
	Initial management: stop aspirin or NSAIDs, large bore IV or central line, group and crossmatch, fluids IV (colloid initially), transfusion, CVP monitoring, irrigate stomach, nil by mouth, correct coagulopathy with FFP and platelets, urine catheter to monitor output; gastro or surgical referral.
Crohn's disease	*Suggested by:* chronic diarrhoea with abdominal pain, weight loss, palpable RLQ mass or fullness, mouth ulcers.
	Confirmed by: **colonoscopy with biopsy, barium studies** show 'skip lesions', string sign in advanced cases.
	Initial management: mild: antimotility drugs (e.g. loperamide); severe: fluids IV, corticosteroids IV or PO, 5-ASA analogues (e.g. mesalazine, sulfasalazine), analgesics, elemental diet ± parenteral nutrition.
Meckel's diverticulum	*Suggested by:* usually asymptomatic, anaemia, rectal bleeding.
	Confirmed by: **technetium-labelled red blood cell scan, laparotomy**.
	Initial management: fluids IV, nil by mouth ± NG tube, transfusion, surgical referral if significant bleeding.
Trauma (in children, possible non-accidental injury)	*Suggested by:* fresh blood, sometimes external signs of trauma.
	Confirmed by: sensitive and careful history, possible surveillance, etc.
	Initial management: analgesia, comforting, etc.
Intussusception	*Suggested by:* child in first 6–18mo of life, acute onset of colicky intermittent abdominal pain, redcurrant 'jelly' PR bleed ± a sausage-shaped mass in upper abdomen.
	Confirmed by: **barium enema** ± reduction of intussusception with appropriate hydrostatic pressure.
	Initial management: fluids IV, NG tube for decompression, analgesics, surgical referral for therapeutic enemas, e.g. hydrostatic reduction.
Also	Ischaemic colitis, infectious colitis, angiodysplasia (lower bowel).

Tenesmus

Intense desire to defaecate, but no stool. Initial investigations (other tests in **bold** below): FBC, CRP or ESR, LFT, sigmoidoscopy or proctoscopy, AXR.

Main differential diagnoses and typical outline evidence, etc.	
Rectal inflammation (proctitis)	*Suggested by:* rectal bleeding, mucus discharge. *Confirmed by:* proctoscopy or **sigmoidoscopy** *reveals* inflamed rectal mucosa. *Initial management:* steroid suppositories or 5-ASA enemas or suppositories in mild disease; fluids IV if vomiting, antibiotics for infection, e.g. ceftriaxone, azithromycin, or doxycycline if *chlamydia*.
Rectal tumour	*Suggested by:* rectal bleeding with defaecation, blood limited to surface of stool. *Confirmed by:* **sigmoidoscopy with rectal biopsy**. *Initial management:* surgical referral.
Tumour of descending colon	*Suggested by:* alternate diarrhoea and constipation. *Confirmed by:* **colonoscopy with biopsy, barium enema**. *Initial management:* surgical referral.
Pelvic inflammatory disease	*Suggested by:* lower abdominal pain, fever, vaginal discharge, dysuria, ↑ESR and CRP, leucocytosis. *Confirmed by:* **high vaginal swab, pelvic US scan ± laparoscopy**. *Initial management:* analgesia, fluids IV if dehydrated, empirical antibiotics, e.g. cefoxitin or other 2nd generation cephalosporin + doxycycline or clindamycin + gentamicin or ofloxacin + metronidazole.

Anorectal pain

Initial investigations (other tests in **bold** below): FBC, CRP or ESR, LFT, sigmoidoscopy or proctoscopy, AXR.

Main differential diagnoses and typical outline evidence, etc.	
Anal fissure	*Suggested by:* skin tag, pain on defaecation, staining of toilet paper following defaecation.
	Confirmed by: physical examination of anal region.
	Initial management: high-fibre diet, stool softeners, warm sitz baths, analgesic cream, glyceryl trinitrate ointment, oral or topical diltiazem, botulinum toxin injection near to the fissures, surgical referral for sphincterotomy if medical therapy fails.
Haemorrhoids (thrombosed pile)	*Suggested by:* rectal bleeding following defaecation, perianal protrusion with pain.
	Confirmed by: digital rectal examination.
	Initial management: high-fibre diet, hydrocortisone for pruritus, surgical referral.
Perianal abscess	*Suggested by:* severe constant throbbing pain, fever, tender lump, redness.
	Confirmed by: digital rectal examination.
	Initial management: analgesics, paracetamol for fever, surgical referral for drainage of abscess.
Proctalgia fugax, coccydynia	*Suggested by:* fleeting pain in rectum or coccyx which may be related to sitting but not defaecation, pain wakes patient at night.
	Confirmed by: physical examination, tenderness of levator muscle.
	Initial management: reassurance, analgesics.
Proctitis	*Suggested by:* rectal bleeding, mucus discharge.
	Confirmed by: proctoscopy or **sigmoidoscopy** revealing inflamed rectal mucosa.
	Initial management: steroid suppositories or 5-ASA enemas or suppositories in mild disease; fluids IV if nausea and vomiting, antibiotics for infection, e.g. ceftriaxone, azithromycin, or doxycycline if *chlamydia*.
Prostatitis (referred pain)	*Suggested by:* rigor, fever, urinary frequency and urgency, dysuria, haemospermia.
	Confirmed by: tender prostate gland on PR examination, **urine microscopy**.
	Initial management: bed rest, NSAIDs for pain control, fluids IV, lactulose, antibiotics, † e.g. cefotaxime or ceftriaxone.
Also	Anal herpes, pilonidal sinus and abscess, caudal equine lesion, anal or rectal malignancy, trauma, referred pain from uterine disease, or pelvic inflammatory disease.

Distended abdomen

Inspect the abdomen from a sitting position next to the bed or couch. Consider the general shape, then look at the skin. Next, consider movement of the abdomen. The causes are the traditional 6 'F's: Fat, Fluid, Flatus, Faeces, Fibroids, Foetus. Initial investigations (other tests in **bold** below): FBC, clotting screen, U&E, CRP or ESR, LFT, AXR, sigmoidoscopy or proctoscopy.

Main differential diagnoses and typical outline evidence, etc.	
Fat (obese)	*Suggested by:* usually sunken umbilicus, dullness to percussion throughout. *Confirmed by:* **CT abdomen.** *Initial management:* lifestyle changes—low-calorie diet, increased physical exercise.
Fluid (ascites)	*Suggested by:* bilateral bulging flanks, shifting dullness, fluid thrill. *Confirmed by:* **US scan liver and abdomen.** *Initial management:* salt restriction, fluid restriction if Na$^+$ <120mmol/L, spironolactone 100–400mg/d ± furosemide 40–120mg/d, thiamine 25–50mg od if alcoholic, daily weight; ascitic tap—paracentesis if gross ascites and symptomatic, treat underlying cause.
Flatus (gas) due to normal dietary variation	*Suggested by:* tympanic sound throughout. Often associated constipation. *Confirmed by:* **AXR** shows normal gas shadow. *Initial management:* diet change.
Small bowel obstruction ('flatus' again)	*Suggested by:* mild distension, early vomiting, central/upper abdominal pain, resonant percussion, increased bowel sounds. Supine AXR showing central gas but no peripheral abdominal large bowel shadow (i.e. without haustra partly crossing) but valvulae conniventes of small intestine entirely crossing the lumen. Fluid levels on erect film. *Confirmed by:* **abdominal US scan and laparotomy findings.** *Initial management:* NG tube + nil by mouth, fluids IV, surgical referral.
Large bowel obstruction	*Suggested by:* severe distension, late vomiting, visible peristalsis, resonant percussion, increased bowel sounds. Supine AXR showing peripheral abdominal large bowel shadow (with haustra partly crossing the lumen). Fluid levels on erect film. *Confirmed by:* **abdominal US scan and laparotomy findings.** *Initial management:* NG tube with suction, nil by mouth, fluids IV, monitor intake and output, preop antibiotics, surgical referral.

Splenic rupture (?delayed)	*Suggested by:* history of trauma (road traffic accident, fall onto left chest wall), bruising over left chest wall or upper abdomen, falling BP, rising pulse, abdominal tenderness, diminished bowel sounds, plain **AXR**—loss of left psoas shadow, **peritoneal tap** demonstrates free blood.
	Confirmed by: CT scan appearance.
	Initial management: large bore IV access, group and crossmatch, fluids IV, colloid ± then blood. NG tube + nil by mouth, urethral catheter to monitor output, analgesics. Surgical referral for splenectomy etc.
Faecal impaction	*Suggested by:* paucity of bowel movement and constipation. **AXR** shows stippled pattern of 'faecal loading'.
	Confirmed by: resolution of swelling with evacuation or partly with flatus tube.
	Initial management: laxatives, enemas ± gentle digital disimpaction.
Fibroids, large ovarian cyst	*Suggested by:* mass in pelvis in middle-aged female.
	Confirmed by: **abdominal US scan** *or* **CT**.
	Initial management: NSAIDs for pain, gynae referral.
Foetus	*Suggested by:* amenorrhoea and mass in pelvis (cannot get below it).
	Confirmed by: +ve **urine pregnancy test** or ↑**plasma hCG**. Also **abdominal US scan**.
	Initial management: arrange antenatal clinic follow-up.

Distended abdominal veins

This suggests that there is an obstruction to normal venous flow and that it is being diverted via superficial veins. Initial investigations (other tests in **bold** below): FBC, clotting screen, U&E, CRP or ESR, LFT, AXR.

Main differential diagnoses and typical outline evidence, etc.	
Portal hypertension	*Suggested by:* veins radiating out from umbilicus (caput medusa) ± ascites ± splenomegaly, other stigmata of chronic liver disease, venous hum over collaterals.
	Confirmed by: **US scan appearance** of liver which is small, cirrhotic with dilated portal veins.
	Initial management: β-blocker, e.g. propranolol, treat complications, e.g. oesophageal varices, ascites.
Superior vena cava obstruction (due to bronchogenic carcinoma, non-Hodgkin's lymphoma, etc.)	*Suggested by:* distended veins with blood flow from chest towards groin when compressed and one end released.
	Confirmed by: **CT thorax**.
	Initial management: elevate the head of the bed, O_2, corticosteroids and diuretics for laryngeal or cerebral oedema, treat underlying cause.
Inferior vena cava obstruction	*Suggested by:* distended veins with blood flow up from groin towards chest when compressed and one end released.
	Confirmed by: **CT abdomen**.
	Initial management: treat cause, e.g. DVT—anticoagulants or thrombolysis.

Abdominal bruits

Abdominal bruising

Also consider the general causes of bruising as indicated in the general examination findings. Initial investigations (other tests in **bold** below): FBC, clotting screen, U&E, LFT, AXR.

Main differential diagnoses and typical outline evidence, etc.	
Retroperitoneal haemorrhage e.g. in acute pancreatitis	*Suggested by:* abdominal tenderness and rigidity, bruises in and around the umbilicus (Cullen's sign), on one or both flanks (Grey Turner's sign). *Confirmed by:* ↑**serum amylase, CT abdomen**. *Initial management:* pain relief, e.g. pethidine, nil by mouth, fluids IV, monitor glucose and Ca^{2+} (if acute pancreatitis), NG tube + nil by mouth for ileus, colloid ± blood.
Ruptured or dissecting abdominal aortic aneurysm	*Suggested by:* hypotension and abdominal pain, tenderness and rigidity, bruises in and around the umbilicus (Cullen's sign), on one or both flanks (Grey Turner's sign). Expansile pulsatile mass >3cm diameter, bruit over the mass. *Confirmed by:* **abdominal US scan** or **CT abdomen**. *Initial management:* pain control with morphine, group and crossmatch, IV access, reduce systolic BP to 100–120mmHg with labetalol IV or propranolol, nitroprusside may be added, intubate if haemodynamically unstable, refer for surgical repair.
Splenic rupture (?delayed)	*Suggested by:* history of trauma (road traffic accident, fall on to left chest wall), bruising over left chest wall or upper abdomen, falling BP, rising pulse, abdominal tenderness, diminished bowel sounds, plain AXR—loss of left psoas shadow, **peritoneal tap** demonstrates free blood. *Confirmed by:* **CT scan** appearance. *Initial management:* large bore IV access, group and crossmatch, fluids IV, colloid ± then blood. NG tube + nil by mouth, urethral catheter to monitor output, analgesics. Surgical referral for splenectomy etc.

Poor abdominal movement

From the sitting position, watch and ask about any areas of tenderness and begin furthest away, palpating gently looking at the patient's face to see if there is any reaction. 'Rigidity' is when there is no initial lack of resistance but reflex rigidity from the outset. Initial investigations (other tests in **bold** below): FBC, clotting screen, U&E, LFT, AXR.

Main differential diagnoses and typical outline evidence, etc.	
Small bowel obstruction	*Suggested by:* mild distension, early vomiting, central/upper abdominal pain, resonant percussion, increased bowel sounds. Supine AXR shows central gas but no peripheral abdominal large bowel shadow (i.e. without haustra partly crossing) but valvulae conniventes of small intestine crossing the entire lumen. Fluid levels on erect film.
	Confirmed by: **abdominal US scan *and* laparotomy findings.**
	Initial management: NG tube + nil by mouth, fluids IV, surgical referral.
Large bowel obstruction	*Suggested by:* severe distension, late vomiting, visible peristalsis, resonant percussion, increased bowel sounds. Supine AXR shows peripheral abdominal large bowel shadow (with haustra partly crossing the lumen). Fluid levels on erect film.
	Confirmed by: **abdominal US scan *and* laparotomy findings.**
	Initial management: NG tube + suction, nil by mouth, fluids IV, monitor intake and output, preop antibiotics, refer to surgical team.
Peritonitis from perforated stomach, duodenum, diverticulum; intraperitoneal haemorrhage or bowel infarction	*Suggested by:* decreased or absent abdominal movement, generalized tenderness and rigidity, absent bowel sounds, and board-like rigidity.
	Confirmed by: **erect AXR *or* CXR** show gas under diaphragm and laparotomy.
	Initial management: analgesics, fluids IV, NG tube + nil by mouth for ileus, broad-spectrum antibiotics—2nd or 3rd generation cephalosporin or quinolone ± metronidazole.

Localized tenderness in the hypogastrium (suprapubic area)

Initial investigations (other tests in **bold** below): FBC, U&E, LFT, urine 'dipstick' testing, MSU culture and sensitivity.

Main differential diagnoses and typical outline evidence, etc.	
Acute bladder distension (due to prostatic hypertrophy in males)	*Suggested by:* suprapubic mass (cannot get below), dull to percussion.
	Confirmed by: **bladder US scan**, **urethral catheterization** and drainage of high volume of urine (e.g. >1L).
	Initial management: urethral or suprapubic catheter, treat underlying cause, e.g. α-blocker for prostatic hypertrophy, urology referral.
Cystitis	*Suggested by:* frequency of urine, dysuria, turbid urine, haematuria on 'dipstick'.
	Confirmed by: excess **WBC** and organisms on microscopy and growth of 'significant' bacterial colonies on **MSU culture**.
	Initial management: fluids to rehydrate (IV if vomiting), provisional antibiotics, e.g trimethoprim, pending sensitivities.

Localized tenderness in the right upper quadrant

Initial investigations (other tests in **bold** below): FBC, U&E, LFT, AXR.

Main differential diagnoses and typical outline evidence, etc.	
Acute cholecystitis	*Suggested by:* fever, guarding and +ve Murphy's sign (abrupt stopping of inspiration when the palpating hand meets the inflamed gallbladder descending with the liver from behind the subcostal margin on the right side—but not on the left side).
	Confirmed by: **US scan gallbladder and biliary ducts.**
	Initial management: nil by mouth, fluids IV, opioid analgesia, antibiotics IV, e.g. metronidazole + cephalosporin.
Acute alcoholic hepatitis	*Suggested by:* history of recent drinking binge, tender hepatomegaly, jaundice.
	Confirmed by: rise and fall in LFT to coincide with binge, –ve **hepatitis serology**.
	Initial management: stop alcohol, no specific treatment in mild illness, folate and thiamine supplements. If hepatic failure: monitor blood glucose, electrolytes, liver function and coagulation profile, IV infusion 5% dextrose (10% if ↓blood glucose), NG tube + nil by mouth, neomycin PO, lactulose, vitamin K IV.
Acute viral hepatitis A (or hepatitis B, C, D, or E)	*Suggested by:* –ve history of recent binge drinking, fever, tender hepatomegaly, jaundice.
	Confirmed by: +ve **hepatitis serology A, B C, D, or E.**
	Initial management: antipyretics, fluids IV, anti-emetics, colestyramine for severe pruritus. If hepatic failure: manage as in acute alcoholic hepatitis.
Acute liver congestion	*Suggested by:* tender hepatomegaly, ↑JVP, leg oedema.
	Confirmed by: **CXR** showing large heart, liver **US scan** showing distension.
	Initial management: salt and fluid restriction, furosemide IV or PO ± K⁺ supplement, treat underlying cause if possible.

Localized tenderness in the left upper quadrant

Initial investigations (other tests in **bold** below): FBC, U&E, LFT, AXR.

Main differential diagnoses and typical outline evidence, etc.	
Pyelonephritis	*Suggested by:* fever, rigor, vomiting, loin pain, tenderness at renal angle, ↑**WCC**, proteinuria, haematuria, leucocytes on **urine testing**.
	Confirmed by: above clinical picture and 'significant' growth of organisms on **urine culture**. US scan for possible anatomical abnormality.
	Initial management: fluids IV, anti-emetic; provisional antibiotics: ampicillin + gentamicin or 3rd generation cephalosporin, e.g. ceftriaxone.
Splenic rupture (?delayed)	*Suggested by:* history of trauma (road traffic accident, fall on to left chest wall), bruising over left chest wall or upper abdomen, falling BP, rising pulse, abdominal tenderess, diminished bowel sounds, plain AXR—loss of left psoas shadow, **peritoneal tap** demonstrates free blood.
	Confirmed by: CT scan appearance.
	Initial management: large bore IV access, group and crossmatch, fluids IV, colloid ± then blood. NG tube + nil by mouth, urethral catheter to monitor output, analgesics. Surgical referral for splenectomy etc.
Splenic infarct	*Suggested by:* presence of predisposing cause, especially sickle cell disease and crisis.
	Confirmed by: **CT abdomen**.
	Initial management: pain control with opioid analgesics or NSAIDs, surgical referral if abscess, haemorrhage, or pseudocyst develops.

Localized tenderness in the epigastrium or central abdomen

Initial investigations (other tests in **bold** below): FBC, U&E, LFT, AXR.

Main differential diagnoses and typical outline evidence, etc.	
Gastritis	*Suggested by:* epigastric pain, dull or burning discomfort, nocturnal pain.
	Confirmed by: **oesophagogastroscopy, barium meal,** *and* **pH study.**
	Initial management: antacids, H₂ blocker or PPI if symptoms persist.
DU	*Suggested by:* epigastric pain, dull or burning discomfort, typically relieved by food, nocturnal pain.
	Confirmed by: **oesophagogastroscopy, barium meal,** and **pH study.** *H. pylori* present in mucosa or **serology.**
	Initial management: antacids, H₂ blocker or PPI for 4wk; *H. pylori* eradication therapy if *H. pylori* +ve: two antibiotics + one PPI, e.g. omeprazole or lansoprazole + metronidazole or amoxicillin + clarithromycin.
GU	*Suggested by:* epigastric pain, dull or burning discomfort, typically exacerbated by food.
	Confirmed by: **oesophagogastroscopy, barium meal,** *and* **pH study.**
	Initial management: antacids, H₂ blocker or PPI for 8wk; *H. pylori* eradication therapy if *H. pylori* +ve (as for DU).
Pancreatitis	*Suggested by:* rigidity or guarding ± bruises, e.g. Cullen or Grey Turner's signs.
	Confirmed by: ↑↑ **serum amylase, CT pancreas** showing enlargement cyst/pseudocyst.
	Initial management: acute: pethidine, nil by mouth, fluids IV, monitor glucose and Ca²⁺, NG tube + nil by mouth if ileus, colloids and blood; chronic: analgesics, pancreatic supplements, monitor blood glucose—?onset diabetes.
Small bowel infarction	*Suggested by:* abdominal distension, absent bowel sounds. Predisposing cause, e.g. atrial fibrillation, extensive atheroma in diabetes.
	Confirmed by: **AXR** showing dilated loop of small bowel with valvulae conniventes but no large bowel (with haustra etc.).
	Initial management: fluids if hypovolaemia, analgesics, broad-spectrum antibiotics, surgical referral.

Ruptured or dissecting abdominal aortic aneurysm	*Suggested by:* hypotension and abdominal pain, tenderness and rigidity, bruises in and around the umbilicus (Cullen's sign), on one or both flanks (Grey Turner's sign). Expansile pulsatile mass >3cm diameter, bruit over the mass.
	Confirmed by: **abdominal US scan** or **CT abdomen.**
	Initial management: morphine, group and crossmatch, IV access, reduce systolic BP to 100–120mmHg with IV labetalol or propranolol ± nitroprusside, NG tube + nil by mouth, surgical referral.

Localized tenderness in the left or right loin

Initial investigations (other tests in **bold** below): FBC, U&E, LFT, AXR.

Main differential diagnoses and typical outline evidence, etc.	
Pyelonephritis	*Suggested by:* fever, rigor, vomiting, loin pain, tenderness at renal angle, ↑**WCC**, proteinuria, haematuria, leucocytes on **urine testing**.
	Confirmed by: clinical picture and 'significant' growth of organisms on **urine culture**. **US scan** for possible anatomical abnormality.
	Initial management: fluids IV, analgesics, anti-emetic; provisional antibiotics pending sensitivities: ampicillin + gentamicin or 3rd generation cephalosporin, e.g. ceftriaxone.
Renal calculus	*Suggested by:* colicky pain beginning in loin and radiating down to lower abdomen. Tenderness at renal angle.
	Confirmed by: haematuria, dilated ureter on **renal US scan**, filling defect on **IVU**.
	Initial management: IV access, opioid analgesics and anti-emetic, urology referral.
Ruptured or dissecting abdominal aortic aneurysm	*Suggested by:* hypotension and abdominal pain, tenderness and rigidity, bruises in and around the umbilicus (Cullen's sign), on one or both flanks (Grey Turner's sign). Expansile pulsatile mass >3cm diameter, bruit over the mass.
	Confirmed by: **abdominal US scan or CT abdomen.**
	Initial management: morphine, group and crossmatch, IV access, reduce systolic BP to 100–120mmHg with labetalol IV or propranolol ± nitroprusside, NG tube + nil by mouth, surgical referral.

Localized tenderness in left or right lower quadrant

Initial investigations (other tests in **bold** below): FBC, U&E, LFT, AXR.

Main differential diagnoses and typical outline evidence, etc.	
Appendicitis	*Suggested by:* abdominal pain, then localized to right lower quadrant (rarely to left in situs inversus), GUARDING +VE, +ve Rovsing's sign (tender on contralateral side), psoas sign (pain from passive extension of right hip), adductor pain (on passive internal rotation of flexed thigh); anterior tenderness on rectal exam.
	Confirmed by: macroscopic and microscopic appearances at **laparotomy**.
	Initial management: nil by mouth, fluids IV, NG tube + nil by mouth if vomiting, analgesics, broad-spectrum antibiotic, e.g. cephalosporin, surgical referral.
Diverticulitis	*Suggested by:* LIF tenderness ± tender mass.
	Confirmed by: **flexible sigmoidoscopy, barium enema**.
	Initial management: mild: clear liquids only, ciprofloxacin PO + metronidazole PO for >7d, then high-fibre diet. Severe: fluids IV, nil by mouth, paracetamol for fever, metronidazole IV + a 3rd generation cephalosporin or a fluoroquinolone.
Mesenteric adenitis (or NSAP)	*Suggested by:* RLQ pain, anorexia, fever.
	Confirmed by: diffuse RLQ tenderness, no guarding, no rebound, no right-sided rectal tenderness, self-limiting outcome.
	Initial management: analgesia.
Ectopic pregnancy	*Suggested by:* enlarged uterus (but often small for dates), vaginal bleeding, faintness/shock in acute rupture.
	Confirmed by: pregnancy test +ve, mass on bimanual examination. **Pelvic US scan** shows empty uterus with thickened decidua.
	Initial management: analgesics, fluid resuscitation if hypotension or shock, urgent referral for surgical therapy.

Hepatomegaly—smooth and tender

Initial investigations (other tests in **bold** below): FBC, coagulation profile, U&E, LFT, US scan.

Main differential diagnoses and typical outline evidence, etc.	
Alcoholic hepatitis	*Suggested by:* history of drinking binge, ↑MCV, jaundice.
	Confirmed by: abnormal **LFT**: ↑AST, ↑ALP, **liver biopsy** later.
	Initial management: no alcohol, folate and thiamine supplements, vitamin K IV if coagulopathy; if acute hepatic failure, monitor blood glucose, U&E, LFT, and coagulation profile. IV infusion 5% dextrose (10% if ↓blood glucose), NG tube + nil by mouth, neomycin PO, lactulose, vitamin K IV.
Infectious hepatitis	*Suggested by:* sharp edge, no or slight splenomegaly, jaundice.
	Confirmed by: abnormal LFT, hepatitis A serology +ve.
	Initial management: antipyretics, fluids IV and anti-emetics if vomiting, colestyramine for pruritus.
Glandular fever (infectious mononucleosis)	*Suggested by:* cervical lymphadenopathy, sharp edge ± splenomegaly ± jaundice.
	Confirmed by: **Paul–Bunnell**, +ve **heterophil antibody test**.
	Initial management: gargles/lozenges, analgesics, paracetamol; if neurological involvement, thrombocytopenia or haemolysis, no aspirin (causes Reye syndrome). Amoxicillin causes rash.
Right heart failure due to pulmonary hypertension, acutely due to pulmonary embolus	*Suggested by:* leg oedema, ↑JVP.
	Confirmed by: large heart on **CXR** and associated large pulmonary arteries or pulmonary oedema if congestive cardiac failure, **echocardiogram**—dilated right ventricle.
	Initial management: stop smoking, salt and fluid restriction, O2, furosemide IV or PO ± K+ supplement, treat underlying cause if possible.
Tricuspid regurgitation with right heart failure	*Suggested by:* pulsatile liver ± jaundice, ↑JVP with big V waves, systolic murmur louder on inspiration.
	Confirmed by: **echocardiogram**—dilated right ventricle.
	Initial management: bed rest during acute phase, stop smoking, salt and fluid restriction, give O_2, furosemide IV or PO ± K+ supplement, treat cause.

Hepatomegaly—smooth but not tender

Initial investigations (other tests in **bold** below): FBC, coagulation profile, U&E, LFT, US scan.

Main differential diagnoses and typical outline evidence, etc.	
Cirrhosis of the liver (early + fatty change)	*Suggested by:* firm, round edge ± splenomegaly, other stigmata of chronic liver disease (e.g. spider naevi). *Confirmed by:* small liver with abnormal parenchyma on **liver US scan and biopsy** appearance. *Initial management:* stop alcohol, treat cause.
Lymphoma (Hodgkin's or non-Hodgkin's)	*Suggested by:* generalized lymphadenopathy, non-tender hepatomegaly, splenomegaly. *Confirmed by:* **lymph node biopsy, bone marrow biopsy, CT thorax/abdomen.** *Initial management:* analgesics, transfusion if symptomatic anaemia, platelet transfusion if platelet count <20,000, broad-spectrum antibiotics IV if febrile and neutropaenia, referral for staging + chemotherapy ± radiotherapy.
Leukaemia	*Suggested by:* anaemia, lymphadenopathy, splenomegaly. *Confirmed by:* abnormal WBC on blood film, **bone marrow examination.** *Initial management:* analgesics, transfusion if symptomatic anaemia, platelet transfusion if platelet count <20,000, broad-spectrum antibiotics if fever and neutropaenia, paracetamol for fever. Referral to oncology management.
Haemochromatosis	*Suggested by:* bronze skin pigmentation, evidence of diabetes mellitus, cardiac failure, arthropathy. *Confirmed by:* ↑**serum ferritin** (>500mcg/L), **liver biopsy with hepatic iron measurement.** *Initial management:* regular venesection (prolongs life) e.g. 1 unit 1–2x per wk, then 1 unit per 3mo when serum iron and ferritin 'normal'.
1° biliary cirrhosis	*Suggested by:* xanthelasmata and xanthomas, scratch marks, arthralgia ± splenomegaly. *Confirmed by:* +ve **anti-mitochondrial antibody, ↑serum IgM, liver biopsy.** *Initial management:* no alcohol, colestyramine to relieve pruritus (or ursodeoxycholic acid).
Amyloidosis in kidneys or heart, nerves, gut, liver, 1° or 2° to rheumatoid, inflammatory bowel disease, TB, etc	*Suggested by:* evidence of underlying chronic infective or inflammatory disease if 2°. *Confirmed by:* **biopsy of rectal mucosa,** stained with Congo red dye. *Initial management:* identify organ failure and treat, including associated illness, e.g. chronic infection, chronic inflammation, or myeloma.

Hepatomegaly—irregular, not tender

Initial investigations (other tests in **bold** below): FBC, coagulation profile, U&E, LFT, US scan.

Main differential diagnoses and typical outline evidence, etc.	
Metastatic carcinoma	*Suggested by:* hard ± nodular liver, cachexia.
	Confirmed by: **liver US scan** *or* **CT** ± **biopsy**.
	Initial management: analgesics, packed cell transfusion if anaemia, hydration and bisphosphonate if hypercalcaemia, FFP and vitamin K for coagulopathy, nutritional support, treat primary if possible.
Hepatoma	*Suggested by:* firm, nodular edge ± arterial bruit, ↑serum alpha-fetoprotein.
	Confirmed by: ↑alpha-fetoprotein, **liver US scan** or CT *and* **biopsy**.
	Initial management: surgical referral, adjunct chemotherapy.
Hydatid cyst	*Suggested by:* sometimes hard, nodular.
	Confirmed by: **liver US scan** *or* **CT** showing cyst and daughter cysts inside, eosinophilia, **serology** (Echinococcus granulosus), **Casoni intradermal test**.
	Initial management: albendazole for six 1-mo cycles separated by 14-d interval, monitor FBC and LFT, surgical referral for resection of the cyst.

Splenomegaly—slight (<3 fingers)

Spleen enlarges diagonally downwards towards the RLQ. Begin there so as not to miss edge of massive enlargement. Initial investigations (other tests in **bold** below): FBC, coagulation profile, U&E, LFT, US scan.

Main differential diagnoses and typical outline evidence, etc.	
Glandular fever	*Suggested by:* cervical lymphadenopathy, hepatomegaly with sharp edge.
	Confirmed by: **Paul–Bunnell,** +ve **heterophil antibody test (Monospot®)**.
	Initial management: gargles/lozenges, analgesics, paracetamol; if neurological involvement, thrombocytopenia, or haemolysis, no aspirin (causes Reye syndrome), amoxicillin causes rash.
Brucella	*Suggested by:* occupation, e.g. farmer, hepatomegaly.
	Confirmed by: **brucella serology**.
	Initial management: doxycycline + rifampicin for 6wk or doxycycline + streptomycin IM for 3wk for osteomyelitis, meningitis, or endocarditis. Prednisolone if CNS is involved.
Hepatitis A, B, C, or D	*Suggested by:* jaundice, tender hepatomegaly, lymphadenopathy
	Confirmed by: abnormal **LFT, hepatitis A, B, C, and D serology**.
	Initial management: antipyretics, fluids IV and anti-emetics if vomiting, colestyramine for pruritus. In hepatic failure: monitor blood glucose, U&E, LFT, coagulation profile, IV infusion 5% dextrose (10% if ↓blood glucose), NG tube + nil by mouth, neomycin PO, lactulose, vitamin K IV.
Bacterial endocarditis	*Suggested by:* splinter haemorrhages, heart murmur, anaemia, microscopic haematuria.
	Confirmed by: **blood cultures, trans-oesophageal echocardiography**.
	Initial management: antibiotics depends on organism and sensitivities, valve surgery.
Amyloidosis in kidneys or heart, nerves, gut, liver, 1° or 2° to rheumatoid, inflammatory bowel disease, TB, etc.	*Suggested by:* evidence of underlying chronic infective or inflammatory disease if 2°.
	Confirmed by: **biopsy of rectal mucosa,** stained with Congo red dye.
	Initial management: identify organ failure and treat, including associated illness, e.g. chronic infection, chronic inflammation or myeloma.

Haemolytic anaemia	*Suggested by:* anaemia, jaundice.
	Confirmed by: FBC showing reticulocytosis, anaemia, **LFT** showing ↑unconjugated bilirubin, ↓haptoglobin.
	Initial management: avoid fava beans in G6PD deficiency ± blood transfusion; surgical referral if splenectomy. Immunization against *H. influenza* and *S. pneumoniae* procedure.

Splenomegaly—moderate (3–5 fingers)

Initial investigations (other tests in **bold** below): FBC, coagulation profile, U&E, LFT, US scan.

Main differential diagnoses and typical outline evidence, etc.	
Lymphoma (Hodgkin's or non-Hodgkin's)	*Suggested by:* generalized lymphadenopathy, non-tender hepatomegaly, splenomegaly.
	Confirmed by: **lymph node biopsy, bone marrow biopsy, CT thorax/abdomen.**
	Initial management: analgesics, transfusion if symptomatic anaemia, platelet transfusion if platelet count <20,000, broad-spectrum antibiotics IV if febrile and neutropaenia, referral for staging + chemotherapy ± radiotherapy.
Chronic leukaemia	*Suggested by:* lymphadenopathy, non-tender hepatomegaly.
	Confirmed by: abnormal FBC and blood film, **bone marrow examination.**
	Initial management: supportive therapy includes analgesics, blood transfusion if symptomatic anaemia, platelet transfusion if platelet count <20,000, broad-spectrum antibiotics IV if febrile and neutropaenia, referral for oncology management.
Cirrhosis ± portal hyper-tension	*Suggested by:* hard, round edge ± hepatomegaly, other stigmata of chronic liver disease.
	Confirmed by: small nodular **liver** on **US scan** ± **biopsy.**
	Initial management: no alcohol, propranolol if portal hypertension, treat underlying cause.

Splenomegaly—massive (>5 fingers)

Spleen enlarges diagonally downwards towards the RLQ. Begin there so as not to miss edge of massive enlargement. Initial investigations (other tests in **bold** below): FBC, coagulation profile, U&E, LFT, US scan.

Main differential diagnoses and typical outline evidence, etc.	
Chronic myeloid leukaemia	*Suggested by:* variable hepatomegaly, bruising, anaemia.
	Confirmed by: presence of **Philadelphia chromosome, ↑↑WCC.**
	Initial management: hydration, avoid antiplatelets, e.g aspirin, packed cell transfusion if symptomatic anaemia, platelet transfusion if platelet count <20,000, broad-spectrum antibiotics IV covering *Pseudomonas* and Gram +ve bacteria if febrile and neutropaenic. Referral for specialist treatment—hydroxycarbamide to control WBC, imatinib 1st line therapy ± bone marrow transplant.
Myelofibrosis	*Suggested by:* anaemia ± **hepatomegaly ± lymphadenopathy.**
	Confirmed by: **bone marrow tap** is usually dry, **bone marrow biopsy** shows fibrosis.
	Initial management: analgesics, blood transfusion if symptomatic anaemia, platelet transfusion if platelet count <20,000, broad-spectrum antibiotics IV if febrile and neutropaenia, referral for specialist treatment.
Malaria	*Suggested by:* anaemia, jaundice, hepatomegaly, paroxysmal rigors.
	Confirmed by: **thick and thin blood films** showing *Plasmodium.*
	Initial management: paracetamol for fever, transfusion for severe anaemia. Antimalarials: chloroquine for *P. vivax, P. ovale, P. malariae,* add primaquine for *P. vivax* and *P. ovale* hepatic phase; mefloquine or pyrimethamine/sulfadoxine if chloroquine resistant; quinine for *P. falciparum,* quinine IV if very ill.
Kala-azar (visceral leish-maniasis)	*Suggested by:* pancytopaenia, hepatomegaly.
	Confirmed by: demonstration of *Leishmania donovani* in **Giemsa-stained smears,** specific **serological test.**
	Initial management: transfusion for bleeding or anaemia, antibiotics for intercurrent infection; specific drugs: pentavalent antimonial compound, e.g. sodium stibogluconate or meglumine antimoniate; or for liposomal form: amphotericin B.

Bilateral masses in upper abdomen

The lower half of normal right kidney is often palpable. A renal mass is bimanually ballotable, moves slightly downwards on inspiration. Initial investigations (other tests in **bold** below): FBC, U&E, LFT, US scan.

Main differential diagnoses and typical outline evidence, etc.	
Polycystic renal disease	*Suggested by:* masses are bimanually ballotable, hypertension. *Confirmed by:* **US scan/CT kidneys.** *Initial management:* keep BP <130/85 (125/75 if proteinuria is present) with ACE inhibitors or angiotensin receptor blockers, monitor renal function and renal US scan yearly, treat UTI, analgesics (avoid NSAIDs), dialysis if end-stage renal failure develops.
Bilateral hydronephroses	*Suggested by:* masses bimanually ballotable, renal impairment. *Confirmed by:* dilated ureters ± renal calyces on **abdominal US scan.** *Initial management:* analgesics, treat infection, urinary catheter if lower tract obstruction, urology referral.
Amyloidosis in kidneys or heart, nerves, gut, liver, 1° or 2° to rheumatoid, inflammatory bowel disease, TB, etc	*Suggested by:* evidence of underlying chronic infective or inflammatory disease if 2°. *Confirmed by:* **biopsy of rectal mucosa,** stained with Congo red dye. *Initial management:* identify organ failure and treat, incuding associated illness, e.g. chronic infection, chronic inflammation, or myeloma.

Unilateral mass in right or left upper quadrant

Initial investigations (other tests in **bold** below): FBC, U&E, LFT, US scan.

Main differential diagnoses and typical outline evidence, etc.	
Renal carcinoma	*Suggested by:* haematuria, pyrexia of unknown origin (PUO) ± polycythaemia.
	Confirmed by: **renal US scan/CT with biopsy.**
	Initial management: surgical referral.
Unilateral hydronephrosis	*Suggested by:* no other symptoms and signs except bimanually ballotable mass.
	Confirmed by: unilateral dilated ureter ± renal calyx on **abdominal US scan.**
	Initial management: referral to urologist for insertion of nephrostomy tube or ureteric stent.
Renal cyst	*Suggested by:* tense, fluctuant feel.
	Confirmed by: cyst on **abdominal US scan.**
	Initial management: antibiotic if UTI is present.
Distended gallbladder (on right side)	*Suggested by:* right-sided, pear-shaped rounded mass that continues with the liver above (Courvoisier's sign—implies extrahepatic biliary obstruction).
	Confirmed by: **US scan gallbladder and biliary ducts.**
	Initial management: analgesics, fluids IV, NG drainage, broad-spectrum antibiotics, surgical referral.

Mass in epigastrium (± umbilical area)

Initial investigations (other tests in **bold** below): FBC, U&E, LFT, US scan.

Main differential diagnoses and typical outline evidence, etc.	
Gastric carcinoma	*Suggested by:* anorexia, weight loss over weeks to months, hard, irregular mass, left supraclavicular node (Virchow's node giving Troisier's sign). *Confirmed by:* **gastroscopy with biopsy**. *Initial management:* NG tube, nil by mouth, fluids IV, analgesics, surgical referral.
Carcinoma of pancreas	*Suggested by:* progressive painless jaundice ± abdominal or back pain later. *Confirmed by:* **ERCP** or **MRCP**. *Initial management:* low-fat and high-protein diet, analgesics, pancreatic supplement, phenothiazine or cholestyramine to reduce pruritus; surgical referral.
Aortic aneurysm	*Suggested by:* >3cm in diameter, pulsatile swelling with bruit. *Confirmed by:* **abdominal US scan** or **CT abdomen**. *Initial management:* BP control, surgical referral.

Mass in right lower quadrant

Initial investigations (other tests in **bold** below): FBC, U&E, LFT, US scan.

Main differential diagnoses and typical outline evidence, etc.	
Appendix mass	*Suggested by:* recent history of fever and right iliac fossa (RIF) pain.
	Confirmed by: **US scan** or **CT abdomen** *and finding at* **laparotomy**.
	Initial management: fluids IV, NG tube + nil by mouth and suction if ileus, broad-spectrum antibiotic, surgical referral.
Crohn's granuloma	*Suggested by:* aphthous ulcers, wasting, anaemia, tender mass, scars of previous surgery, anal fissures, fistulae.
	Confirmed by: **barium follow-through** and **small bowel enema, colonoscopy with biopsy**.
	Initial management: analgesics, haematinics, nutritional support.
Carcinoma of caecum	*Suggested by:* asymptomatic right iliac fossa mass, iron-deficiency anaemia.
	Confirmed by: **colonoscopy with biopsy**.
	Initial management: iron supplement, transfusion if severe anaemia; fluids IV, nil by mouth, NG tube + nil by mouth if bowel obstruction is present; surgical referral.
Transplanted kidney	*Suggested by:* obvious history of transplant and scar over mass, usually in iliac fossa.
	Confirmed by: **abdominal US scan**.
Other causes	Intussusception, carcinoma of ascending colon, caecal volvulus.

Mass in hypogastrium (suprapubic region)

Initial investigations (other tests in **bold** below): FBC, U&E, LFT, US scan.

Main differential diagnoses and typical outline evidence, etc.	
Distended bladder	*Suggested by:* suprapubic dullness, resonance in flank, tender mass and acute retention of urine.
	Confirmed by: mass disappears on **bladder US scan** *and* **catheterization, abdominal/pelvic US scan.**
	Initial management: urethral or suprapubic catheter to relieve retention, treat cause or urology referral.
Pregnant uterus	*Suggested by:* suprapubic dullness, resonance in flank.
	Confirmed by: **pregnancy test** +ve, bimanual examination, **abdominal/pelvic US scan.**
	Initial management: antenatal clinic referral.
Uterine fibroid	*Suggested by:* asymptomatic, hard, rounded, non-tender mass on bimanual palpation.
	Confirmed by: **pelvic examination and US scan.**
	Initial management: analgesia, gynae referral.
Uterine neoplasm	*Suggested by:* postmenopausal bleeding, bloodstained vaginal discharge, irregular bleeding.
	Confirmed by: pelvic examination *and* **pelvic US scan.**
	Initial management: gynae referral.
Ovarian cyst	*Suggested by:* tense, fluctuant feel, fluid thrill if cyst is large.
	Confirmed by: pelvic examination and **US scan of ovary.**
	Initial management: analgesia, gynae referral.

Mass in left lower quadrant

Initial investigations (other tests in **bold** below): FBC, U&E, LFT, US scan.

Main differential diagnoses and typical outline evidence, etc.	
Diverticular abscess	*Suggested by:* fever, tender mass.
	Confirmed by: **US scan/CT abdomen/pelvis**.
	Initial management: fluids IV, nil by mouth, paracetamol for pain and fever, antibiotics, e.g. metronidazole IV + a 3rd generation cephalosporin or a fluoroquinolone.
Carcinoma of descending or sigmoid colon	*Suggested by:* hard mass, not tender.
	Confirmed by: **barium enema, colonoscopy with biopsy**.
	Initial management: NG tube + nil by mouth with suction if obstructed, fluids IV, monitor intake and output, preop antibiotics; surgical referral.
Faecal impaction	*Suggested by:* paucity of bowel movement and constipation. **AXR** shows stippled pattern of 'faecal loading'.
	Confirmed by: resolution of swelling with evacuation or partly with flatus tube.
	Initial management: laxatives, enemas ± digital disimpaction.

Central dullness, resonance in flank

Initial investigations (other tests in **bold** below): FBC, U&E, LFT, US scan.

Main differential diagnoses and typical outline evidence, etc.	
Distended bladder	*Suggested by:* suprapubic mass, tender in acute retention of urine.
	Confirmed by: mass disappears on **bladder US scan and catheterization**.
	Initial management: urethral or suprapubic catheter to relieve retention, α-blocker for prostatism, treat cause, urology referral.
Pregnant uterus	*Suggested by:* suprapubic mass.
	Confirmed by: **pregnancy test** +ve, pelvic/**abdominal US scan**.
	Initial management: arrange antenatal clinic referral.
Massive ovarian cyst	*Suggested by:* tense, fluctuant feel, fluid thrill.
	Confirmed by: **pelvic/abdominal US scan**.
	Initial management: analgesia, gynae referral.

Shifting dullness

Implies ascites. Initial investigations (other tests in **bold** below): FBC, U&E, LFT, US scan.

Main differential diagnoses and typical outline evidence, etc.	
Carcinomatosis with spread to peritoneum	*Suggested by:* cachexia. *Confirmed by:* **diagnostic paracentesis** including **cytology, liver US scan with biopsy.** *Initial management:* analgesia, paracentesis if massive ascites, packed cells if anaemia, hydration, FFP and vitamin K for coagulopathy, nutritional support, look for 1°.
Cirrhosis	*Suggested by:* stigmata of chronic liver disease ± splenomegaly. *Confirmed by:* **paracentesis, liver US scan with biopsy.** *Initial management:* no alcohol, propranolol if portal hypertension, paracentesis if massive ascites, spironolactone PO ± furosemide PO, treat underlying cause.
Congestive cardiac failure	*Suggested by:* ↑JVP, leg oedema ± tender hepatomegaly. *Confirmed by:* **LFT**, FBC, **diagnostic paracentesis, CXR, echocardiogram.** *Initial management:* salt and fluid restriction, O$_2$, furosemide IV or PO ± K$^+$ supplement, spironolactone PO, look for cause.
Nephrotic syndrome	*Suggested by:* generalized oedema, including face on rising from bed. *Confirmed by:* **proteinuria, hypoalbuminaemia.** *Initial management:* monitor BP, intake and output, fluid restriction to 1L/d, furosemide IV, monitor renal function; low protein, phosphate, and potassium diet; ACE inhibitor if hypertension. Establish cause, e.g. if glomerulonephritis, consider prednisolone.

Silent abdomen with no bowel sounds

Initial investigations (other tests in **bold** below): FBC, U&E, LFT, AXR.

Main differential diagnoses and typical outline evidence, etc.	
Peritonitis e.g. due to bowel perforation	*Suggested by:* decreased or absent abdominal movement, generalized tenderness with 'board-like' rigidity.
	Confirmed by: **AXR**, erect **CXR** shows gas under diaphragm.
	Initial management: analgesia, fluids IV, NG tube + nil by mouth if ileus, broad-spectrum antibiotics—e.g. 2nd or 3rd generation cephalosporin or quinolone ± metronidazole. Surgical referral for repair of perforation.
Bowel infarction due to embolus, e.g. from fibrillating atrium or atheroma, e.g. in diabetic	*Suggested by:* decreased or absent abdominal movement, generalized tenderness with 'board-like' rigidity.
	Confirmed by: **AXR**, erect **CXR** shows no gas under diaphragm.
	Initial management: fluids if hypovolaemia, analgesia, broad-spectrum anibiotics. Surgical referral for possible resection of infarcted bowel.

High-pitched bowel sounds

Initial investigations (other tests in **bold** below): FBC, U&E, LFT, AXR.

Main differential diagnoses and typical outline evidence, etc.	
Small bowel obstruction	*Suggested by:* mild distension, early vomiting, central/upper abdominal pain, resonant percussion, increased bowel sounds. Supine AXR showing central gas but no peripheral abdominal large bowel shadow (i.e. without haustra partly crossing) but valvulae conniventes of small intestine entirely crossing the lumen. Fluid levels on erect film.
	Confirmed by: **abdominal US scan and laparotomy** findings.
	Initial management: NG tube + nil by mouth, fluids IV, surgical referral for initial defunctioning ileostomy.
Large bowel obstruction	*Suggested by:* severe distension, late vomiting, resonant percussion, increased bowel sounds. Supine AXR showing peripheral abdominal large bowel shadow (with haustra partly crossing the lumen). Fluid levels on erect film.
	Confirmed by: **abdominal US scan and laparotomy** findings.
	Initial management: NG tube + suction, nil by mouth, fluids IV, monitor intake and output, preop antibiotics, surgical referral for initial defunctioning colostomy.
Hernial orifice strangulation	*Suggested by:* hernia visible, not reducible, very ill, peritonism, **signs of bowel obstruction**.
	Confirmed by: **laparotomy** findings.
	Initial management: NG tube with suction, fluids IV, monitor intake and output, preop antibiotics, surgical referral.
Sigmoid volvulus	*Suggested by:* **signs of severe bowel obstruction**. Supine AXR showing U-shaped gas shadow.
	Confirmed by: **sigmoidoscopy** and **reduction with flatus tube** and **laparotomy** findings.
	Initial management: analgesia, fluids IV, NG tube + nil by mouth; rigid sigmoidoscopic decompression, surgical referral for laparotomy and resection if gangrenous segment.
Irritable bowel syndrome	*Suggested by:* slight distension, history of abdominal pain and small hard motions.
	Confirmed by: abdominal US scan and spontaneous resolution.
	Initial management: high-fibre diet; symptomatic treatment, e.g. metoclopramide, mebeverine, loperamide, lactulose; reassurance.
Faecal impaction	*Suggested by:* paucity of bowel movement and constipation. Hard faeces on rectal examination. **AXR** shows stippled pattern of 'faecal loading'.
	Confirmed by: resolution of swelling with evacuation or partly with flatus tube.
	Initial management: laxatives and enemas ± digital disimpaction.

Abdominal/loin bruit

Initial investigations (other tests in **bold** below): FBC, U&E, LFT, US.

Main differential diagnoses and typical outline evidence, etc.	
Aortic aneurysm	*Suggested by:* systolic bruit in the epigastrium (over mass), expansile pulsatile swelling.
	Confirmed by: **US scan/CT abdomen.**
	Initial management: BP control, referral for surgical repair.
Renal artery stenosis	*Suggested by:* systolic bruit in the RUQ, hypertension.
	Confirmed by: **renal arteriography—spiral CT or MR angiography.**
	Initial management: BP control (ACE inhibitors contraindicated), refer for renal angioplasty ± stenting.
Dissecting aorta	*Suggested by:* tearing abdominal pain radiating to back, hypertension (severe hypotension is a grave prognostic indicator). Brachial–ankle gradient and pulse delay.
	Confirmed by: urgent **US scan/CT abdomen.**
	Initial management: BP control with oral propranolol, or labetalol IV, or sodium nitroprusside IV; surgical referral.

Lump in the groin

Initial investigations (other tests in **bold** below): FBC, U&E, LFT, US scan.

Main differential diagnoses and typical outline evidence, etc.	
Lymph node inflammation	*Suggested by:* enlarged, tender, mobile, nodes, usually multiple.
	Confirmed by: above clinical examination.
	Initial management: analgesics, treat underlying cause.
Inguinal hernia	*Suggested by:* origin horizontally just above and medial to pubic tubercle, impulse on coughing or bearing down, reducible.
	Confirmed by: above clinical examination and surgery.
	Initial management: surgical referral for herniorrhaphy.
Femoral hernia	*Suggested by:* origin horizontally just below and lateral to pubic tubercle, cough impulse rarely detectable, usually irreducible (because of narrow femoral canal).
	Confirmed by: above clinical examination and surgery.
	Initial management: surgical referral for hernia repair.
Strangulated hernia	*Suggested by:* irreducible, tense and tender, red, followed by symptoms and signs of bowel obstruction.
	Confirmed by: above clinical examination and surgery.
	Initial management: analgesia, fluids IV, nil by mouth and NG tube + nil by mouth if obstruction, urgent surgical referral.
Lymphoma (Hodgkin's or non-Hodgkin's)	*Suggested by:* fixed nodes when infiltrated by tumour.
	Confirmed by: **US scan, exploration of groin.**
	Initial management: analgesics, transfusion if symptomatic anaemia, platelet transfusion if platelet count <20,000, broad-spectrum antibiotics IV if febrile and neutropaenia, referral for staging + chemotherapy ± radiotherapy.
Femoral artery aneurysm	*Suggested by:* lump lies below the midpoint of the inguinal ligament, expansile pulsation.
	Confirmed by: above clinical examination. **Duplex US scan.**
	Initial management: surgical referral for elective repair or reconstruction.
Saphena varix (dilatation of long saphen-ous vein in the groin)	*Suggested by:* soft and diffuse swelling that lies below inguinal ligament, empties with minimal pressure and refills on release, disappears on lying down, cough impulse.
	Confirmed by: above clinical examination.
	Initial management: avoid prolonged standing, avoid wearing anything which constricts the limb, treat complications, e.g. phlebitis, ulceration, etc; treat underlying cause.
Cold abscess of psoas sheath	*Suggested by:* fluctuant, tender swelling arising below the inguinal ligament.
	Confirmed by: **US scan, exploration of groin.**
	Initial management: surgical referral for drainage or by CT guided percutaneous catheter, followed by antibiotics.
Also	Sebaceous cyst, local abscess, retractile testicle, lipoma, etc.

Scrotal swelling

Initial investigations (other tests in **bold** below): FBC, U&E, LFT, US scan.

Main differential diagnoses and typical outline evidence, etc.	
Inguinal hernia descended into scrotum	*Suggested by:* inability to get above it. Does not transilluminate.
	Confirmed by: above clinical examination.
	Initial management: surgical referral for hernia repair.
Hydrocoele	*Suggested by:* non-tender, unilateral mass in scrotal sac.
	Confirmed by: above clinical and demonstration of transillumination.
	Initial management: surgical referral if it gets larger and causes discomfort.
Epididymal cyst	*Suggested by:* non-tender nodule in the head of epididymis, adjacent to inferior pole of testis and transillumination.
	Confirmed by: above clinical examination and demonstration of transillumination.
	Initial management: surgical referral for spermatocoelectomy if large or enlarges or causes discomfort.
Testicular torsion	*Suggested by:* exquisitely tender, unilateral mass in the scrotal sac, cord thickened, opposite testis lies horizontally (bell clapper testis).
	Confirmed by: above clinical examination, **US scan** reveals ↓blood flow.
	Initial management: emergency! Skilled manual detorsion of testicle immediately.
Haematocoele	*Suggested by:* history of trauma or scrotal surgery. Tenderness.
	Confirmed by: above history and examination, US scan.
	Initial management: surgical referral for exploration and evacuation of haematoma.
Varicocoele (90% on the left)	*Suggested by:* non-tender, unilateral fleshy mass that feels like a bag of worms, decreases in size with scrotal elevation.
	Confirmed by: above clinical examination (patient must be examined while standing).
	Initial management: scrotal support ± surgical referral for varicocoelectomy.
Acute epididymitis	*Suggested by:* diffuse tenderness in the epididymis, marked redness and oedema.
	Confirmed by: **urine microscopy and culture** (white cells and organisms).
	Initial management: elevation of scrotum, cold packs to the scrotum regularly, analgesia, antibiotic, e.g. doxycycline or a cephalosporin.

Acute orchitis	*Suggested by:* large and tender testes, fever.
	Confirmed by: above history and examination.
	Initial management: elevation of scrotum, cold packs for comfort, analgesia, e.g. NSAIDs or opiate, oral antibiotics, e.g. ciprofloxacin or a cephalosporin.
Chronic epididymitis	*Suggested by:* chronic, diffuse scrotal tenderness.
	Confirmed by: identification of infecting organism by **urine cultures or culture of urethral discharge** after prostatic massage.
	Initial management: analgesia, e.g. NSAIDs, antibiotics, e.g. doxycycline or a cephalosporin ± epididymectomy.
Spermatocoele	*Suggested by:* non-tender, small nodules posterior to the head of the epididymis.
	Confirmed by: above clinical examination, may or may not transilluminate.
	Initial management: surgical referral for spermatocoelectomy if enlarging or causes discomfort.
Seminoma	*Suggested by:* firm, non-tender, non-transilluminable nodule or mass adjacent to a testis.
	Confirmed by: **US scan of scrotal contents** showing a solid testicular mass, **direct surgical examination**, normal **serum alpha-fetoprotein**.
	Initial management: referral for radiotherapy ± chemotherapy and orchidectomy.
Teratoma	*Suggested by:* firm, non-tender, non-transilluminable nodule or mass adjacent to a testis.
	Confirmed by: **US scan of scrotal contents** showing a solid testicular mass, **direct surgical examination**, ↑*serum* alpha-fetoprotein.
	Initial management: surgical referral for resection, followed by chemotherapy.

Anal swelling

The rectal examination (with a chaperone) begins with an examination of the anus by parting the buttocks with the patient lying in the left lateral position with knees flexed. Initial investigations (other tests in **bold** below): FBC, U&E, LFT.

Main differential diagnoses and typical outline evidence, etc.	
Prolapsed internal haemorrhoids	*Suggested by:* segmental, plum-coloured rectal protrusion.
	Confirmed by: proctoscopy.
	Initial management: high-fibre diet, hydrocortisone suppositories for pruritus, surgical referral.
Acute anal fissure	*Suggested by:* acute pain during defaecation, exquisite anal tenderness. Mucosal fissure with skin tag if chronic (sentinel pile).
	Confirmed by: above history and clinical **examination under anaesthesia.**
	Initial management: high-fibre diet, stool softeners, warm sitz baths, analgesic cream, nitroglycerin ointment, oral or topical diltiazem, botulinum toxin injection near to the fissures, surgical referral for sphincterotomy if medical therapy fails.
Spontaneous perianal haematoma	*Suggested by:* blue-black lump in the skin near the anal margin.
	Confirmed by: above history and examination.
	Initial management: ice or cold packs.
Perianal abscess	*Suggested by:* tender, fluctuant, perianal mass.
	Confirmed by: above clinical examination.
	Initial management: analgesics, paracetamol for fever, surgical referral for incision and drainage of abscess.
Rectal prolapse	*Suggested by:* smooth, elongated, rectal protrusion continuous with anal skin.
	Confirmed by: above clinical examination.
	Initial management: local perianal analgesia, reduction with digital pressure, treat constipation.

Enlargement of prostate

The rectal examination continues by feeling for a prostatic protrusion anteriorly and sweeping around for other masses including impacted faeces. Initial investigations (other tests in **bold** below): FBC, U&E, LFT.

Main differential diagnoses and typical outline evidence, etc.	
Prostatitis	*Suggested by:* smooth, enlarged and tender.
	Confirmed by: +ve **urine culture, culture of prostatic secretions.**
	Initial management: fluids IV if vomiting and dehydration, analgesia, e.g. NSAIDs, stool softener, antibiotics, e.g. cephalosporins.
Benign prostatic hypertrophy	*Suggested by:* smooth, enlarged, firm, non-tender usually with a palpable median groove.
	Confirmed by: normal or slightly ↑**serum prostatic-specific antigen (PSA), prostatic biopsy.**
	Initial management: ↓fluid intake before bedtime, α-blocker, e.g. terazosin, alfuzosin to relieve symptoms, 5-α-reductase inhibitor, e.g. finasteride, dutasteride, urology referral if severe symptoms.
Prostatic carcinoma	*Suggested by:* irregular, hard, sometimes obliteration of median groove, non-tender.
	Confirmed by: ↑↑**serum PSA, prostatic biopsy.**
	Initial management: supportive therapy, consult urologist.

Melaena on finger

The rectal examination ends by inspecting the faecal smear on the examining gloved finger for colour, especially bright red blood or tarry melaena. Initial investigations (other tests in **bold** below): FBC, U&E, LFT.

Main differential diagnoses and typical outline evidence, etc.	
Bleeding DU	*Suggested by:* epigastric pain and tenderness, nausea.
	Confirmed by: **oesophagogastroscopy** showing bleeding ulcer.
	Initial management: large bore IV or central line, fluids IV, colloid initially ± transfusion, CVP monitoring, NG tube + nil by mouth + irrigation, urinary catheter to monitor output, surgical referral. H_2 blocker or PPI for 4wk; *H. pylori* eradication therapy if *H. pylori* +ve.
Bleeding GU	*Suggested by:* epigastric pain, dull or burning discomfort, nocturnal pain.
	Confirmed by: appearance of ulcer on **oesophagogastroscopy** and **pH study** showing hyperacidity.
	Initial management: treat acute severe bleed as DU; antacid; H_2 blocker or PPI for 8wk; *H. pylori* eradication therapy if *H. pylori* +ve.
Gastric erosion	*Suggested by:* history of NSAIDs or alcohol ingestion, epigastric pain, dull or burning discomfort, nocturnal pain.
	Confirmed by: appearance of erosion on **oesophagogastroscopy** and **pH study** showing hyperacidity.
	Initial management: treat acute bleed as DU; stop aspirin, NSAIDs, alcohol; antacids, H_2 blocker or PPI.
Oesophageal varices	*Suggested by:* liver cirrhosis, splenomegaly, prominent upper abdominal veins.
	Confirmed by: **oesophagogastroscopy** showing varicose mucosa and blood, distally and in stomach.
	Initial management: if bleeding stopped, propranolol or long-acting nitrate. Still bleeding: large bore IV or central line, fluids IV (colloid initially) ± transfusion, CVP monitoring, NG tube + nil by mouth + irrigation, urinary catheter to monitor output, correct coagulopathy with FFP and vitamin K IV. Surgical or gastro referral for banding or sclerotherapy.
Mallory–Weiss tear	*Suggested by:* preceding marked vomiting, later bright red blood.
	Confirmed by: **oesophagogastroscopy** showing tear.
	Initial management: monitor vital signs, Hb, fluids IV, nil by mouth, surgical referral if persistent bleeding requiring blood transfusion, treat underlying cause.

Oesophageal carcinoma	*Suggested by:* progressive dysphagia with solids which sticks, weight loss.
	Confirmed by: **barium swallow, fibreoptic gastroscopy with mucosal biopsy** showing malignant tissue.
	Initial management: treat severe bleed as DU. Nil by mouth, fluids IV, analgesics ± blood transfusion if bleeding continues ± antibiotic prophylaxis, surgical referral for oesophageal dilatation or stent insertion by endoscopy.
Gastric carcinoma	*Suggested by:* marked anorexia, fullness, pain, Troisier's sign (enlarged left supraclavicular lymph (Virchow's) node).
	Confirmed by: **oesophagogastroscopy with biopsy** showing malignant tissue.
	Initial management: NG tube + nil by mouth, fluids IV, analgesics ± transfusion, treat severe bleed as DU, surgical referral.
Gastro-oesophageal reflux	*Suggested by:* heartburn worse when lying flat, anorexia, nausea ± regurgitation of gastric content.
	Confirmed by: appearance of erosion on **oesophagoscopy, barium meal**, and **pH study** showing ↑acidity.
	Initial management: treat severe bleed as in DU. Small meals, no food before bed, raise head of bed, antacids; moderate to severe: nil by mouth, fluids IV, H_2 blocker or PPI, antibiotics to eradicate *H. pylori* if ulceration.
Hiatus hernia	*Suggested by:* heartburn, worse with stooping, relieved by antacids.
	Confirmed by: herniation of stomach into chest on plain X-ray or barium meal, appearance of erosion on **oesophagoscopy** and **pH study** showing hyperacidity.
	Initial management: treat severe bleed as DU. Reduce weight, avoid stooping, semi-sitting position for sleep, correct constipation, antacids or H_2 blockers for pain.
Ingestion of corrosives	*Suggested by:* history of ingestion, etc.
	Confirmed by: **oesophagogastroscopy** showing severe erosions.
	Initial management: removal of offending agent, fluids IV ± blood transfusion if hypotension or bleeding, laryngoscopy ± tracheostomy if respiratory distress; broad-spectrum antibiotics if infection, steroids to reduce stricture formation.
Meckel's diverticulum	*Suggested by:* no haematemesis, usually asymptomatic, anaemia, rectal bleeding.
	Confirmed by: **technetium-labelled red blood cell scan**, showing isotopes in gut lumen and laparotomy.
	Initial management: fluids IV, nil by mouth ± NG tube, transfusion if significant bleeding, surgical referral.

(Continued)

Melaena on finger *(continued)*

Main differential diagnoses and typical outline evidence, etc. *(continued)*

False haematemesis	*Suggested by:* swallowed nose bleed or haemoptysis.
	Confirmed by: normal **oesophagogastroscopy** and **bleeding source** identified in nose.
	Initial management: treat underlying cause.
Bleeding diathesis	*Suggested by:* symptoms or signs of bleeding elsewhere (or bruising), drug history of warfarin, etc.
	Confirmed by: abnormal clotting screen and/or low platelets and/or improvement on withdrawal of a potentially causal drug (NB. Possibility of another cause).
	Initial management: discontinue warfarin, treat underlying cause.
Also	Angiodysplasia.

Fresh blood on finger on rectal examination

Usually suggestive of lower GI bleeding, but occasionally from massive upper GI bleeding passing through rapidly without alteration. Initial investigations (other tests in **bold** below): FBC, U&E, LFT.

Main differential diagnoses and typical outline evidence, etc.

Haemorrhoids	*Suggested by:* rectal bleeding follows defaecation, perianal protrusion with pain.
	Confirmed by: anal inspection and **proctoscopy** (haemorrhoids drop over edge of proctoscope as it is withdrawn).
	Initial management: high-fibre diet, hydrocortisone suppositories for pruritus ± surgical referral.
Rectal carcinoma	*Suggested by:* rectal bleeding with defaecation, blood often limited to surface of stool.
	Confirmed by: **sigmoidoscopy with rectal biopsy.**
	Initial management: surgical referral for resection.
Colonic carcinoma	*Suggested by:* alternate diarrhoea and constipation with red blood.
	Confirmed by: **colonoscopy with biopsy, barium enema**.
	Initial management: surgical referral.
Ulcerative colitis	*Suggested by:* loose bloodstained stools, anaemia ± arthropathy, uveitis, and iritis.
	Confirmed by: **colonoscopy with biopsy, barium studies.**
	Initial management: mild: prednisolone PO and mesalazine ± prednisolone enemas. Moderate: prednisolone + 5-ASA ± prednisolone enemas. Severe: fluids IV + hydrocortisone, antibiotics, NG tube + nil by mouth, transfusion if severe anaemia, surgical referral if toxic megacolon.
Angiodysplasia	*Suggested by:* chronic recurrent GI bleeding.
	Confirmed by: **endoscopy, mesenteric angiography**.
	Initial management: fluids IV ± blood transfusion if symptomatic anaemia, correct coagulopathy, surgical referral.
Diverticulitis	*Suggested by:* history of red 'splash' in the toilet pan, LIF tenderness ± tender mass.
	Confirmed by: **flexible sigmoidoscopy, barium enema**.
	Initial management: fluids IV, nil by mouth, transfusion if significant bleeding occurs, surgical referral.
Ischaemic colitis	*Suggested by:* left-sided abdominal pain, loose stools, dark clots.
	Confirmed by: **barium enema** (may show 'thumb printing' sign), **colonoscopy**.
	Initial management: analgesia, fluids IV, nil by mouth, O2, NG tube + nil by mouth if ileus ± broad-spectrum antibiotics. Surgical referral.

Meckel's diverticulum	*Suggested by:* usually asymptomatic, anaemia, rectal bleeding.
	Confirmed by: **technetium-labelled red blood cell scan, laparotomy.**
	Initial management: fluids IV, nil by mouth, transfusion if significant bleeding, surgical referral.
Intussusception (in children or elderly)	*Suggested by:* child, usually between 6–18mo of life, acute onset of colicky intermittent abdominal pain, redcurrant 'jelly' PR bleed ± a sausage-shaped mass in upper abdomen.
	Confirmed by: **barium or air enema**, may reduce the intussusceptions with appropriate hydrostatic pressure.
	Initial management: fluids IV, NG tube + nil by mouth for decompression, analgesics, therapeutic enemas, e.g. hydrostatic reduction.
Mesenteric infarction (acute occlusion)	*Suggested by:* acute abdominal pain, generalized tenderness, shock, profuse diarrhoea (patient often in atrial fibrillation).
	Confirmed by: **mesenteric angiography, exploratory laparotomy.**
	Initial management: fluids if hypovolaemia, analgesics, broad-spectrum antibiotics, surgical referral.
Massive upper GI bleed	*Suggested by:* bright or dark red 'maroon'-coloured stool.
	Confirmed by: **upper GI endoscopy.**
	Initial management: stop aspirin or NSAIDs, large bore IV or central line, group and crossmatch, fluids IV (colloid initially), transfusion, CVP monitoring, NG tube + nil by mouth, irrigate stomach, nil by mouth, correct coagulopathy with FFP and platelets, urine catheter to monitor output; gastro or surgical referral.
Crohn's disease	*Suggested by:* aphthous ulcers, anaemia, tender mass, scars of previous surgery, anal fissures, fistulae.
	Confirmed by: **colonoscopy with biopsy, barium studies.**
	Initial management: mild: antimotility drugs (e.g. loperamide. Acute attack: fluids IV, corticosteroids IV or PO, high dose 5-ASA analogues (e.g. mesalazine, sulfasalazine), analgesics, elemental diet ± parenteral nutrition.
Trauma	*Suggested by:* pain, history or physical signs of trauma (e.g. sexual assault).
	Confirmed by: sigmoidoscopy.
	Initial management: counselling if sexual assault.

Urological and gynaecological symptoms and physical signs

Urinary frequency ± dysuria

This is a very common presentation and may pass unnoticed by the patient, especially in the elderly. A urine 'dipstick' test should be done at the slightest suspicion. Initial investigations (other tests in **bold** below): urine 'dipstick' ± MSU, FBC.

	Main differential diagnoses and typical outline evidence, etc.
Urinary tract infection with cystitis	*Suggested by:* vomiting, fever, abdominal pain, blood in urine, nitrites, white cells, and blood on urine 'dipstick'.
	Confirmed by: **MSU** microscopy and culture. **US scan** for possible anatomical abnormality.
	Initial management: increased fluid intake, cranberry juice, and regular bladder emptying. Provisional 1st line antibiotic pending MSU result, e.g. trimethoprim, cefalexin for 5d; 2nd line, e.g. ciprofloxacin bd for 5d.
Bladder or urethral calculus	*Suggested by:* suprapubic pain, macroscopic or microscopic haematuria.
	Confirmed by: **US scan** of bladder showing urethral dilation, **plain X-ray** showing radio-opaque calculus, **IVU** showing filling defect.
	Initial management: immediate analgesia, e.g. diclofenac (IM or suppository) or pethidine IM with metoclopramide IM + antibiotics. Emergency surgery if renal tract obstruction proved on imaging.
Uterine prolapse	*Suggested by:* incontinence of urine, 'feeling like something coming down'.
	Confirmed by: pelvic examination: cervix observed in lower vagina.
	Initial management: weight reduction, smoking cessation. Treating coexisting conditions, e.g. COPD, constipation. Ring pessary for frail patients. Surgical correction of prolapse.
Prostatic hypertrophy	*Suggested by:* hesitancy, poor stream, urgency, incontinence, nocturia, acute retention of urine, large prostate on rectal examination.
	Confirmed by: ↑prostatic-specific antigen (PSA), **US scan of prostate gland**, and response to transurethral resection of prostate (TURP).
	Initial management: catheter for acute retention. α-blockers, e.g. tamsulosin, then trial without catheter. 5α-reductase inhibitors, e.g. finasteride, TURP.
'Spastic' bladder due to upper motor neurone lesion	*Suggested by:* weakness, increased tone, and reflexes in lower limbs.
	Confirmed by: small bladder on **US scan**.
	Initial management: antibiotics for infections, catheterization.

Incontinence of urine alone (not faeces)

This symptom may be hidden because of embarrassment; a hint of ammonia smell on the patient's clothing during the examination should prompt gentle questioning. Initial investigations (other tests in **bold** below): urine 'dipstick' ± MSU, FBC.

Main differential diagnoses and typical outline evidence, etc.	
Prostatic hypertrophy	*Suggested by:* hesitancy, poor stream, urgency, incontinence, nocturia, acute retention of urine, large prostate on rectal examination.
	Confirmed by: ↑PSA, **US scan of prostate gland**, and response to TURP.
	Initial management: catheter for acute retention. α-blockers, e.g. tamsulosin, then trial without catheter. 5α-reductase inhibitors, e.g. finasteride. TURP.
Uterine prolapse	*Suggested by:* incontinence of urine, 'feeling like something coming down'.
	Confirmed by: pelvic examination: cervix observed in lower vagina.
	Initial management: weight reduction, smoking cessation. Treating coexisting conditions, e.g. COPD, constipation. Ring pessary for frail patients. Surgical correction of prolapse.
Urinary tract infection with cystitis	*Suggested by:* vomiting, fever, abdominal pain, blood in urine, nitrites, white cells, and blood on urine 'dipstick'.
	Confirmed by: **MSU** microscopy and culture. US scan for possible anatomical abnormality.
	Initial management: increased fluid intake, cranberry juice, and regular bladder emptying. Provisional 1st line antibiotic pending MSU result, e.g. trimethoprim, cefalexin for 5d; 2nd line, e.g. ciprofloxacin bd for 5d.
Weakness of pelvic floor muscles	*Suggested by:* incontinence during coughing, sneezing, laughing.
	Confirmed by: **urodynamic studies**.
	Initial management: pelvic floor exercises.

Incontinence of urine and faeces

Again this symptom may be hidden because of embarrassment; a hint of ammonia or faecal soiling on the patient's clothing during the examination should prompt gentle questioning. Initial investigations (other tests in **bold** below): Urine 'dipstick' ± MSU, FBC.

Main differential diagnoses and typical outline evidence, etc.	
'Neurogenic' bladder	*Suggested by:* paresis, low tone and diminished reflexes in lower limbs, sensory loss in anal region.
	Confirmed by: small and spastic bladder (upper motor neurone) or large and hypotonic bladder (lower motor neurone) on **US scan**.
	Initial management: infection. Wearing pads. Catheterization.
Epileptic fits	*Suggested by:* history of loss of consciousness, tongue biting, jerking movements (may be subtle).
	Confirmed by: clinical history, electroencephalogram **(EEG)**.
	Initial management: carbamazepine, lamotrigine, or topiramate in focal fits; valproate or lamotrigine for generalized fit.
Dementia (Alzheimer's, cerebrovascular disease with multi-infarct dementia, B12 or folate deficiency, hypothyroidism)	*Suggested by:* chronic worsening confusion, especially in elderly, previous strokes.
	Confirmed by: low mental score ± cerebral atrophy on **CT head scan**.
	Initial management: a care management plan and family support. Cholinesterase inhibitors for Alzheimer's disease. Treat any cause.
Severe depression	*Suggested by:* severe lack of motivation, low mood, tearfulness, precipitating event, e.g. bereavement.
	Confirmed by: continence improvement in response to treatment of depression.
	Initial management: counselling. Anti-depression agents.
Faecal impaction with 'overflow'	*Suggested by:* hard, rock-like faeces in rectum.
	Confirmed by: response to evacuation of faeces.
	Initial management: laxatives: large doses of Movicol®, phosphate enema. Manual evacuation.

Painful haematuria (with dysuria)

Initial investigations (other tests in **bold** below): Urine 'dipstick', MSU, FBC, U&E.

Main differential diagnoses and typical outline evidence, etc.	
Urinary tract infection with cystitis	*Suggested by:* vomiting, fever, abdominal pain, blood in urine, nitrites, white cells, and blood on urine 'dipstick'.
	Confirmed by: **MSU** microscopy and culture. US scan for possible anatomical abnormality.
	Initial management: increased fluid intake, cranberry juice, and regular bladder emptying. Provisional 1st line antibiotic pending MSU result, e.g. trimethoprim, cefalexin for 5d; 2nd line, e.g. ciprofloxacin bd for 5d.
Renal calculus	*Suggested by:* dysuria, spasmodic loin to groin pain, no fever.
	Confirmed by: **MSU** showing RBC, **renal US scan** showing ureteric dilatation, **IVU** showing filling defect in contrast medium.
	Initial management: immediate analgesia, e.g. diclofenac (IM or suppository) or pethidine IM with metoclopramide a IM + antibiotics. Emergency surgery if renal tract obstruction proved on imaging.
Trauma (due to urethral catheterization, traumatic sexual intercourse)	*Suggested by:* dysuria, history of urethral catheterization, or recent painful sexual intercourse.
	Confirmed by: history, normal **MSU**, **renal US scan**, **IVU**.
	Initial management: analgesia, e.g. paracetamol, alkalinization of urine (e.g. cranberry juice, 'Mist. Pot. Cit.').

Painless haematuria

In females, care has to be taken to distinguish between haematuria, vaginal, and anorectal bleeding. This may depend on the result of pelvic and rectal examination. Initial investigations (other tests in **bold** below): FBC with platelets, clotting tests, US scan of abdomen.

Main differential diagnoses and typical outline evidence, etc.	
Renal tumour	*Suggested by:* palpable mass, fever (often previously of unknown origin).
	Confirmed by: **US scan or CT of abdomen/kidney**, **IVU** showing renal mass.
	Initial management: nephrectomy for local disease. Immunotherapy for metastatic disease.
Ureteric tumour	*Suggested by:* colicky pain if obstructed.
	Confirmed by: **US scan or CT abdomen/kidney**, **IVU** showing ureteric mass.
	Initial management: referral for stenting to relieve obstruction ± resection of tumour with or without nephrectomy or cystectomy depending on site.
Bladder tumour	*Suggested by:* pelvic pain, pelvic mass, recurrent urine infections, dysuria, haematuria.
	Confirmed by: positive **urine cytology**, **cystoscopy**, **IVU** shows filling defects of bladder.
	Initial management: depends on staging. T1 local excision by transurethral cystoscopy and diathermy, followed by intravesicular chemotherapeutic agents, e.g. mitomycin. T2–3 radical cystectomy with post-operative chemotherapy. T4 palliative chemo- or radiotherapy.
Bleeding diathesis	*Suggested by:* anticoagulant therapy, easy bruising, or other bleeding sites.
	Confirmed by: abnormal **clotting screen** ± FBC: ↓platelets.
	Initial management: if on warfarin and INR >3.5, stop or adjust dose; if INR >>3.5, vitamin K therapy. Otherwise, detailed assessment of clotting or platelet abnormality and appropriate treatment.
Urinary tract infection with cystitis	*Suggested by:* vomiting, fever, abdominal pain, blood in urine, nitrites, white cells, and blood on urine 'dipstick'.
	Confirmed by: **MSU** microscopy and culture. **US scan** for possible anatomical abnormality.
	Initial management: increased fluid intake, cranberry juice and regular bladder emptying. Provisional 1st line antibiotic pending MSU result, e.g. trimethoprim, cefalexin for 5d; 2nd line, e.g. ciprofloxacin bd for 5d.

Secondary amenorrhoea

Absence of menstruation for >3mo. Initial investigations (other tests in **bold** below): pregnancy test, FSH, LH, testosterone, and sex hormone binding globulin (SHBG), prolactin.

Main differential diagnoses and typical outline evidence, etc.	
Pregnancy	*Suggested by:* presentation during childbearing age.
	Confirmed by: **pregnancy test** +ve, **pelvic US scan**.
	Initial management: refer to the community maternity health team.
Normal menopause	*Suggested by:* >40y of age, hot flushes.
	Confirmed by: ↑**FSH**.
	Initial management: hormone replacement therapy (HRT) to ease menopausal symptoms and prevent osteoporosis after counselling the patient about benefits and risks.
Premature ovarian failure	*Suggested by:* hot flushes, <40y of age, and no signs of other endocrine disease (adrenal failure, hypothyroidism, etc.).
	Confirmed by: ↑**LH**, ↑**FSH**, ↓**oestradiol**, **ovarian biopsy**: atrophic.
	Initial management: HRT until the age of 50y, then review after counselling.
Polycystic ovary syndrome	*Suggested by:* oligo-/amenorrhoea, hirsutism, head hair thinning, acne, obesity, impaired fasting glucose or type 2 diabetes mellitus, acanthosis nigricans, skin tags, infertility.
	Confirmed by: ↑testosterone, ↓SHBG, ↑LH, LH>FSH, cystic ovaries on **pelvic US scan**.
	Initial management: Co-cyprindiol (for hirsutism, acne) + cyclical progesterone (to induce monthly withdrawal bleed). Metformin for insulin resistance. Clomifene to induce ovulation.
Hyperprolactinaemia due to macro- or micro-adenoma, or idiopathic (no apparent adenoma)	*Suggested by:* galactorrhoea, amenorrhoea. Headache or bitemporal visual field defect (if large prolactinoma).
	Confirmed by: ↑serum prolactin. Expanded pituitary fossa on **skull X-ray** or **CT scan**. **MRI scan**: visible micro- (<10mm) or macro-adenoma (>10mm).
	Initial management: dopamine agonists, e.g. bromocriptine or cabergoline. Surgical referral if >10mm, field defect, pressure effects not changed by dopamine agonist, or pregnancy planned.

Thyrotoxicosis due to Graves's disease, single or multiple toxic nodules	*Suggested by:* amenorrhoea alone, anxious-looking, thin, lid retraction and lag, tremor, hyper-reflexic, diffuse goitre in Graves's, visible or palpable nodule(s) if toxic nodules.
	Confirmed by: ↓**TSH** and ↑**T3** or ↑**T4** or both. **Thyroid antibodies** +ve if Graves's. **US scan** or **isotope scan** appearance.
	Initial management: propranolol 40–80 mg 8 hourly to control symptoms. Carbimazole 40mg od, reduced to 5–15mg od over 1–3mo period with regular TFT monitoring; continue treatment for 6–18mo. Radioiodine therapy if hot nodule(s) or relapse of Graves's disease after full course of carbimazole.

Excessive menstrual loss: menorrhagia

Menorrhagia can be due to uterine or systemic disorders. Initial investigations (other tests in **bold** below): FBC, TSH, US scan of abdomen/pelvis.

Main differential diagnoses and typical outline evidence, etc.	
Fibroids	*Suggested by:* menorrhagia alone ± urinary frequency, pelvic pain, constipation, recurrent miscarriage, infertility. Mass on bimanual pelvic examination.
	Confirmed by: **US scan or CT** appearance.
	Initial management: antiprostaglandin agents, e.g. mefenamic acid, or antifibrinolytic agents, e.g. tranexamic acid to control bleeding. GnRH to shrink fibroids, e.g. prior to surgery (long-term use may cause osteoporosis). Hysterectomy, myomectomy to preserve fertility.
Endometrial carcinoma	*Suggested by:* abnormal uterine bleeding, bloodstained vaginal discharge, postmenopausal bleeding.
	Confirmed by: **pelvic US scan**, **hysteroscopy** with tissue sampling of endometrium.
	Initial management: depends on stage of the cancer and fitness, e.g. total abdominal hysterectomy with bilateral salpingo-oophorectomy + radiotherapy if tumour stage >1b.
Pelvic endometriosis	*Suggested by:* dysmenorrhoea, heavy periods, abdominal pains, dyspareunia, infertility, pelvic mass.
	Confirmed by: appearance of peritoneal deposits at **laparoscopy**.
	Initial management: combined pill, e.g. norethisterone, danazol, etc. or GnRH analogues. Removal of deposits + abdominal hysterectomy + bilateral salpingo-oophorectomy.
Chronic pelvic inflammatory disease	*Suggested by:* lower abdominal pain, fever, vaginal discharge, dysuria. ↑**ESR** and ↑**CRP**, leucocytosis.
	Confirmed by: organisms on **high vaginal swab**, adhesions on **pelvic US scan** ± **laparoscopy**.
	Initial management: long-term antibiotics ± surgical restoration of normal anatomy.
Intrauterine contraceptive device (IUCD)	*Suggested by:* history of its insertion, painful periods.
	Confirmed by: symptoms subsiding after removal of IUCD.
1° hypothyroidism	*Suggested by:* menorrhagia alone ± cold intolerance, tiredness, constipation, bradycardia.
	Confirmed by: ↑**TSH**, ↓**FT4**.
	Initial management: thyroxine replacement.

Bleeding diathesis	*Suggested by:* anticoagulant therapy, easy bruising, or other bleeding sites.
	Confirmed by: abnormal **clotting screen** ± **FBC**: ↓platelets.
	Initial management: if on warfarin and INR >3.5, stop or adjust dose; if INR >>3.5, vitamin K therapy. Otherwise, detailed assessment of clotting or platelet abnormality and appropriate treatment.

Intermenstrual or post-coital bleeding

Expert pelvic examination is required. Initial investigations (other tests in **bold** below): pelvic US scan.

Main differential diagnoses and typical outline evidence, etc.	
Endometrial carcinoma of the uterus	*Suggested by:* abnormal uterine bleeding, bloodstained vaginal discharge, postmenopausal bleeding.
	Confirmed by: **pelvic US scan**, **hysteroscopy** with tissue sampling of endometrium.
	Initial management: depends on stage of the cancer and fitness, e.g. total abdominal hysterectomy with bilateral salpingo-oophorectomy + radiotherapy if tumour stage >1b.
Carcinoma of cervix	*Suggested by:* irregular vaginal bleeding, offensive, watery or bloodstained vaginal discharge, obstructive uropathy, and back pain in late stage.
	Confirmed by: appearance on vaginal speculum examination, **biopsy of cervix**.
	Initial management: in micro-invasive disease and family not complete: cone biopsy; later, total hysterectomy after completion of family. If invasive, radical hysterectomy and radiotherapy.
Cervical or intrauterine polyps	*Suggested by:* intermenstrual spotting or postmenstrual staining.
	Confirmed by: appearance on vaginal speculum examination, **hysteroscopy**, histology of resection specimen.
	Initial management: resection.

Vulval skin abnormalities

Initial investigations (other tests in **bold** below): urine 'dipstick' for glucose and blood, vulval swab for microsopy and culture.

Main differential diagnoses and typical outline evidence, etc.	
Thrush: *Candida albicans* (often in pregnancy, contraceptive, and steroids, immunodeficiencies, antibiotics and diabetes mellitus)	*Suggested by:* vulva and vagina red, fissured, and sore. *Confirmed by:* mycelia or spores on **microscopy and culture.** *Initial management:* clotrimazole cream + treatment of any underlying condition.
Allergy	*Suggested by:* being worse after contact with some substances, e.g. nylon underwear, chemicals, and soap. *Confirmed by:* response to avoidance of precipitants. *Initial management:* emollient, with or without steroid creams or ointments.
Lichen sclerosis	*Suggested by:* being intensely itchy. Bruised, red, purpuric appearance. Bullae, erosions, and ulcerations. Later, white, flat, and shiny with an hourglass shape around the vulva and anus. *Confirmed by:* above clinical appearance and **biopsy**. *Initial management:* biopsy of any suspicious lesion. Topical steroids. Vulvectomy in advanced cases, if not responding to medical treatment. Follow-up to ensure resolution or re-investigation.
Leukoplakia	*Suggested by:* itchiness and white vulval patches due to skin thickening and hypertrophy. *Confirmed by:* above clinical appearance and histology on **biopsy**. *Initial management:* if non-atrophic biopsy appearance: topical steroids. If atrophic histology: topical oestrogen or testosterone. Surgical treatment if suspicious histology.
Carcinoma of the vulva	*Suggested by:* an indurated ulcer with an everted edge. *Confirmed by:* appearance **biopsy**. *Initial management:* surgical resection (5-y survival rate 95%).
Other rarer causes	Obesity, incontinence, diabetes mellitus, psoriasis, lichen planus, scabies, pubic lice, threadworms.

Ulcers and lumps of the vulva

The diagnoses depend on examination and biopsy of lesions, and thus requiring specialist skills. Initial investigations (other tests in **bold** below): urine 'dipstick'.

Main differential diagnoses and typical outline evidence, etc.	
Vulval warts (condylomata acuminata) due to human papilloma virus	Suggested and *Confirmed by*: warts on vulva, perineum, anus, vagina, or cervix (florid in pregnancy or if immunosuppressed). *Initial management*: if single wart, not pregnant, Podophyllin paint applied weekly by a nurse and washed after 6h (or liquid applied bd for 3d as self-treatment). If multiple warts: cryotherapy, laser, or diathermy under general anaesthesia. Annual **cervical smears,** and checking of the vulva and anus.
Urethral carbuncle caused by meatal prolapse	Suggested and *Confirmed by*: small, red swelling at the urethral orifice. Tender and pain on micturition. *Initial management*: topical oestrogen. Surgical resection if no resolution.
Bartholin's cyst and abscess caused by blocked duct	Suggested and *Confirmed by*: extreme pain (cannot sit) and red, hot, swollen labium. *Initial management*: antibiotics in early stage. If no response, incision and drainage ('marsupialization').
Herpes simplex (herpes type II) complicated by urinary retention	Suggested and *Confirmed by*: vulva ulcerated and exquisitely painful. *Initial management*: topical aciclovir, PO if severe. Topical or systemic antibiotics if 2° infection.
Other causes	Local varicose veins, boils, sebaceous cysts, keratoacanthomata, condylomata, latent syphilis, primary chancre, molluscum contagiosum, abscess, uterine prolapse or polyp, inguinal hernia, varicocoele, carcinoma. Also causes of vulval ulcers: syphilis, herpes simplex, chancroid, lymphogranuloma venereum, granuloma inguinale, TB, Behçet's syndrome, aphthous ulcers, Crohn's disease.

Lumps in the vagina

The clinical assessment depends on special examination techniques. Initial investigations (other tests in **bold** below): urine 'dipstick'

Main differential diagnoses and typical outline evidence, etc.	
Cystocoele	*Suggested by:* frequency and dysuria. Bulging, upper front wall of the vagina.
	Confirmed by: **cystogram** showing residual urine within the cystocoele.
	Initial management: surgical anterior vaginal repair (colporrhaphy)
Urethrocoele	*Suggested by:* stress incontinence (e.g. 'leaks' when laughing or coughing). Bulging of the lower anterior vaginal wall.
	Confirmed by: **micturating cystogram** showing displaced urethra and impaired sphincter mechanisms.
	Initial management: surgical referral for repair.
Rectocoele	*Suggested by:* patient may have to reduce herniation prior to defaecation by putting a finger in the vagina. Bulging, middle posterior wall.
	Confirmed by: **barium enema** *or* **MRI scan** showing rectum bulging through weak levator ani.
	Initial management: surgical referral for vaginal posterior repair (colporrhaphy)
Enterocoele	*Suggested by:* bulging of upper posterior vaginal wall.
	Confirmed by: **barium enema** *or* **MRI scan** showing loops of intestine in the pouch of Douglas.
	Initial management: surgical referral for vaginal posterior repair (colporrhaphy)
Uterine prolapse (made worse by obesity, chronic bronchitis, or COPD)	*Suggested by:* 'dragging' or 'something coming down', worse by day. Frequency, stress incontinence, and difficulty in defaecation.
	Confirmed by: cervix well down in the vagina (1st degree prolapse) or protruding from the introitus when standing or straining (2nd degree) or the keratinized uterus lying outside vagina, the cervix ulcerated (3rd degree prolapse or procidentia).
	Initial management: weight reduction, smoking cessation. Ring pessary for frail patients. Surgical correction of prolapse. Treat aggravating factors.
Vaginal carcinoma	*Suggested by:* vaginal bleeding, mass in the upper third of the vagina.
	Confirmed by: squamous cell carcinoma on **biopsy**.
	Initial management: surgical referral in early cases, otherwise radiotherapy.

Ulcers and lumps in the cervix

The clinical assessment depends on special examination techniques. Initial investigations (other tests in **bold** below): urine 'dipstick'.

Main differential diagnoses and typical outline evidence, etc.	
Cervical ectropion ('erosion' innocuous)	*Suggested by:* red ring of soft glandular tissue around cervical opening often found with puberty, combined pill, during pregnancy ± bleeding, producing excess mucus, or infected.
	Confirmed by: (in cases of doubt) **histology** showing columnar epithelium.
	Initial management: cauterization.
Nabothian cysts	*Suggested and Confirmed by:* appearance of smooth spherical cyst (mucus retention).
	Initial management: cauterization.
Cervical polyps	*Suggested by:* increased mucus discharge or post-coital bleeding.
	Confirmed by: **histology** of resected, pedunculated, benign tumour arising from endocervical junction.
	Initial management: resection.
Cervicitis	*Suggested by:* increased mucus discharge or post-coital bleeding. Very red swollen cervix with overlying mucus and blood.
	Confirmed by: **histology** showing follicular or mucopurulent changes. Vesicles in herpes. **Culture** *showing* chlamydia, gonococci, etc.
	Initial management: antibiotics for *chlamydia* or gonococcus. Cauterization.
Cervical intraepithelial neoplasia (CIN)	*Suggested by:* overlying cervicitis, in older woman, smoker, underprivileged background, prolonged pill use, high parity, many sexual partners or a partner having many other partners, early first coitus, past sexually transmitted diseases.
	Confirmed by: **Papanicolaou smear** showing dyskaryosis; no malignancy on **cervical biopsy**.
	Initial management: small localized lesions of CIN1 and CIN2: cryocautery. More severe lesions: laser or loop wedge excision. Cone biopsy is for more advanced lesions. Hysterectomy if symptomatic, recurrent abnormal smears, and family complete.
Carcinoma of cervix	*Suggested by:* irregular vaginal bleeding, offensive, watery or bloodstained vaginal discharge, obstructive uropathy, and back pain in late stage. Firm or friable mass which bleeds on contact.
	Confirmed by: appearance on vaginal speculum examination, **biopsy of cervix**.
	Initial management: in micro-invasive disease and family not complete: cone biopsy; later, total hysterectomy after completion of family. If invasive, radical hysterectomy and radiotherapy.

Tender or bulky mass (uterus, Fallopian tubes or ovary) on pelvic examination

The clinical assessment depends on special examination techniques. Initial investigations (other tests in **bold** below): urine 'dipstick', pregnancy tests, US scan of pelvis.

Main differential diagnoses and typical outline evidence, etc.	
Pregnancy	*Suggested by:* amenorrhoea in sexually active woman. Uterus at 6wk of pregnancy is like an egg, at 8wk like a peach, at 10wk like a grapefruit, and at 14wk, it fills the pelvis.
	Confirmed by: **pregnancy test** +ve, pregnancy sac seen on abdominal or **transvaginal US scan**.
	Initial management: refer to community midwife.
Ovarian mass (benign tumour, functional cysts, theca-lutein cysts, epithelial cell tumours (serous and mucinous), cystadenomas, mature teratomas, fibromas malignant cystadenomas, germ cell or sex cord malignancies, 2°s from the uterus or stomach, Krukenberg tumours spreading via the peritoneum)	*Suggested by:* painless pelvic mass, often to one side ± amenorrhoea.
	Confirmed by: **abdominal or transvaginal US scan** appearances.
	Initial management: analgesia, provisional antibiotics for associated infections. Surgical referral.
Endometritis (uterine infection) after abortion and childbirth, IUCD insertion, or surgery. May involve Fallopian tubes and ovaries. Low-grade infection is often due to *chlamydia*	*Suggested by:* lower abdominal pain and fever, uterine tenderness on bimanual palpation.
	Confirmed by: **transvaginal US scan, endocervical swabs**, and **blood cultures**.
	Initial management: analgesics for pain, provisional antibiotics, then change according to results of culture and sensitivity.
Endometrial proliferation due to oestrogen stimulation	*Suggested by:* heavy menstrual bleeding and irregular bleeding (dysfunctional uterine bleeding), and polyps.
	Confirmed by: 'cystic glandular hyperplasia' in specimen after **dilatation and curettage**.
	Initial management: combined contraceptive pill for the young age group; antiprostaglandin agents, e.g. mefenamic acid, or antifibrinolytic agents, e.g. tranexamic acid, to control bleeding. Surgical referral for endometrial ablation and hysterectomy.

Pyometra (uterus distended by pus, associated with salpingitis or 2° to outflow blockage)	*Suggested by:* lower abdominal pain and fever, uterine tenderness on bimanual palpation. *Confirmed by:* **transvaginal US scan, cervical swabs, and blood cultures**. *Initial management:* analgesia. Antibiotic according to culture and sensitivity; surgical evacuation ± total hysterectomy ± bilateral salpingo-oophorectomy.
Haematometra due to imperforate hymen in the young, carcinoma, iatrogenic cervical stenosis after cone biopsy	*Suggested by:* lower abdominal pain and uterine tenderness on bimanual palpation. *Confirmed by:* no fever, WCC normal. **Transvaginal US scan** appearance. *Initial management:* surgical referral to gynaecology.
Endometrial tuberculosis (also affects the Fallopian tubes with pyosalpinx)	*Suggested by:* infertility, pelvic pain, amenorrhoea, oligomenorrhoea. *Confirmed by:* **transvaginal US scan, cervical swabs**, and +ve smear or **cultures for AFB**. *Initial management:* antituberculosis treatment, e.g. isoniazid + rifampicin + pyrazinamide + ethambutol for 2mo (initial phase), followed by combined isoniazid + rifampicin for another 4mo (continuation phase).
Ectopic pregnancy	*Suggested by:* abdominal pain or bleeding in a sexually active woman with a history of a missed period. Gradually increasing vaginal bleeding, shoulder-tip pain (diaphragmatic irritation), and pain on defecation and passing water (due to pelvic blood). Sudden severe pain, peritonism, and shock with rupture. *Confirmed by:* **hCG** >6000IU/L and an intrauterine gestational sac not seen on pelvic US scan, or if **hCG** 1000–1500IU/L and no sac is seen on **transvaginal US scan**. *Initial management:* IV access, crossmatch blood, correct shock and Hb. Emergency gynaecology surgical referral for laparotomy ± preliminary laparoscopy.
Fibroids (uterine leiomyomata)	*Suggested by:* heavy and prolonged periods, infertility, pain, abdominal swelling, urinary frequency, oedematous legs and varicose veins, or cause retention of urine. *Confirmed by:* normal **hCG** and **transvaginal US scan** showing discrete lump(s) in the wall of the uterus or bulging out to lie under the peritoneum (subserosal) or under the endometrium (submucosal) or pedunculated. *Initial management:* if menorrhagia, small fibroids, and subfertility, GnRH analogues in short term. Hysterectomy (or myomectomy to retain fertility).

(Continued)

Tender or bulky pelvic mass (continued)

Main differential diagnoses and typical outline evidence, etc. *(continued)*

Acute salpingitis often associated with endometritis, peritonitis, abscess, and chronic infection

Suggested by: being unwell, with pain, fever, spasm of lower abdominal muscles (more comfortable lying on back with legs flexed). Cervicitis with profuse, purulent or bloody vaginal discharge. Cervical excitation and tenderness in the fornices bilaterally, but worse on one side. Symptoms vague in subacute infection.

Confirmed by: **laparoscopy**.

Initial management: analgesia. Fluids IV. Provisional broad-spectrum antibiotics to cover *Chlamydia trachomatis* and *Neisseria gonorrhoea*. Contact tracing and treatment of the sexual partner.

Chronic salpingitis (un-resolved, unrecognised, or inadequately treated acute salpingitis) leading to fibrosis and adhesions, pyosalpinx, or hydrosalpinx

Suggested by: pelvic pain, menorrhagia, secondary dysmenorrhoea, discharge, deep dyspareunia, depression. Palpable tubal masses, tenderness, and fixed retroverted uterus.

Confirmed by: **laparoscopy** to differentiate between infection and endometriosis.

Initial management: analgesia. Surgical referral.

Vaginal discharge

The clinical assessment depends on special examination techniques. Initial investigations (other tests in **bold** below): urine 'dipstick', high vaginal swab.

Main differential diagnoses and typical outline evidence, etc.	
Excessive normal secretion	*Suggested by:* women of reproductive age, milky white, or mucoid discharge.
	Confirmed by: normal investigations.
	Initial management: explanation and reassurance.
Vaginal thrush	*Suggested by:* pruritis vulvae with a white discharge in a well patient.
	Confirmed by: **high vaginal swab**.
	Initial management: clotrimazole cream or pessaries or fluconazole PO (not in pregnancy).
Bacterial vaginosis	*Suggested by:* fishy odour discharge, itching, irritation.
	Confirmed by: **high vaginal swab + wet saline microscopy shows presence of cells.**
	Initial management: oral or vaginal metronidazole, amoxicillin in pregnancy.
Cervical erosions (ectropion)	*Suggested by:* no other obvious symptoms.
	Confirmed by: **speculum examination.**
	Initial management: colposcopy and cryo- or electrocautery of the affected area.
Endocervicitis (gonococcus, chlamydia)	*Suggested by:* symptoms in partner of urethritis.
	Confirmed by: inflamed cervix on **speculum examination** and **endocervical swab** result.
	Initial management: broad-spectrum antibiotics. Contact tracing and treatment of sexual partner. Referral to the Genitourinary medicine team.
Carcinoma of cervix	*Suggested by:* bloodstained discharge, irregular vaginal bleeding, obstructive uropathy, and back pain in late stage.
	Confirmed by: **cervical smear, cytology, colposcopy with biopsy.**
	Initial management: discuss diagnosis and treatments. Pain relief. Cone biopsy for stage 1a if family not yet complete (applies to squamous cell carcinoma only). Radical surgery + radiotherapy.
Foreign body	*Suggested by:* bloodstained discharge, use of ring pessary, intrauterine contraceptive device, tampon.
	Confirmed by: **speculum examination** or colposcopy or hysteroscopy.
	Initial management: removal of foreign body.

Endometrial polyp	*Suggested by:* bloodstained discharge, intermenstrual spotting, postmenstrual staining.
	Confirmed by: **hysteroscopy**.
	Initial management: surgical excision.
Trichomonas vaginitis	*Suggested by:* profuse, greenish yellow, frothy discharge, dysuria, dyspareunia.
	Confirmed by: protozoa and WBC on **smear**.
	Initial management: metronidazole for 1wk. If pregnant, lower dose for 5d. Treat the partner.
Gonococcal cervicitis	*Suggested by:* purulent discharge, lower abdominal pain, fever, cervix appears red and bleeds easily.
	Confirmed by: **Gram stain of cervical or urethral exudates** shows intracellular Gram –ve diplococci.
	Initial management: cefixime or ciprofloxacin. Azithromycin or doxycycline for possible associated *chlamydia*. Trace contacts and treat sexual partner. No alcohol or intercourse during treatment.
Chlamydia cervicitis	*Suggested by:* purulent discharge, lower abdominal pain, fever, cervix appears red and bleeds easily.
	Confirmed by: **endocervical swab**.
	Initial management: doxycycline or erythromycin at standard doses for 7–10d. Higher doses in addition to metronidazole for complicated infections. Trace contacts and treat sexual partner. No intercourse and alcohol for 4 weeks.

Enlargement of prostate

The rectal examination includes feeling for a prostatic protrusion anteriorly and sweeping around for other masses, including impacted faeces. Initial investigations (other tests in **bold** below): urine 'dipstick', MSU, FBC, PSA.

Main differential diagnoses and typical outline evidence, etc.	
Prostatitis	*Suggested by:* smooth, enlarged, and tender.
	Confirmed by: **+ve urine culture, culture of prostatic secretions.**
	Initial management: ciprofloxacin for 4wk.
Prostatic hypertrophy	*Suggested by:* hesitancy, poor stream, urgency, incontinence, nocturia, acute retention of urine, smooth, enlarged, firm, non-tender, usually with a palpable median groove.
	Confirmed by: ↑ **serum PSA, US scan of prostate gland**, and response to TURP.
	Initial management: catheter for acute retention. α-blockers, e.g. tamsulosin, then trial without catheter. 5α-reductase inhibitors, e.g. finasteride, TURP.
Prostatic carcinoma	*Suggested by:* irregular, hard, sometimes obliteration of median groove, non-tender.
	Confirmed by: ↑↑ **serum PSA, prostatic biopsy.**
	Initial management: for local disease, radical prostatectomy or radiotherapy combined with hormonal treatment. For metastatic disease, endocrine therapy.

Joint, limb, and back symptoms and physical signs

Muscle stiffness or pain

Usually worse in the early morning, often with pain and stiffness. Initial investigations (others in **bold** below): FBC, ESR, or CRP.

Main differential diagnoses and typical outline evidence, etc.	
Normal response to strenuous exercise	*Suggested by:* fit, healthy, unaccustomed exercise 1–2d before.
	Confirmed by: spontaneous resolution.
	Initial management: explanation and reassurance.
Polymyalgia rheumatica	*Suggested by:* abrupt onset of symptoms, severe morning stiffness and limb girdle pain, tender proximal muscles. Fatigue, night sweats, and fever in elderly person.
	Confirmed by: ↑↑**ESR** and **CRP**, ↓**Hb**, **rheumatoid factor** –ve, prompt response to prednisolone, no other cause (e.g. infection on follow-up).
	Initial management: NSAIDs if not contraindicated, analgesics, advise exercises, low dose prednisolone, e.g. 20–30mg daily—reduced gradually over a period of weeks or months. Can resolve spontaneously, even without treatment.
Rheumatoid arthritis	*Suggested by:* early morning stiffness, fatigue and joint pain, and swelling. Fingers showing 'swan neck' or 'boutonnière' deformities. Thumbs show Z-deformities. Metacarpophalangeal (MCP) joints and wrists— subluxed giving ulnar deviation. Knees—valgus or varus deformity and popliteal 'Baker's' cysts. Feet—subluxation of metatarsal heads with hallux valgus, clawed toes.
	Confirmed by: **rheumatoid factor** +ve, **anti-IgG auto-antibody, cryoglobulins. FBC:** normochromic anaemia, ↑**ESR** and ↑**CRP** when active.
	Initial management: supportive physiotherapy and occupational therapy, NSAIDs with gastric protection, analgesics. Disease-modifying drugs, e.g. methotrexate. Immunotherapy, e.g. infliximab.
Ankylosing spondylitis	*Suggested by:* onset over months or years. Spinal pain and stiffness with progressive loss of spinal movement. Kyphosis and spinal extension.
	Confirmed by: 'bamboo' spine on **back X-ray** and loss of sacroileal joint space. **Rheumatoid factor** –ve, **HLA-B27** +ve. ↑IgA.
	Initial management: exercise, physiotherapy, NSAIDs, and analgesics. Dramatic response to immunotherapy using anti-tumour necrosis factor (TNF) drugs, e.g. infliximab.

1° muscle disease	*Suggested by:* onset over weeks to years. Predominant weakness of proximal muscles mainly, seasonal variation of symptoms ± symptoms of an associated malignancy.
	Confirmed by: ↑**CPK**, **electromyography (EMG)**, **MRI scan**, and **muscle biopsy**.
	Initial management: investigate a possible underlying malignancy. Physiotherapy, high dose steroids, immunosuppressants, e.g. methotrexate.
1° hypothyroidism	*Suggested by:* onset over weeks to months. Predominant fatigue. Also cold intolerance, depression.
	Confirmed by: ↑**TSH**, ↓**FT4**.
	Initial management: thyroid replacement treatment.
Early manifestation of occult malignancy	*Suggested by:* onset over weeks or months. Weight loss, anorexia.
	Confirmed by: subsequent appearance of malignancy, especially spinal 2° deposits.
'Fibromyalgia'	*Suggested by:* variable onset—weeks to years. Fatigue, diffuse pain, muscles stiffness and tender points, but no features of specific diagnosis.
	Confirmed by: no 'subsequent' development of features of another diagnosis, normal **ESR**, **rheumatoid factor** –ve, **CPK** normal, **TSH** and **FT4** normal.
	Initial management: education and reassurance, exercise, relaxation techniques, tricyclic antidepressants (e.g. amitriptyline), selective serotonin reuptake inhibitors—SSRIs (e.g. fluoxetine), muscle relaxants (e.g. tizanidine).

Monoarthritis

One joint affected by pain, swelling, overlying erythema, stiffness, and local heat (± fever). Initial investigations (others in **bold** below): FBC, ESR or CRP, rheumatoid factor.

Main differential diagnoses and typical outline evidence, etc.	
Acute septic arthritis	*Suggested by:* extremely painful, red hot joint, high fever.
	Confirmed by: ↑↑WCC. Joint **aspiration**: synovial fluid turbid. **Culture** growing *staphylococcus* or *streptococcus* or *pseudomonas* or gonococci or TB, etc.
	Initial management: aspiration of joint, culture and sensitivity, analgesics, NSAIDs, antimicrobial according to culture and sensitivity results, Urgent orthopaedic referral for possible washout.
Gout	*Suggested by:* one acutely inflamed joint (usually small especially big toe) at a time, but other joints in hands, arms, legs, and feet deformed. Tophi on ears and tendon sheaths.
	Confirmed by: ↑**serum urate** (not always). Urate crystals (negatively birefringent in plane-polarized light) present on **joint aspiration**. **X-rays** showing damage to cartilage and bones.
	Initial management: appropriate diet, avoiding food high in purines, plenty of fluids, reduce alcohol consumption, lose weight, analgesics, NSAIDs, colchicines. Allopurinol to prevent future attacks.
Pseudogout (Ca^{2+} pyrophosphate arthropathy/ chondrocalcinosis) Hyperparathyroidism, myxoedema, osteoarthritis, dialysis or trauma, haemochromatosis, acromegaly	*Suggested by:* one painful joint (usually knee), especially in elderly or history of associated condition. Occasionally, family history of the condition.
	Confirmed by: **X-rays of joint** *show chondrocalcinosis.* **Joint aspiration:** synovial calcium pyrophosphate crystal deposits, positively bifringent in plane-polarized light.
	Initial management: joint aspiration to ease pain, analgesics, NSAIDs, intra-articular joint injection, colchicine, and in severe cases, systemic steroids.

Reiter's disease	*Suggested by:* monoarthritis, urethritis, conjunctivitis—especially in a young man—or a history of diarrhoea (dysentery). Also suggested by associated iritis, keratoderma blenorrhagica (brown, aseptic abscesses on soles and palms), mouth ulcers, circinate balanitis (painless, serpiginous penile rash), plantar fasciitis, achilles tendonitis, and aortic incompetence.
	Confirmed by: **rheumatoid factor** –ve (i e. 'seronegative'), ↑**ESR**, +ve culture for *chlamydia*. **X-rays** show spondylitis and sacroiliitis. Urinalysis: first glass of a 2-glass urine test shows debris in urethritis.
	Initial management: bed rest, exercise, analgesics, NSAIDs, local intra-articular steroid injections, antibiotics for proved infections, e.g. *chlamydia*. Immunosuppression in severe cases.
Psoriasis	*Suggested by:* acutely inflamed terminal interphalangeal (IP) joint, but other joints deformed, especially terminal IP joints, and pitting and thickening of fingernails.
	Confirmed by: psoriatic plaques on elbows and extensor surfaces of limbs, scalp, behind ears, and around navel. **Rheumatoid factor** –ve (i.e. 'seronegative').
	Initial management: analgesics, NSAIDs, and in intractable cases, immunosuppressants, e.g. methotrexate.
Rheumatoid arthritis	*Suggested by:* early morning stiffness. Fingers: 'swan neck' or 'boutonnière' deformities. Thumbs have Z-deformities. MCP joints and wrists: subluxation acquiring ulnar deviation. Knees: valgus or varus deformity and popliteal 'Baker's' cysts. Feet: subluxation of metatarsal heads with hallux valgus, clawed toes, and calluses.
	Confirmed by: **rheumatoid factor** +ve (i e. 'seropositive'), ↑**anti-IgG autoantibody**. **FBC**: normochromic anaemia, ↑ESR when active.
	Initial management: supportive physiotherapy and occupational therapy, NSAIDs with stomach protection, analgesics. Disease-modifying drugs, e.g. methotrexate. Immunotherapy, e.g. infliximab.

(Continued)

Monoarthritis (continued)

Main differential diagnoses and typical outline evidence, etc. *(continued)*

Traumatic haemarthrosis	*Suggested by:* acutely inflamed joint after trauma.
	Confirmed by: **joint aspiration:** aspiration of blood from joint.
	Initial management: analgesia ± joint aspiration.
Leukaemic joint deposits	*Suggested by:* acutely inflamed joint.
	Confirmed by: leukaemic picture on **peripheral film** and **bone marrow**.
	Initial management: analgesics, NSAIDs, and treatment of the original problem.
Reactive arthritis (aseptic) due to venereal or enteric infection, *Yersinia, Chlamydia trachomatis, Campylobacter, Salmonella/Shigella* and *Chlamydia pneumoniae, HIV, Vibrio parahaemolyticus, Borrelia burgdorferi, Clostridium difficile*	*Suggested by:* asymmetric mono- or oligoarthritis developing about 1wk after infection elsewhere. Previous history of food poisoning or another intestinal illness.
	Confirmed by: ↑**ESR**, **HLA-B27** +ve, microbiological investigations (see 'causes').
	Initial management: heat-cold application for temporary easing of pain, analgesics, NSAIDs, appropriate antibiotics, exercise, and in severe cases, DMARDs.

Polyarthritis

Several joints affected by pain, swelling, overlying redness, stiffness, and local heat (± fever). Initial investigations (others in **bold** below): FBC, ESR or CRP, rheumatoid factor.

Main differential diagnoses and typical outline evidence, etc.	
Viruses	*Suggested by:* several acutely inflamed joints. History of recent rubella or mumps or hepatitis A or Epstein–Barr viral infection, etc.
	Confirmed by: ↑**viral titres**, rheumatoid factor –ve ('seronegative').
	Initial management: analgesia and reassurance.
Rheumatoid arthritis	*Suggested by:* history of early morning stiffness. Fingers: 'swan neck' or 'boutonnière' deformities. Thumbs have Z-deformities. MCP joints and wrists: subluxation acquiring ulnar deviation. Knees: valgus or varus deformity and popliteal 'Baker's' cysts. Feet: subluxation of metatarsal heads with hallux valgus, clawed toes, and calluses.
	Confirmed by: **rheumatoid factor +ve**, ↑**anti-IgG autoantibody**. ↑**ESR** when active.
	Initial management: supportive physiotherapy and occupational therapy, NSAIDs with stomach protection, analgesics. DMARDs, e.g. methotrexate. Immunotherapy, e.g. infliximab.
Sjögren's syndrome associated diabetes mellitus, hypothyroidism	*Suggested by:* several acutely inflamed joints and diminished lacrimation, causing dry eyes and dry mouth. Enlarged salivary glands.
	Confirmed by: Schirmer's test +ve (ability to wet a small test strip put under the eye), **rheumatoid factor +ve**, and **anti-Ro** (SS-A) and **anti-La** (SS-B) antibodies present. Salivary gland biopsy.
	Initial management: symptomatic. For dry eyes, artificial tears, eye lubricants, or cicilosporin eye drops. For dry mouth, artificial saliva, lemon drops, and salivary gland stimulants, e.g. pilocarpine—if not contraindicated ± hydroxychloroquine. For severe cases with vasculitis, immunosuppressants, e.g. prednisolone or azathioprine.
Rheumatic fever (reactive arthritis to earlier infection with Lancefield Group A B-haemolytic streptococci)	*Suggested by:* flitting polyarthritis (a major 'Jones criterion').
	Confirmed by: evidence of recent streptococcal infection plus 1 more major revised Jones criterion or 2 more minor criteria. Evidence of streptococcal infection = scarlet fever or positive throat swab or increase in **ASOT** >200 or ↑**DNase B** titre. (Major criteria = carditis or flitting polyarthritis or subcutaneous nodules or erythema marginatum or Sydenham's chorea. Minor criteria = fever or ↑**ESR/CRP**, arthralgia (but not if arthritis is one of the major criteria), prolonged PR interval on ECG (but not if carditis is a major criterion), previous rheumatic fever.) **Rheumatoid factor –ve.**
	Initial management: bed rest, penicillin to eradicate streptococcal infection, NSAIDs. Treat chorea with benzodiazepines or haloperidol.
Systemic lupus erythematosus	*Suggested by:* polyarthritis with periarticular and tendon involvement, muscle pain, proximal myopathy.
	Confirmed by: ↑↑**double-stranded DNA antibodies** titre. **ANA +ve** and **rheumatoid factor +ve.**

	Initial management: analgesics and NSAIDs, sunscreens to protect skin, oral steroids for acute exacerbations, hydroxychloroquine to improve joint and skin symptoms, immunosuppressants, e.g. methotrexate, for resistant cases.
Ulcerative colitis	*Suggested by:* large joint polyarthritis, sacroiliitis, ankylosing spondylitis, background of gradual onset of diarrhoea with blood and mucus, and crampy abdominal discomfort. *Confirmed by:* **rheumatoid factor** –ve. **FBC:** ↓Hb and ↑**ESR**. Inflamed, friable mucosa on **sigmoidoscopy** and biopsy shows inflammatory infiltrate, goblet cell depletion, etc. *Initial management:* analgesics and antidiarrhoeic agents, topical anti-inflammatory agents (e.g. mesalazine), systemic anti-inflammatory agents (e.g. oral steroids), and immunosuppressants (e.g. azathioprine and methotrexate) for the more severe cases. Surgical intervention after many years when risk of colon cancer increases.
Crohn's disease	*Suggested by:* large joint polyarthritis, sacroiliitis, ankylosing spondylitis, background of gradual onset of diarrhoea, abdominal pain, weight loss. *Confirmed by:* **rheumatoid factor** –ve. **Contrast studies** showing ileal strictures, proximal dilatation, inflammatory mass or fistula, e.g. **barium enema:** 'cobblestoning', 'rose thorn' ulcers, colonic strictures with rectal sparing. *Initial management:* advise healthy, balanced and high-fibre content diet. Analgesics and antidiarrhoeic agents, oral anti-inflammatory agents (e.g. mesalazine, oral prednisolone) or immunosuppressants (e.g. azathioprine) in more severe cases. Surgical referral for intractable symptoms not controlled medically.
Drug reaction	*Suggested by:* several acutely inflamed joints. History of suspicious drug. *Confirmed by:* **rheumatoid factor** –ve and improvement on withdrawing drug. *Initial management:* withdrawing suspect drug(s).
Reiter's syndrome	*Suggested by:* polyarthritis, urethritis, conjunctivitis—especially in a young man—or a history of diarrhoea (dysentery). Also suggested by associated iritis, keratoderma blenorrhagica (brown, aseptic abscesses on soles and palms), mouth ulcers, circinate balanitis (painless, serpiginous penile rash), plantar fasciitis, achilles tendonitis, and aortic incompetence. *Confirmed by:* **rheumatoid factor** –ve. **Urinalysis:** first glass of a 2-glass urine test shows debris in urethritis. *Initial management:* bed rest, exercise, analgesics, NSAIDs, local intra-articular steroid injections, antibiotics for proved infections, e.g. *chlamydia*. Immunosuppression in severe cases.
Psoriasis	*Suggested by:* several acutely inflamed joints (usually terminal IP and other joints deformed, especially terminal IP joints, with pitting and thickening of fingernails. *Confirmed by:* psoriatic plaques on elbows and extensor surfaces of limbs, scalp, behind ears, and around navel. **Rheumatoid factor** –ve. *Initial management:* analgesics, NSAIDs, or immunosuppressants, e.g. methotrexate.

Pain or limitation of movement in the hand

Ask patient to flex and extend fingers, and then wrists. Observe opening and closing. Note buttons degree of movement, any limitation, or pain. Initial investigations (others in **bold** below): X-ray hand and wrist.

Main differential diagnoses and typical outline evidence, etc.	
Carpal tunnel syndrome Associated hypothyroidism, acromegaly, or pregnancy.	*Suggested by:* pain, numbness, and weakness of hand. Symptoms worse early hours of morning, waking up patient from sleep. Shaking the hand eases symptoms. *Confirmed by:* nerve conduction studies showing a delay at the wrist. *Initial management:* analgesics, night splints, local injection of steroids, or surgery.
Dupuytren's contracture usually familial or associated with alcohol, anti-epileptic therapy, or diabetes mellitus	*Suggested by:* progressive flexion deformity of base ring and little fingers, mainly with palmar fibrosis (often bilateral, familial). *Confirmed by:* fixed flexion at MCP joints first, then IP joints (inability to place hand on flat surface = severe). *Initial management:* wait and see if the palm only is affected. Surgical intervention if fingers affected.
Ganglion	*Suggested by:* painless, spherical swelling around wrist. *Confirmed by:* fluctuant, soft sphere. Disappears spontaneously leave alone, if persists or after blow, e.g. from a book. *Initial management:* aspiration and local steroid injection.
Rheumatoid arthritis	*Suggested by:* 'swan neck' or 'boutonnière' deformities of fingers. Thumbs have Z-deformities. MCP joints and wrists: subluxation acquiring ulnar deviation. Nodules on elbows and extensor tendons. *Confirmed by:* **rheumatoid factor** +ve. **↑anti-IgG autoantibody**. *Initial management:* supportive physiotherapy and occupational therapy, NSAIDs with stomach protection, analgesics. DMARDs, e.g. methotrexate. Immunotherapy. e.g. infliximab.
Psoriasis	*Suggested by:* several acutely inflamed joints (usually terminal IP) and other joints deformed, especially terminal IP joints with pitting and thickening of fingernails. *Confirmed by:* psoriatic plaques on extensor surfaces of limbs, scalp, behind ears, and around navel. **Rheumatoid factor** –ve. *Initial management:* analgesics, NSAIDs or immunosuppressants, e.g. methotrexate.

Trigger finger due to nodule sticking in tendon sheath	*Suggested by:* fixed flexion at the ring or little finger with no fibrosis in palm. Patient unable to extend finger spontaneously.
	Confirmed by: 'click' as fingers passively extended. Nodule, then palpable on flexor surface of finger.
	Initial management: orthopaedic referral for possible division of the sheath at the level of MP joint.
De Quervain's syndrome— stenosing tenosynovitis	*Suggested by:* pain at the wrist, e.g. when lifting teapot. History of forceful hand use, e.g. wringing clothes. Weakness of grip.
	Confirmed by: pain over radial styloid process, made worse by forced adduction and flexion of thumb into palm.
	Initial management: orthopaedic referral for possible dividing of lateral wall of tendon sheath.
Volkmann's ischaemic contracture due to ischaemia flexor muscles of thumb and fingers (supplied by brachial artery)	*Suggested by:* flexion deformity at the thumb, fingers, wrist, and elbow with forearm pronation. History of trauma or surgery near to brachial artery, or plaster of Paris applied too tightly to forearm.
	Confirmed by: cold, dark, ischaemic arm, no pulse at the wrist, and pain when fingers extended.
	Initial management: orthopaedic referral for possible surgical release of pressure.
Soft tissue injury or fracture	*Suggested by:* history of recent impact and acute pain and/ or loss of function, tenderness, deformity, swelling, crepitus.
	Confirmed by: acute pain and deformity clinically and on **X-ray**.
	Initial management: analgesia; orthopaedic referral if fracture ± physiotherapy.

Pain or limitation of movement at the elbow

Ask the patient to straighten arms, and compare for deformity and deviation from the normal valgus angle. Ask the patient to flex elbow, and to supinate and rotate normally over 90°. Note degree of movement, any limitation, or pain. Initial investigations (others in **bold** below): FBC, ESR, rheumatoid factor, X-ray elbow.

Main differential diagnoses and typical outline evidence, etc.	
Epicondylitis: tennis elbow (tenoperiostitis)	*Suggested by:* preceding repetitive strain, e.g. use of screwdriver, tennis racquet. Pain worse when patient asked to flex fingers and wrist, and pronate hand. Difficulty in holding a heavy object at arm's length. The arm feels stiff, heavy, and weak.
	Confirmed by: pain when patient's extended wrist pulled. Improvement after avoidance of preceding repetitive movement.
	Initial management: avoid suspected triggering activity, analgesics, and NSAIDs. RICE (Rest, Ice, Compression, and Elevation), physiotherapy, arm brace or tape, or local injections.
Osteoarthritis	*Suggested by:* joint deformity, intermittent pain and swelling, past history of injury, e.g. fracture or dislocation. 'Locking' if loose bodies.
	Confirmed by: impairment of flexion and extension, but rotation full. **Elbow X-ray** showing osteoarthritic changes and might show loose bodies.
	Initial management: analgesics, NSAIDs, physiotherapy, local injections of steroids or hyaluronic acid. Arthroscopy to remove inflammatory tissues or loose bodies, and to smooth out irregular surfaces. Orthopaedic referral for possible joint replacement.
Old trauma	*Suggested by:* history of impact, fracture, deformity.
	Confirmed by: deformity and related **elbow X-ray**.
	Initial management: analgesia and physiotherapy.
Soft tissue injury or fracture	*Suggested by:* recent impact and acute pain and/or loss of function, tenderness, deformity, swelling, crepitus.
	Confirmed by: **X-ray** appearance.
	Initial management: analgesia; orthopaedic referral if fracture ± physiotherapy.

Pain or limitation of movement at the shoulder

Ask patients to put their arms behind their head, and note angle at which any restriction and pain occurs. Initial investigations (others in **bold** below): FBC, ESR or CRP, X-ray shoulder.

Main differential diagnoses and typical outline evidence, etc.	
Impingement syndrome	*Suggested by:* pain on shoulder abduction, e.g. when throwing. Pain worse at night.
	Confirmed by: painful arc of movement between 70° and 120° abduction. Neer's impingement test: pain is triggered when forcibly internally rotating the shoulder while flexed to 90°. **MRI** studies of shoulder joint.
	Initial management: rest and reduced activities, analgesics and NSAIDs, physiotherapy, local injection of steroids. Surgery with decompression of subacromial space in non-responding cases.
Rotator cuff tears of the supraspinatus tendon or adjacent subscapularis or infraspina-tus tendons	*Suggested by:* limitation and/or pain on abduction at the shoulder to the first 60° range (achieved by scapular rotation), the pain is recurrent for several months. History of trauma at the time of onset.
	Confirmed by: passive movement pain-free and spontaneous above 90°. **MRI** showing connection between joint capsule and subacromial bursa.
	Initial management: analgesics, NSAIDs, and physiotherapy. Surgical repair in selected cases.
Chronic supraspinatus inflammation ± calcification	*Suggested and Confirmed by:* acute and continued limitation and/or pain on abduction at the shoulder in the final 60° to 90° range. Acutely painful, tender, swollen, and warm shoulder.
	Further confirmation by: any calcification in muscle on **shoulder X-ray**.
	Initial management: analgesics and NSAIDs. Joint aspiration and local injection.
Cervical spondylosis (pain is re-ferred to shoulder), very common cause of shoulder pain	*Suggested by:* pain and tenderness on the same side of the neck, occipital headache.
	Confirmed by: any positive neurological signs, e.g. absent arm reflexes, muscle weakness, and sensory impairment. **Neck X-ray and MRI scan.**
	Initial management: analgesics, NSAIDs, cervical collar, and physiotherapy. Surgical decompression of nerve root if intractable pain.
Biceps tendonitis	*Suggested by:* repetitive overhead activity, pain in front of the shoulder aggravated by contraction of the biceps.
	Confirmed by: above clinical findings.
	Initial management: resting arm, change of activity or sport, NSAIDs, physiotherapy. Orthopaedic referral for possible arthroscopic surgery.

Rupture of long head of biceps	*Suggested by:* sudden pain in front of the shoulder during an activity, a snapping sensation felt.
	Confirmed by: pain aggravated by contraction of the biceps, and a lump (contracting muscle belly) appears between the shoulder and elbow, possibly with some bruising.
	Initial management: a sling to rest shoulder, NSAIDs, occupational therapy and physiotherapy, surgical repair for patients who need arm strength.
Frozen shoulder—adhesive capsulitis	*Suggested by:* pain worse at night, marked reduction in active and passive movement with less than 90° abduction. Difficulty in brushing hair or putting on shirts or bra.
	Confirmed by: above clinical findings and normal **shoulder X-ray**.
	Initial management: NSAIDs, analgesics, exercises, physiotherapy, and intra-articular steroid injections. Surgical intervention, e.g. manipulation under anaesthesia and arthroscopic capsular release.
Osteoarthritis of acromio-clavicular (AC) joint	*Suggested by:* pain and swelling at the AC joint.
	Confirmed by: very well localized tenderness to the AC joint. Positive **X-ray** and **MRI** appearance.
	Initial management: analgesics, NSAIDs, physiotherapy. Surgical intervention if intractable.
Rheumatoid arthritis	*Suggested by:* history of early morning stiffness. Multiple joint involvement, small joints affected. Fingers: 'swan neck' or 'boutonnière' deformities. Thumbs have Z-deformities.
	Confirmed by: **rheumatoid factor** +ve, **↑anti-IgG autoantibody**. **↑ESR** when active.
	Initial management: supportive physiotherapy and occupational therapy, NSAIDs with gastric protection, e.g. PPI. DMARDs, e.g. methotrexate. Immunotherapy, e.g. infliximab.
Soft tissue injury or fracture	*Suggested by:* recent impact and acute pain and/or loss of function, tenderness, deformity, swelling, crepitus.
	Confirmed by: **X-ray** appearance.
	Initial management: analgesia; support and immobilize. Orthopaedic referral if fractured ± physiotherapy.
Septic arthritis	*Suggested by:* acutely, painful, red hot joint, with very restricted movements. High temperature with sweats and shivering.
	Confirmed by: **↑WCC**, **↑ESR**, **↑CRP**, joint aspirate positive for culture and sensitivity.
	Initial management: antibiotics as per culture and sensitivity results.
Osteoarthritis of the gleno-humeral joint. Very rare	*Suggested by:* history of avascular necrosis of head of humerus, following an injury to the proximal humerus.
	Confirmed by: **X-ray** appearance, **arthroscopy**.
	Initial management: analgesics, e.g. NSAIDs, local injection of steroids, joint replacement for severe cases.

Pain or limitation of movement at the neck

Look from the side to see if there is normal cervical (and lumbar) lordosis. Ask the patient to tilt head: move ear towards shoulder. Note angle at which any restriction and pain occurs. Initial investigations (others in **bold** below): FBC, ESR, X-ray of cervical spine.

Main differential diagnoses and typical outline evidence, etc.	
Neck pain due to an abnormal posture	*Suggested by:* a sedentary job, long hours on computer or driving. Loss of normal neck curvature.
	Confirmed by: history, full range of neck movements, and normal **cervical X-rays**.
	Initial management: analgesics, NSAIDs, postural exercises for the neck, eliminating bad posture, and a good support neck pillow for sleeping.
Whiplash (rapid extension and flexion movement) and extension injuries	*Suggested by:* history of road traffic accident (RTA) (rear end car crashes) with rapid extension and flexion movement of neck. Pain and stiffness of neck and the arms.
	Confirmed by: typical history.
	Initial management: soft cervical collar, analgesics, NSAIDs, and physiotherapy. Encourage early return to work.
Spasmodic torticollis (cervical dystonia) (anterocollis (tilts forwards), retrocollis (tilts backwards), laterocollis (tilts to one side))	*Suggested by:* recurrent involuntary contraction of neck muscles causing pain and the turning of the head to one side.
	Confirmed by: presence of tremor, stiffness of neck muscles, and elevation of shoulder on the affected side. Absence of root compression pattern pain or paresis.
	Initial management: analgesics for pain. GABA-regulating drugs (e.g. lorazepam or baclofen), dopamine agonists (e.g. bromocriptine), or anticonvulsants (e.g. carbamazepine), all used individually or in combination. Botulinum toxin or surgery for non-responding cases.
Infantile torticollis due to birth damage of sternomastoid	*Suggested by:* onset early childhood (up to 3y). Head tilted to shoulder with restricted neck movements, and retarded growth of the cranium or face on the affected muscle side (plagiocephaly). Presence of associated muscle or skeletal disorder, e.g. hip dysplasia.
	Confirmed by: palpable nodule in muscle on affected side. **Biopsy of nodule**: fibrous only and no gangliocytoma.
	Management: physiotherapy consisting of positioning, gentle range of movements, and strengthening by the stimulation of head and trunk muscles. Cervical collars and cranial remoulding orthosis in cases of plagiocephaly. Botulinum toxin and surgery for intractable cases.

Cervical rib with compression of lower brachial plexus affecting median and ulnar nerves, and brachial artery (thoracic outlet syndrome)	*Suggested by:* weakness and numbness in forearm and hand, usually on ulnar side. Wasting of the intrinsic hand muscles. Arm cyanosis and absent pulse. *Confirmed by:* symptoms exacerbated by abduction and external rotation of shoulder. **Cervical rib neck X-ray** (may be no rib—fibrous band instead). *Initial management:* analgesics, NSAIDs, physiotherapy, and local injections of trigger points. Referral to surgical specialist for possible intervention.
Cervical spondylosis	*Suggested by:* pain and stiffness of neck. Occipital headache, shoulder and arm pain due to radiation. Symptoms of nerve root or spinal cord involvement. *Confirmed by:* **X-ray** and **MRI** appearances. *Initial management:* analgesics and NSAIDs, physiotherapy, and local injections. Trial of traction. Surgical referral for intractable symptoms.
Posterior prolapsed (cervical disc, usually C5/C6 disc and C6/C7 disc pressure on nerve roots)	*Suggested by:* torticollis, stiffness and pain in neck over side of disc lesion. Pain, numbness in arm and tip of little or middle finger or thumb. *Confirmed by:* loss of biceps or supinator reflexes. Loss of sensation in medial or lateral borders of hand. **MRI scan** shows posterior protrusion. *Initial management:* analgesics and NSAIDs, physiotherapy, and local injections. Trial of traction. Surgical referral for possible intervention for weakness, severe pain, or suspected cord compression.
Anterior prolapsed cervical disc (usually C5/C6 disc and C6/C7 disc pressure on spinal cord)	*Suggested by:* torticollis, stiffness and pain in neck over side of disc lesion. Numbness and weakness in leg. Unsteadiness of gait, walking problems, and impaired bladder and bowel function. *Confirmed by:* flaccid first, then spastic paresis of leg. Loss of knee, ankle reflexes, and extensor plantar response. Loss of vibration sense, touch and pain with sensory level. **MRI scan** shows protrusion. *Initial management:* analgesics and NSAIDs, physiotherapy, and local injections. Trial of traction. Surgical intervention if weakness, severe pain, or suspected cord compression.

Pain or limitation of movement of the back: with sudden onset over seconds to hours originally

Look from the side to see if there is normal lumbar lordosis. Ask patients to touch their toes and watch for movement of spine (?rounded) and hips. Ask the patient to arch backwards, bend to each side, and rotate trunk from side to side. Lie patient down and measure length of legs. Raise each straight leg for any restriction before 45°. Initial investigations (others in **bold** below): FBC, ESR or CRP, rheumatoid factor.

Main differential diagnoses and typical outline evidence, etc.	
Mechanical pain (strains, tear, or crushing of ligaments, discs, vertebrae with normal healing)	*Suggested by:* recent onset over minutes of pain and restriction of movement in lower back in a young person. History of lifting a heavy weight or a head-on impact RTA. *Confirmed by:* recovery with minimal loss of function over days or weeks. *Initial management:* analgesics, NSAIDs, and physiotherapy. Encourage back to work early.
Posterior lumbar disc prolapse	*Suggested by:* onset over seconds of severe back pain on coughing, sneezing, or twisting after earlier strain. Radiation to buttock, thigh, or calf if prolapse compresses posterior root. *Confirmed by:* back flexed and extension restricted. Straight leg raising stopped before 45° by pain. Loss of sensation lateral foot (L4/5). Loss of ankle jerk and sensation sole of foot (S1). **MRI scan**. *Initial management:* bed rest, analgesics, NSAIDs, muscle relaxants, and physiotherapy. If these fail, then surgical referral.
Anterior lumbar disc prolapsed	*Suggested by:* onset over seconds of severe back pain on coughing, sneezing, or twisting after earlier strain (if large, prolapse compresses cauda equina, with leg weakness, incontinence, and numbness around perineum). *Confirmed by:* flaccid paresis of leg(s). Loss of knee, ankle reflexes, and extensor plantar response. Loss of vibration sense, touch, and pain with sensory level. **MRI scan** shows protrusion. *Initial management:* bed rest, analgesics, NSAIDs, muscle relaxants, and physiotherapy. If these fail, then surgical referral.
Spondylolisthesis due to spondylolysis, congenital malformation of articular process, osteoarthritis of posterior facet joints	*Suggested by:* positive family history. Sudden onset over minutes of back pain with or without sciatica in adolescence. *Confirmed by:* **plain back X-ray** shows forward displacement of vertebra over one below. *Initial management:* analgesics, NSAIDs, avoidance of sports, and the use of a corset support. Surgical referral for intractable symptoms.

Central disc protrusion	*Suggested by:* sudden onset over minutes or hours with bilateral sciatica, disturbance of bladder or bowel function. Saddle or perineal anaesthesia.
	Confirmed by: history and compression of cord visible on **MRI scan**.
	Initial management: pain control and referral to neurosurgery.

Pain or limitation of movement of the back: with onset over days to months originally

Look from the side to see if there is normal lumbar lordosis. Ask the patient to touch toes, and watch for movement of spine (?rounded) and hips. Ask to arch backwards, bend to each side, and rotate trunk from side to side. Lie patient down and measure length of legs. Raise each straight leg for any restriction before 45°. Initial investigations (others in **bold** below): FBC, ESR, rheumatoid factor.

Main differential diagnoses and typical outline evidence, etc.	
Lumbar spinal stenosis due to facet joint osteoarthrosis	*Suggested by:* onset of pain over months, worse on walking with ache and weakness in one leg. *Confirmed by:* pain on extension of back. Straight leg raising normal. Few CNS signs (but may appear shortly after exercise). **MRI scan**. *Initial management:* analgesics. If pain intractable, surgical referral for possible spinal decompression.
Spinal tumours 1° arising in spinal cord, meninges, nerve roots; 2° usually lung, breast, prostate, thyroid, kidney; Lymphoma, myeloma	*Suggested by:* onset of back pain over months with progressive pain or paresis in one or both legs. (Physical signs depend on part of cord or nerve roots affected). *Confirmed by:* 'hot spot' on bone scan with erosion or sclerosis on **plain X-ray** of 'hot spot'. Space-occupying lesion on **MRI** or **CT scan** and *histology on biopsy*. *Initial management:* effective analgesia and control of other symptoms, e.g. vomiting. Radiotherapy, chemotherapy, and surgery, individually or in combination.
Pyogenic spinal infection usually of disc space due to *staphylococcus*, *Salmonella typhi*, etc.	*Suggested by:* onset of pain over days or weeks. Little or no fever, tenderness or ↑WCC. ↑ESR. Background debilitation, surgery, or diabetes. *Confirmed by:* bone rarefaction or erosion with joint space narrowing on **back X-ray**. 'Hot spot' on **isotope bone scan** and space-occupying lesion on **MRI** or **CT scan**. *Initial management:* analgesics, NSAIDs, and antibiotics.
Spinal TB with abscesses and cord compression (Pott's para-plegia), psoas abscess.	*Suggested by:* onset of weeks or months. Low grade fever, tenderness or ↑WCC. ↑ESR. Background debilitation, diabetes. *Confirmed by:* bone rarefaction or erosion with joint space narrowing, then wedging of vertebrae. Space-occupying lesion on **MRI and CT scan**. Tubercle baccilli on stains or **culture** *of drainage material*. *Initial management:* standard antituberculous treatment.

Pain or limitation of movement of the back: with onset over years

This is a notoriously poor lead. Look from the side to see if there is normal lumbar lordosis. Ask the patient to touch toes and watch for movement of spine (?rounded) and hips. Ask the patient to arch backwards, bend to each side, and rotate trunk from side to side. Lie patient down and measure length of legs. Raise each straight leg for any restriction before 45°. Initial investigations (others in **bold** below): FBC, ESR, rheumatoid factor, back X-ray (A–P and lateral).

Main differential diagnoses and typical outline evidence, etc.	
Kyphotic pain	*Suggested by:* poor posture with a hump appearance of the back (hunchback). Onset over years usually, exacerbated over days with wedge fracture. Spinal curvature visible from the side. Associated neuromuscular disease.
	Confirmed by: **back X-ray** appearance suggestive of congenital deformity, Scheuermann's or Calve's osteochondritis, wedge fracture from osteoporosis or carcinoma, ankylosing spondylitis.
	Initial management: analgesics and OBAS (Observation, Bracing And Surgery).
Scoliotic pain, poliomyelitis, syringomyelia, etc (see under 'Suggested by')	*Suggested by:* lateral curvature visible from the back and associated rib prominence apparent from the front. Head appears off centre, and a hip or shoulder is higher than the other side. Known to have past poliomyelitis, syringomyelia, torsion dystonia, spinal tumours, spondylolisthesis, arthrogryphosis, enchondromatosis, osteogenesis imperfecta, neurofibromatosis, Chiari malformation, Duchenne muscular dystrophy, Friedreich's ataxia, Marfan's syndrome, Pompe's disease.
	Confirmed by: history and **X-ray** appearance of bony congenital anomaly.
	Initial management: treat underlying causes. Otherwise analgesics and OBAS.
Idiopathic scoliosis of thoracic or lumbar spine	*Suggested by:* progressive loss over years of horizontal alignment of shoulders and hips with age, usually in adolescent girls more than boys.
	Confirmed by: **X-ray** appearance. Increased scoliosis with growth.
	Initial management: OBAS.

Pain or limitation of movement of the hip

Assess activity. Test flexion (normal >120°) by grasping ankle in one hand and iliac crest in the other to eliminate pelvic rotation. Test abduction (normal 30–40°), preventing pelvic tilt. Test abduction in flexion (normal >70°) and adduction (normal >30°) by moving one foot over the other, internal and external rotation. Measure true length of legs from anterior superior iliac spines to medial malleoli. Trendelenburg test is positive if hip drops when foot on that same side is lifted from ground. Initial investigations (others in bold below): FBC, ESR, X-ray (A–P and lateral).

Main differential diagnoses and typical outline evidence, etc.	
Osteoarthritis	*Suggested by:* elderly, overweight and overwork. Onset over months or years. Pain, often causing a disturbed sleep, with stiffness and limitation of movement, initially of internal rotation. Difficulties in putting on stockings and cutting the toenails. *Confirmed by:* **A–P and lateral X-rays** *of hips* show loss of joint space, deformity of head and acetabulum with osteophytes and sclerosis. *Initial management:* advise weight reduction, analgesics, NSAIDs, physiotherapy. Orthopaedic referral for possible hip replacement/resurfacing.
Coxa vara caused by congenital slipped upper femoral epiphyses, fracture with malunion or non-union, osteomalacia or Paget's disease	*Suggested by:* pain and stiffness, limp with Trendelenburg 'dip' to affected side. True shortening of leg. *Confirmed by:* angle between neck and femur <125° on **X-ray**. *Initial management:* surgical referral for possible correction.
Transient synovitis (most common cause of hip pain in children)	*Suggested by:* hip pain in a child, usually a boy, with a limp and sometimes history of a preceding minor trauma. Restricted extension and internal rotation of hip. Usually no temperature. *Confirmed by:* **X-ray** and **US scan** showing synovitis. *Initial management:* symptomatic treatment with analgesics and NSAIDs ± bed rest for up to 6wk. If slow to respond, check stool culture for *Campylobacter*, and treat accordingly.
Soft tissue injury or fracture	*Suggested by:* recent impact and acute pain and/or loss of function, tenderness, deformity, swelling, crepitus. *Confirmed by:* **A–P and lateral X-ray** appearance. *Initial management:* analgesia; orthopaedic referral if fracture ± physiotherapy.

Perthes' disease	*Suggested by:* pain in hip or knee with limp with onset over months from age 3–11y. Limitation of hip movement in all ranges ± thin affected leg.
	Confirmed by: **A–P and lateral X-rays** of hips show widening of joint space and ↓size of femoral head, patchy density and later, collapse. **US scan** shows capsular distension due to synovial thickening, usually bilateral.
	Initial management: analgesics, NSAIDs, rest and traction + physiotherapy. If it is difficult to preserve mobility, then plaster casts, bracing, and surgery (to put the femoral head back in the socket).
Slipped femoral epiphysis sometimes associated with 1° hypothyroidism	*Suggested by:* typically an overweight boy with pain in groin, front of thigh or knee, and limping with onset over minutes or weeks to months. Limitation of flexion, abduction, and medial rotation. Pain usually comes with exercise and sports. Affected leg turns outwards and might be shorter than other side. Both hips might be affected.
	Confirmed by: displacement of growth plate visible on **lateral X-ray view of hip** (not A–P) or avascular necrosis and chondrolysis.
	Initial management: exclude associated conditions, e.g. hypothyroidism. If suspected, admit straight away. Traction initially; early orthopaedic referral.
Tuberculous arthritis	*Suggested by:* fever and night sweats. Pain and limp in 2–5y old, especially from poor country. Pain at night. Pain and spasm in all directions of movement with progressive muscle wasting.
	Confirmed by: rarefaction of bone on **X-ray,** then fuzziness of joint margin, then erosions. AFB in **biopsy ± culture of synovial membrane** (or in cultures from aspirates).
	Initial management: rifampicin + isoniazid + pyrazinamide for 2mo, followed by rifampicin and isoniazid for another 2mo in addition to bed rest and traction. Surgical referral if deformity.
Developmental dysplasia (still referred to as congenital dislocation of the hip)	*Suggested by:* pain, stiffness and ↓movement in childhood or adolescence; undiagnosed hip dislocation early in life. Waddling gait with hyperlordosis in bilateral hip involvement.
	Confirmed by: positive Ortolani test (palpable clunk when hip is reduced in and out of acetabulum) or Barlow test (clunk is felt when gentle pressure is applied to the adducted hip) in the newborn. Shallow acetabulum with or without current dislocation on **A–P and lateral X-ray of hips** (ultrasound in neonate).
	Initial management: bracing (Pavlick harness) if under 6y old. Closed reduction preceded by traction for the 'over 6y old'. If >2y or failed previous treatment, open reduction or various procedures depending on age.

(Continued)

Pain or limitation of movement of the hip (continued)

Main differential diagnoses and typical outline evidence, etc. *(continued)*	
Post-total hip replacement problems (dislocation, prosthesis failure, prosthesis loosening, and infection)	*Suggested by:* pain, difficult or impossible weight-bearing. Limb shorter and externally rotated in the case of dislocation. General ill heath, high temperature, and night sweats in cases of infection
	Confirmed by: radiological appearances. +ve culture and sensitivity if infection.
	Initial management: analgesia. Antibiotics. Orthopaedic referral for possible re-replacement.

Pain or limitation of movement of the knee

Look for quadriceps wasting ability to weight bear, deformity of the knee or swelling. Feel for swelling with palm of other hand pressing above patella. Compare flexion and extension on both sides. Abduct and adduct tibia with knee flexed at 30° to test medial and lateral ligaments. With knee flexed at 90°, pull and push tibia to test anterior and posterior cruciate ligaments. Initial investigations (others in **bold** below): FBC, ESR, or CRP, X-ray of knee (P–A and lateral).

Main differential diagnoses and typical outline evidence, etc.	
Osteoarthritis	*Suggested by:* old age, overweight or overwork. onset of months or years, worse in cold and damp. Deformity (especially varus—bow-legged) and swelling. Crepitus on passive movement.
	Confirmed by: above history and examination. Loss of joint space on **X-ray** with deformity, osteophytes, and sclerosis.
	Initial management: weight reduction, analgesics, NSAIDs, physiotherapy. Orthopaedic referral, e.g. for total knee replacement in advanced cases.
Chondromalacia patellae	*Suggested by:* patella aching after sitting or walking on slopes or stairs in a young adult, typically females. Patellar tenderness.
	Confirmed by: above history and examination, and 'fibrillation' of patellar cartilage on **arthroscopy or MRI**.
	Initial management: restrict activities which aggravate symptoms, analgesics, and physiotherapy. Orthopaedic referral if no response.
Recurrent patella subluxation	*Suggested by:* jumping-type sports, e.g. basketball or volleyball. Knee often giving way (especially in knocked-kneed girls).
	Confirmed by: increased lateral movement of patella.
	Initial management: orthopaedic referral for possible stabilization.
Patella tendinopathy (jumper's knee)	*Suggested by:* jumping-type sports. Pain on forceful movement of knee in sport.
	Confirmed by: tenderness over patellar tendon. **X-rays** show normal bones.
	Initial management: rest, NSAIDs, analgesics, physiotherapy to build up quadriceps, hamstrings and calf muscles. Orthopaedic referral if no response.
Ileotibial band syndrome	*Suggested by:* long distant runners and cyclists, pain when active. Rest eases the pain.
	Confirmed by: tenderness over lateral femoral condyle.
	Initial management: RICER regime (Rest, Ice, Compression, Elevation and Referral). If no response, advise different sporting activity.

Medial shelf syndrome	*Suggested by:* repetitive stress, single blunt trauma, anterior knee pain, knee clicking or brief locking. Symptoms made worse by activity, prolonged standing or stair climbing.
	Confirmed by: inflamed synovial fold above medial meniscus on **arthroscopy**.
	Initial management: analgesics, NSAIDs, and physiotherapy. If no response, possible arthroscopic resection of inflamed medial band.
Hoffa's fat pad syndrome	*Suggested by:* history of major acute or chronic repetitive trauma. Brief locking of knee with pain and swelling under patella.
	Confirmed by: hypertrophic pad between articular surfaces on **MRI** or **arthroscopy**.
	Initial management: analgesics, NSAIDs, ice, and rest in the acute stage ± physiotherapy. If no response, arthroscopic resection of inflamed fat pad.
Acute arthritis due to sepsis, gout or rheumatoid arthritis	*Suggested by:* onset hours, days of pain and swelling.
	Confirmed by: aspiration, microscopy, and culture. ↑**urate** in gout. **Rheumatoid factor** +ve in rheumatoid arthritis.
	Initial management: analgesics, NSAIDs; treat cause, e.g. antibiotics, and urgent orthopaedic referral for septic arthritis.
Medial collateral ligament (MCL) tear	*Suggested by:* a blow on the outer surface of the knee or an injury forcing the leg outwards. Pain and swelling over the injured ligament. Pain triggered by stretching ligament. Unstable knee, feeling that the knee may give way or buckle.
	Confirmed by: pain and excessive laxity when gentle pressure is applied to the outside of the knee. **X-ray** and **MRI scan**.
	Initial management: rest, ice, compression, analgesics, and NSAIDs. Wearing knee immobilizer; avoid weight-bearing. Orthopaedic referral and possible repair for very severe injuries.
Lateral collateral ligament (LCL) tear	*Suggested by:* an injury causing a direct impact to the inner surface of the knee. Pain and swelling over the injured ligament. Pain is triggered or made worse by stretching the ligament. In severe injuries, the knee is very unstable.
	Confirmed by: pain and laxity when gentle pressure is applied to the inside of the knee. **X-ray** and **MRI scan**.
	Initial management: rest, ice, compression, analgesics and NSAIDs. Wearing of a knee immobilizer and avoiding weight-bearing for about 2wk in more severe injuries. Surgical repair for very severe injuries with persisting instability.

(Continued)

Pain or limitation of movement of the knee (continued)

Main differential diagnoses and typical outline evidence, etc. *(continued)*

Anterior cruciate ligament (ACL) tears	*Suggested by:* history of a posterior blow or a rotational force when foot fixed to ground. Sudden swelling and pain in the knee. Hearing a 'pop' at the time of the injury and/or a sensation that the knee will 'give way'.
	Confirmed by: tibia moves forward when pulled after effective analgesia or anaesthesia (Lachman's test). **X-ray** and **MRI scan**.
	Initial management: RICE, analgesics, and NSAIDs. Reconstruction of ACL if instability persists
Posterior cruciate ligament (PCL) tears	*Suggested by:* history of a direct impact on the shin when the knee is bent. Pain and swelling with a feeling that the knee will 'give way'.
	Confirmed by: tibia moves backward when pulled after effective analgesia or anaesthesia (reverse Lachman's test). **X-ray** and **MRI scan**.
	Initial management: RICE, analgesics, and NSAIDs. Reconstruction of PCL if persistent instability.
Meniscal tears	*Suggested by:* history of twisting, pivoting, and decelerating of the knee. Stiffness, swelling, locking, and buckling of the knee. A popping sensation at the time of injury.
	Confirmed by: **X-ray** and **MRI scan**.
	Initial management: RICE, analgesics, and NSAIDs. Arthroscopic trimming of damaged meniscus.
Meniscal cyst	*Suggested by:* history of a blow on the side of the knee. Variable swelling, worse when knee flexed to 60°, less when flexed further. Knee clicking and giving way.
	Confirmed by: cyst present on **MRI scan**.
	Initial management: aspiration to give temporary relief. Definitive treatment is excision with or without meniscectomy.
Osteochondritis dessicans (juvenile and adult types)	*Suggested by:* history of repetitive stress as in competitive sports. Pain and swelling of knee. A snapping, catching feeling, or locking when the knee is moved.
	Confirmed by: defect on articular surface with or without a loose body on **X-ray**.
	Initial management: in the juvenile, suspending exercise and sports, using crutches, or wearing a cast for 2mo (until symptoms subside) followed by physiotherapy. If bone growth ceased, orthopaedic referral for correction.

Loose bodies due to osteo-chondritis dessicans, osteoarthritis, chip fractures, synovial chondromatosis	*Suggested by:* locking of knee during extension and flexion. Swelling and effusion. *Confirmed by:* seeing loose bodies on **arthroscopy**. *Initial management:* arthroscopic or open surgical removal if symptomatic.
Bursitis (without or with infection) due to pre-patellar bursitis (housemaid's knee), etc.	*Suggested by:* localized pain and swelling over site of bursa (e.g. below patella). *Confirmed by:* localized pain and swelling over site of bursa. Improvement with rest, analgesia, and physiotherapy. *Initial management:* analgesics and antibiotics if infected. Aspiration and local steroid injection if no infection. Orthopaedic referral for possible excision.

Pain or limitation of movement of the foot

Watch gait, examine wear on shoe sole and print on floor of damp foot. Ask to extend or dorsiflex (normal >25°), flex (normal 30°). Evert and invert. Ask to extend toes (normal >60°) and stand on tiptoe. Initial investigations (others in **bold** below): FBC, ESR, rheumatoid factor, X-ray.

Main differential diagnoses and typical outline evidence, etc.	
Hallux valgus associated with bunion and osteoarthritis	*Suggested by:* the first metatarsal is deviated medially and the big toe deviated laterally. Painful motion of joint and/or difficulty with footwear. *Confirmed by:* above clinical appearance (big toe deviated laterally). **X-ray** to assess joint pathology and measure angular deformity. *Initial management:* analgesics, NSAIDs, adapting footwear, and functional orthotic therapy. Orthopaedic referral to correct the deformity.
Pes planus	*Suggested by:* loss of medial foot arch, (appearance of damp surface in contact with floor, normal in early childhood) causing the foot to roll inwards. Pain if foot and heel everted. *Confirmed by:* above clinical appearance and response to exercises, and medial heel shoe wedges in some cases. *Initial management:* use of orthotics (special insoles), combined with supportive footwear that fit the foot correctly and contains a firm low heel. Orthopaedic referral if these measures fail.
Pes cavus normal variant, hereditary, idiopathic, or due to spina bifida, past polio	*Suggested and Confirmed by:* accentuated foot arches and other neurological disorders, e.g. spina bifida. The ankle may be rolled out slightly and the toes may appear clawed. *Confirmed by:* above clinical appearanc e. *Initial management:* foot orthotics (insoles), pads to get pressure off painful areas, proper fitting of footwear, treatment of associated corns and calluses.
Hammer toes	*Suggested by:* tip of a lesser toe points downwards. *Confirmed by:* toe extended at the metatarsophalangeal (MTP) joint, flexed at the proximal IP joint but extended at the distal IP joint. *Initial management:* wide fitted, low-heeled shoes, non-medicated pads to take pressure off corns and hard skin, moisturizing creams to keep skin soft, silicon toe prop to prevent further contracture. In rigid deformities, surgical interventions, e.g. arthroplasty or arthrodesis.
Claw toes	*Suggested by:* tip of a lesser toe points down and back. *Confirmed by:* toe extended at the MTP joint, flexed at the proximal IP and distal ip joint. *Initial management:* same as in hammer toes

Mallet toes	*Suggested by:* tip of a lesser toe points downwards.
	Confirmed by: toe is extended at the MTP and proximal IP joints, and flexed at the distal IP joint.
	Initial management: same as in hammer toes.
Trigger toe	*Suggested by:* tip of the big toe points downwards.
	Confirmed by: big toe is extended at MTP joint and flexed at the IP joint.
	Initial management: same as in hammer toes
Hallux rigidus	*Suggested by:* pain and stiffness localized to big toe, aggravated by cold damp weather. Difficulties with running and squatting.
	Confirmed by: tenderness and swelling of 1st MTP joint. **X-ray** may show a distal ring of osteophytes.
	Initial management: shoe modifications, e.g. wide fitting shoes, orthotic devices, analgesics, NSAIDs, physiotherapy, local steroid injections. Orthopaedic referral for intervention in advanced cases.
Metatarsalgia due to shoe pressure, previous trauma, rheumatoid arthritis, sesamoid fracture, synovitis	*Suggested by:* pain in the ball of the foot, the part of the sole just behind the toes worse on standing or running. Feeling as if walking on pebbles. Patient typically does high impact sport or overweight.
	Confirmed by: tenderness of heads of metatarsals. **X-ray** to exclude other conditions, e.g. stress fracture.
	Initial management: rest, ice packs on the affected areas, analgesics and NSAIDs, proper shoes, shock-absorbing insoles, metatarsal pads. Orthopaedic referral for intervention if these measures fail.
Morton's metatarsalgia due to interdigital neuroma	*Suggested by:* intermittent pain, burning sensation or numbness on the bottom of the foot radiating to the 3rd and 4th toes. A description of 'as if walking on marbles'.
	Confirmed by: tenderness on compression of site of neuroma between metatarsals (e.g. squeezing the forefoot together triggers pain) and massaging offers significant relief.
	Initial management: soft-soled shoes with a wide toe box and low heel. Plantar pad to elevate metatarsal head adjacent to neuroma preventing compression. Orthopaedic referral if refractory case.
March fracture	*Suggested by:* localized foot pain after excessive walking.
	Confirmed by: tenderness of 2nd or 3rd metatarsals. **X-ray** showing fracture.
	Initial management: analgesics, NSAIDs.
Calcaneum disease; arthritis of subtalar joint; tear of calcaneal tendon; post calcaneal bursitis; plantar fasciitis, etc.	*Suggested by:* localized heel pain.
	Confirmed by: **X-ray** and **MRI scan** appearance.
	Initial management: analgesics, NSAIDs, physiotherapy. Orthopaedic referral if refractory

(Continued)

Pain or limitation of movement of the foot (continued)

Main differential diagnoses and typical outline evidence, etc. *(continued)*
Soft tissue injury or fracture	*Suggested by:* recent impact and acute pain and/or loss of function, tenderness, deformity, swelling, crepitus.
	Confirmed by: **X-ray** appearance.
	Initial management: analgesia; orthopaedic referral if fracture ± physiotherapy

Psychiatric and neurological symptoms and physical signs

Neurological and psychiatric symptoms and signs

Neurological and psychiatric symptoms (e.g. stroke and depression) are more damaging to self-confidence than symptoms in the other systems. Self-confidence is central to the way in which we interact with our environment, both social and physical. It was emphasized on page 20 that there are three areas over which our bodies try to exercise control:

- the internal milieu,
- the structure of our bodies and,
- our environment, social, and physical.

We are unaware of the first two when we are healthy, but when we become ill, we become actively involved in supplementing them. We are aware of the third from our earliest experience. Difficulties with the way we interact with people and our environment blend into a continuum with neurological and mental illness. The diagnosis and treatment of neurological and psychiatric conditions has to focus on how patients can learn how to adapt to their circumstances and how those around them can help, including those who work in health and social services.

Psychiatric signs may have been noted during the history and examination. The patient may have complained of 'anxiety' or 'depression', but in order to arrive at diagnoses, a number of attributes have to be present, some of which are observed rather than reported by the patient.

The idea that a diagnosis is an envelope that encloses patients with different requirements which share a common mechanism is particularly applicable to psychiatry. For example, patients within the 'envelope' of depression will contain subgroups, some who benefit from cognitive therapy alone (especially if mild), others who benefit from antidepressant medication (especially of the depression is moderate); in severe cases, they may require electroconvulsive treatment (ECT).

Inability to carry out the activities of daily living

This is the patient's failure to exercise the most basic control over his or her personal space and immediate environment due to mental or physical disability. The patient's family, neighbours, or community may provide support to compensate (which can place enormous demands and burdens upon them). Failing this, it has to be provided by salaried personnel from a funded source. Each disability will then need to be identified specifically so that it can be supported properly.

Main differential diagnoses and typical outline evidence, etc.	
Mildly impaired activities of daily living	*Suggested by:* inability without assistance to: get out of bed or chair or dress or use toilet or wash or bathe or prepare food or eat it or shop or maintain a home or go outside or earn a living.
	Confirmed by: formal documentation of **at least one** of the above disabilities.
	Initial management: arrange assistance for each specific disability in patient's own home.
Moderately impaired activities of daily living	*Suggested by:* inability without assistance to: get out of bed or chair or dress or use toilet or wash or bathe or prepare food or eat it or shop or maintain a home or go outside or earn a living
	Confirmed by: formal documentation of **many of the above** disabilities, which require **constant supervision** but no additional skilled nursing assistance.
	Initial management: arrange admission to residential home or constant supervision in patient's home.
Severely impaired activities of daily living	*Suggested by:* inability without assistance to: get out of bed or chair or dress or use toilet or wash or bathe or prepare food or eat it or shop or maintain a home or go outside or earn a living
	Confirmed by: formal documentation of many of the above disabilities, which require constant supervision **and additional skilled nursing assistance.**
	Initial management: arrange admission to institution providing skilled nursing or constant supervision and skilled nursing assistance in patient's home.

General anxiety

Anxiety is a common experience; when patients seek advice, it is usually because it has been severe or prolonged. The history, examination, and tests are directed at confirming or excluding secondary causes. Initial investigations (other tests in **bold** below): FBC, U&E, LFT, TSH, FT4.

Main differential diagnoses and typical outline evidence, etc.	
Generalized anxiety disorder	*Suggested by:* long history of fearful anticipation, restlessness, inability to relax, irritability, sensitivity to noise, restlessness, poor concentration, worrying thoughts, insomnia, nightmares, depression, obssessions, depersonalization and derealization, dry mouth, difficulty swallowing, tremor, dizziness, headache, parasthesiae, tinnitus, epigastric discomfort, excessive wind, frequent or loose motions, constriction/discomfort in the chest, difficulty breathing or hyperventilation, palpitations and awareness of missed beats, frequency or urgency of micturition, erectile dysfunction, menstrual problems. Panic attacks, depression, and alcohol dependence.
	Confirmed by: no evidence of thyrotoxicosis or hypoglycaemia or Cushing's disease or phaeochromocytoma.
	Initial management: listening, reassurance about nature of symptoms, cognitive behaviour therapy, anxiolytics (e.g. diazepam), or antidepressants (e.g. selective serotonin reuptake inhibitors (SSRIs)).
Panic disorder	*Suggested by:* intense feeling of apprehension or impending disaster. Developing quickly and unexpectedly without a recognizable trigger. Shortness of breath and sensation of smothering, nausea, abdominal pain, depersonalization and derealization, choking, numbness, tingling, palpitations, flushes, trembling, shaking, chest discomfort, fear of dying, sweating, dizziness, faintness.
	Confirmed by: 4 symptoms of panic attack in one episode and 4 attacks in a month, or a persistent fear of attacks. No evidence of thyrotoxicosis or hypoglycaemia or Cushing's disease or phaeochromocytoma, and no other physical cause of symptoms.
	Initial management: reassurance about nature of symptoms, cognitive behaviour therapy, anxiolytics (e.g. diazepam), or antidepressants (e.g. SSRIs).
Alcohol withdrawal	*Suggested by:* recent heavy alcohol intake (usually superimposed on habitually high intake). Visual hallucinations imply 'delirium tremens', tremor, agitations, paranoid delusions and intense fright, sleep disturbance, ↓MCV, abnormal **LFT**, **EEG** changes.
	Confirmed by: alcohol history, subsequent episodes in similar circumstances.
	Initial management: sedation and alcohol detoxification (e.g. chlordiazepoxide) with tailing off over days.

Thyrotoxicosis	*Suggested by:* heat intolerance, tremor, nervousness, palpitation, frequent bowel movements, goitre.
	Confirmed by: ↓**TSH**, ↑**FT4**.
	Initial management: non-selective β-blocker, e.g. propranolol, to control symptoms if no contraindication, e.g. asthma, carbimazole, or propylthiouracil to suppress thyroid hormone production.
Hypoglycaemia	*Suggested by:* preceded by seconds or minutes by anxiety, fear, chest tightness, sweating, hunger, and darkening of vision. Usually in diabetic, usually on insulin.
	Confirmed by: ↓**blood glucose** (<2mmol/L).
	Initial management: if unconscious, glucose IV or glucagon IM or buccal glucose gel. If safe to swallow, glucose by mouth, then carbohydrate snack.
Phaeochromo-cytoma	*Suggested by:* abrupt episodes of anxiety, fear, chest tightness, sweating, headaches, and marked rises in BP.
	Confirmed by: catecholamines (↑**VMA**, ↑**HMMA**) or ↑free **metadrenaline** in urine and blood soon after episode.
	Initial management: α-blocker followed by β-blocker.

Anxiety in response to specific issues

The cause of the anxiety is established from the history and the inappropriate emotional response is managed by cognitive therapies.

Main differential diagnoses and typical outline evidence, etc.	
Anorexia nervosa	*Suggested by:* self-induced weight loss, body image distortion, intense fear of gaining weight though underweight. Amenorrhoea in women for ≥3mo. and diminished sexual interest. Bingeing and vomiting, purging or excessive exercise. Depression and social withdrawal, sensitivity to cold, delayed gastric emptying, constipation, low BP, bradycardia, hypothermia.
	Confirmed by: (BMI <17.5kg/m^2) and many of above clinical features.
	Initial management: if no cooperation with keeping food diary, restoration of nutritional balance, correction of electrolyte and other deficiencies and weight falling, seek psychiatric help, and admit to specialist unit. Cognitive behavioural therapies, analytic therapy, interpersonal therapy, supportive therapy, family therapy, antidepressants (e.g. SSRIs), may need specialist feeding.
Bulimia nervosa	*Suggested by:* preoccupation with eating and irresistible craving for food, fear of gaining weight, recurrent episodes of binge eating far beyond normally accepted amounts of food, self-induced vomiting, use of laxatives, diuretics ± appetite suppressants, often previous history of anorexia nervosa.
	Confirmed by: some of above features and normal menses and normal weight.
	Initial management: keeping food diary, cognitive behavioural therapy, SSRI antidepressants, fluoxetine.
Dissociation (hysteria)	*Suggested by:* amnesia, depersonalization, dissociative identity disorder (displaying multiple personalities), or fuge (inability to recall past, formation of new identity).
	Confirmed by: absence of physical findings.
	Initial management: exploration of any precipitating causes and associated psychiatric disorders.
Somatization disorder (Briquet's syndrome)	*Suggested by:* long history of numerous unsubstantiated physical complaints with no adequate physical explanation and refusal to be reassured.
	Confirmed by: absence of physical findings.
	Initial management: reassurance that no serious underlying illness, explanation of mechanisms of symptoms, treat any underlying psychiatric disorder, e.g antidepressants if indicated by other features, cognitive behaviour therapy.

Simple (specific) phobia	*Suggested by:* evoked anxiety in specific situations, avoidance of phobic situation, symptoms and signs of generalized anxiety disorder.
	Confirmed by: inappropriate anxiety in the presence of particular circumstances, e.g. enclosed spaces (claustrophobia), spiders (arachnophobia).
	Initial management: behavioural therapy, e.g. systematic desensitization therapy, exposure, flooding, implosion therapy, anti-anxiety medications (e.g benzodiazepine), or antidepressant.
Social phobia (social anxiety)	*Suggested by:* anxiety with intense and persistent fear of being scrutinized or negatively evaluated by others in comparatively small groups, resulting in fear and avoidance of social situations (e.g. meeting people in authority, using a telephone, speaking in front of a group). Fear of specific social situations.
	Initial management: cognitive behavioural therapy ± antidepressants, e.g. SSRI, paroxetine, fluoxetine.
Agoraphobia	*Suggested by:* fear of open spaces, crowds, or situations where escape is difficult. Staying at home, will not visit doctors ± depression, and obsessional thoughts may be present but not dominant.
	Initial management: cognitive behavioural therapy ± anti-anxiety medications, antidepressants, e.g. SSRI, paroxetine, fluoxetine.
Post-traumatic stress disorder caused by experiencing a traumatic event, e.g. major accident, fire, assault, military combat	*Suggested by:* memories, nightmares, flashbacks, numbing of emotions, anxiety and irritability, insomnia, poor concentration, hypervigilance and depression, anxiety and alcohol/other substance abuse and dependence. Delayed response arising within 6mo of an exceptional traumatic event.
	Initial management: psychotherapy, trauma-focused cognitive therapy, antidepressants, e.g. paroxetine if depressive component and with somatic symptoms.

Depression

Depression is a common experience; it is its duration and severity that make patients to seek advice. This is also what is used to select the appropriate treatment. The diagnosis and selection of treatment is based on the history and mental state examination.

Main differential diagnoses and typical outline evidence, etc.	
Major depression	*Suggested by:* depressed mood ± loss of interest and enjoyment, reduced energy causing easy tiredness and reduced activity, change in appetite or weight, psychomotor agitation or retardation, insomnia or hypersomnia, sense of worthlessness or guilt, fatigue or loss of energy, diminished appetite, recurrent thoughts of death, low self-esteem, poor attention and concentration, hopelessness, suicidal and self-harm preoccupations.
	Confirmed by: presence of approximately 5 or more of above symptoms. Duration of at least 2wk.
	Initial management: reassurance, cognitive behavioural therapy. Antidepressant, especially if somatic symptoms. ECT if severely depressed, especially with delusions and poor response to medications alone. Admission if suicidal ideas and isolation.
Mild to moderate depression	*Suggested by:* depressed mood ± loss of interest in pleasure, change in appetite or weight, psychomotor agitation or retardation, insomnia or hypersomnia, sense of worthlessness or guilt, fatigue, loss of energy, recurrent thoughts of death or suicide.
	Confirmed by: presence of about 5 or more of above 7 symptoms
	Initial management: cognitive therapy if mild. Antidepressant, especially if somatic symptoms.
Depression 2° or partly due to other conditions	*Suggested by:* history of any other illness that undermines self-confidence, e.g. physical illness but especially anxiety disorders, alcohol abuse, substance abuse.
	Confirmed by: improvement when underlying condition alleviated.
	Initial management: treatment of identifiable cause. Antidepressant, especially if somatic symptoms.
Depression 2° or partly to medication	*Suggested by:* history of taking β-blockers, α-blockers, anticonvulsants, calcium channel blockers, corticosteroids, oral contraceptives, opiates, drugs used for Parkinson's disease (e.g. levodopa).
	Confirmed by: improvement if drug stopped or changed.
	Initial management: stopping potential cause.
Seasonal affective disorder	*Suggested by:* 'winter blues'—depression of mood + ↑sleep, ↑food intake (with carbohydrate craving) and weight gain, sometimes with opposite mood swings in summer.
	Initial management: reassurance, antidepressant, especially if somatic symptoms.

Delusions

Delusions are strongly held beliefs, held despite evidence to the contrary.

Main differential diagnoses and typical outline evidence, etc.	
Mania and hypomania Unipolar or bipolar disorder (i.e. manic depression)	*Suggested by:* persistently high or euphoric mood out of keeping with circumstances, pressure of speech, no insight, over-assertiveness, ↑energy and activity, grandiose delusions, spending spree, ↑appetite, hallucinations, disinhibition, ↑sexual desire, labile mood, elation, self-important ideas, ↓pain threshold, irritability, poor concentration, hostility when thwarted, ↓desire or need for sleep. *Confirmed by:* inability to lead normal life because of above symptoms. *Initial management:* antipsychotics (e.g. olanzapine) or mood stabilizer (e.g. valproate), admission for supervision of care if danger to self or others, treat potential precipitating cause, e.g. infection, hyperthyroidism, etc. Stop potential precipitating drug, e.g. amphetamine, cocaine, antidepressants, glucocorticoids, etc.
Acute schizophrenia	*Suggested by:* delusions (usually bizarre), hallucinations, especially somatic and auditory hallucinations, thought disorder, e.g. insertion ± withdrawal, thought broadcasting, primary delusions (in addition to thought delusions, passivity feelings, thought echo, or hearing voices referring to the patient in the 3rd person), including blunting of affect. *Confirmed by:* at least one of the above Schneider 1st rank symptoms present for most of the time for a month or more. Symptoms occur in clear consciousness. *Initial management:* antipsychotics, preferably atypicals, e.g. olanzapine, risperidone to avoid side effects. Typical antipsychotics, e.g. chlorpromazine or haloperidol (if extrapyramidal side effects, reduce dose, add anticholinergic, e.g. procyclidine, or use atypical antipsychotics, e.g. clozapine—specialist treatment). Admission for supervision of care if danger to self or others.
Major psychotic depression	*Suggested by:* depressed mood ± loss of interest in pleasure, change in appetite or weight, psychomotor agitation or retardation, insomnia or hypersomnia, sense of worthlessness or guilt, fatigue or loss of energy, recurrent thoughts of death, poor concentration suicide. Concurrent psychotic symptoms, e.g. delusions and hallucinations. *Confirmed by:* diagnosis of depression and presence of psychotic symptoms. *Initial management:* combined antipsychotic and antidepressant medication. Admission to hospital if symptoms are severe, suicidal ideas, and isolation. Consider adding ECT if poor response to medication.

Acute confusion

Onset over hours/days, fluctuating conscious level (typically worse at night), impaired memory, disorientation in time and place, drowsy ± withdrawn or hyperactive and agitated, disordered thinking, (slow and muddled ± delusions, e.g. accusing relatives of taking things), hallucinations (particularly visual), mood swings.

Diagnostic approach: look for other leads in history and examination. Initial investigations (other tests in **bold** below): FBC, U&E, ABG, blood glucose , urine and blood cultures, LFT, CXR, ECG, CT scan.

Main differential diagnoses and typical outline evidence, etc.	
Bacteraemia or septicaemia due to urinary tract infection (UTI), upper respiratory tract infection (URTI)	*Suggested by:* fever, rigors, associated cough, chest signs, dysuria, frequency, urine 'dipstick' +ve if UTI, ↑WCC. *Confirmed by:* blood or urine culture growing bacteria. Resolution of confusion on antibiotics. *Initial management:* provisional antibiotics depending on suspected source (e.g. trimethoprim for UTI), then definitive antibiotics depending on sensitivities.
Hypoxia	*Suggested by:* history or signs of lung or heart disease. Central cyanosis. *Confirmed by:* ↓P_aO_2. ↓P_aCO_2 on **blood gas analysis** in type 1 respiratory failure or right-to-left pulmonary shunt, ↑P_aCO_2 in type 2 respiratory failure due to ventilator failure. *Initial management:* controlled O_2 <28% if ↑P_aCO_2.
Alcohol withdrawal	*Suggested by:* tremor, visual hallucinations, ↑MCV, abnormal LFT. *Confirmed by:* history of heavy alcohol intake with sudden decrease. *Initial management:* sedation (e.g. chlordiazepoxide) with tailing off over days.
Post-ictal state	*Suggested by:* history of previous fits, evidence of injury from clonic movements, tough biting, incontinence. *Confirmed by:* recovery of minutes to hours and subsequent history of fit from witness. *Initial management:* neurological observations. Restoration of anti-epileptic treatment of already established, manage as 'first fit' if not.
Thiamine deficiency	*Suggested by:* history of poor diet, ataxia, nystagmus, ocular palsies. *Confirmed by:* ↓**red cell ketolase**, response to treatment. *Initial management:* thiamine IV initially, then PO.

Hypothyroidism	*Suggested by:* puffy features, sleepy, cold intolerant, slow-relaxing ankle (and other) jerks.
	Confirmed by: ↓T4, ↑TSH (if primary thyroid failure), ↓TSH or normal (if 2° to pituitary failure).
	Initial management: low dose liothyronine initially if severe.
Thyrotoxicosis	*Suggested by:* tremor, sweating, lid retraction or lag, ± goitre, tachycardia, hyper-reflexia.
	Confirmed by: ↑T4 or ↑T3, ↓↓TSH.
	Initial management: non-selective β-blocker, e.g. propranolol followed by carbimazole or propylthiouracil.
Hypoglycaemia	*Suggested by:* confusion, ataxia, sweating, tachycardia.
	Confirmed by: ↓blood glucose (<2mmol/L).
	Initial management: if unconscious, 10% glucose IV or glucagon IM or buccal glucose gel. If safe to swallow, glucose by mouth, then carbohydrate snack.
Adrenal failure due to 1° adrenal disease (Addison's disease) or 2° to ACTH deficiency	*Suggested by:* lethargy, weakness, dizziness, buccal and scar pigmentation if Addison's, hypotension.
	Confirmed by: ↓9 a.m plasma cortisol and impaired response to **short Synacthen test**.
	Initial management: if ↓BP, fluids IV or colloids; if glucose, 10% dextrose IV. If ill, hydrocortisone IV, (otherwise PO) + fludrocortisone.
Frontal lobe lesion: ischaemia, tumour, abscess	*Suggested by:* personality change, emotional lability, features of dementia, recent epilepsy.
	Confirmed by: **CT** or **MRI scan** of brain.
	Initial management: assess for feasibility of surgical removal.
Drug effect	*Suggested by:* presence drug which can potentially cause acute confusion.
	Confirmed by: resolution by stopping drug.
	Initia l management: stopping drug.

Chronic confusion or cognitive impairment

Patient admitting to 'being a bit forgetful', but relatives complain of loss of short-term memory and inability to perform normally simple tasks or failure to cope at home or self-neglect. Established with Mini Mental State Examination (MMSE) with scores: place and date (10), registering three named objects (3), calculation (5), recall above three objects (3), naming two objects (2), repeating a phrase (1), three-stage command (3), reading (1), writing (1), copying (1), interpretation: <10/30—severe cognitive impairment, <17/30—moderate, <23/30—mild.

Diagnostic approach: history and examination for more diagnostic leads.

Initial investigations (other tests in **bold** below): FBC, ESR or CRP, LFT, calcium etc., TSH, FT4, CT scan.

Main differential diagnoses and typical outline evidence, etc.	
Alzheimer's disease	*Suggested by:* MMSE <10 with dysphasia, dyspraxia, agnosia, and inability to plan strategically.
	Confirmed by: by absence of features of vascular (multi-infarct) dementia or parkinsonism. CT: reduced brain mass and ↑ventricles.
	Initial management: assess care requirements at home or need for institutional care.
Vascular (multi-infarct) dementia	*Suggested by:* stepwise progression of dementia with each infarct. Associated neurological defects, e.g. hemiparesis, pseudobulbar palsy, etc.
	Confirmed by: by multiple lacunar infarcts or larger strokes on CT scan.
	Initial management: aspirin, statin, control of BP to prevent progression, assess care requirements.
Lewy body dementia	*Suggested by* and *Confirmed by:* fluctuating but persistent dementia with parkinsonism ± hallucinations.
	Initial management: assess care requirements. Treatment of associated parkinsonism, etc.
Huntington's disease	*Suggested by* and *Confirmed by:* cognitive impairment in 3rd or 4th decade with psychomotor slowing, personality change, apathy and depression. Involuntary choreiform movements of the face, shoulders, upper limbs, and gait.
	Initial management: assess care requirements.
Creutzfedt–Jakob disease (CJD) and variant CJD	*Suggested by:* progressive dementia, myoclonus, depression, diplopia, supranuclear palsy, field defects, hallucinations, cortical blindness. Aged <50 and slower progress suggests variant CJD.
	Suggested by and *Confirmed by:* clinical progress, tonsillar biopsy, **MRI scan** appearance.
	Initial management: assess care requirements.

Headache—acute, new onset

Onset over seconds to hours. Initial investigations (other tests in **bold** below): FBC, ESR or CRP, CT scan.

Main differential diagnoses and typical outline evidence, etc.	
Meningitis viral or bacterial	*Suggested by:* photophobia, fever, neck stiffness, vomiting, Kernig's sign. Petechial or purpuric rash (in meningococcal meningitis).
	Confirmed by: **CT brain** to exclude abscess if neurological signs present, **lumbar puncture**—viral meningitis: CSF clear, ↑lymphocytes, ↑protein, normal glucose). Bacterial meningitis: CSF with ↑neutrophils, ↑protein, ↓glucose ↑visible bacteria on Gram stain.
	Initial management: benzylpenicillin IM or IV while awaiting confirmation of diagnosis, culture and sensitivity. Analgesia.
Low CSF pressure	*Suggested by:* worsening or recurrence of headache after lumbar puncture (usually for suspected meningitis) made worse by sitting up.
	Confirmed by: spontaneous resolution after few days.
	Initial management: bed rest for 24h until CSF reforms. Analgesia.
Subarachnoid haemorrhage	*Suggested by:* sudden occipital headache (often described as 'like a blow to the head'), variable degree of consciousness ± neck stiffness, subhyaloid haemorrhage ± focal neurological signs.
	Confirmed by: **CT or MRI brain scan. Lumbar puncture:** bloodstained CSF that does not clear in successive bottles, presence of xanthochromia in CSF (up to 2wk after the haemorrhage).
	Initial management: neuro obs until stable enough for neurosurgery if indicated by imaging results. Analgesia. Dexamethasone if ↑intracranial pressure.
Intracranial haemorrhage	*Suggested by:* focal neurological signs.
	Confirmed by: **CT/MRI brain scan**.
	Initial management: nil by mouth and fluids IV if dysphagia. Speech and Language therapist (SALT) assessment. DVT prophylaxis: stockings/LMW heparin (if no bleed). If haemorrhage: treat severe hypertension (systolic >200mmHg), neuro obs until stable enough for neurosurgery (if indicated by imaging results). Analgesia. Dexamethasone if ↑intracranial pressure.

Head injury with cerebral contusion	*Suggested by:* history of trauma, cuts/bruises, ↓conscious level, lucid period, amnesia. *Confirmed by:* **skull X-ray, CT head** normal or showing oedema but no subdural haematoma or extradural haemorrhage. *Initial management:* neuro obs until stable enough for neurosurgery if indicated by imaging results. Analgesia. Dexamethasone if ↑intracranial pressure.
Acute closed angle glaucoma	*Suggested by:* red eyes, haloes, ↓visual acuity due to corneal clouding, pupil abnormality. *Confirmed by:* ↑**intra-ocular pressure.** *Initial management:* pilocarpine 2–4% eye drops 1 hourly. Acetazolamide PO or IV. Stepwise analgesia.
Sinusitis	*Suggested by:* fever, facial pain, mucopurulent nasal discharge, tender over sinuses ± URTI. ↑WCC suggest bacterial infection. *Confirmed by:* **X-ray of sinuses or CT scan:** mucosal thickening, a fluid level or opacification. *Initial management:* analgesia. Antibiotic if strong suspicion of bacterial infection.
Tension headache	*Suggested by:* generalized or bilateral, continuous, tight bandlike, worsens as the day progresses, associated with stress or tension ± aggravated by eye movement. *Confirmed by:* spontaneous improvement with simple analgesia. *Initial management:* reassurance regarding benign nature. Simple analgesia.
Bilateral migraine	*Suggested by:* bilateral, throbbing ± vomiting, aura ± visual or other neurological disturbances with precipitating factor, e.g. premenstrual. *Confirmed by:* resolution over hours in dark room and analgesics, helped by sleep. *Initial management:* simple analgesia. Bed rest in darkened room. Plan prophylaxis.

Headache—subacute onset

Onset over hours to days. Initial investigations (other tests in **bold** below):
FBC, ESR or CRP, CT scan.

Main differential diagnoses and typical outline evidence, etc.	
Raised intracranial pressure due to tumour, hydrocephalus, cerebral abscess, etc.	*Suggested by:* dull headache, worse on waking, vomiting, aggravated by, for example, cough, sneezing, bending; look for papilloedema, ↑BP, ↓pulse rate, progressive focal neurological signs. *Confirmed by:* **CT/MRI brain scan**. *Initial management:* analgesia. Dexamethasone if ↑intracranial pressure.
Encephalitis	*Suggested by:* fever, confusion, ↓conscious level. *Confirmed by:* CSF microscopy, serology or PCR. *Initial management:* analgesia. Provisional antibiotics after discussion with microbiologist while awaiting culture results. Aciclovir if virus suspected. Dexamethasone if ↑intracranial pressure.
Temporal/giant cell or cranial arteritis	*Suggested by:* scalp tenderness, jaw claudication, loss of temporal arterial pulsation, sudden loss of vision, ↑↑ESR. *Confirmed by:* **temporal artery biopsy** (may be done shortly after starting prednisolone). *Initial management:* high dose prednisolone.

Headache—chronic and recurrent

Onset over weeks to months. Initial investigations (other tests in **bold** below): FBC, ESR or CRP, U&E, LFT, CT scan.

Main differential diagnoses and typical outline evidence, etc.	
Tension headache	*Suggested by:* generalized or bilateral, continuous, tight bandlike, worsens as the day progresses, associated with stress or tension, often aggravated by eye movement.
	Confirmed by: spontaneous improvement with simple analgesia.
	Initial management: simple analgesia.
Migraine	*Suggested by:* typically unilateral, throbbing ± vomiting, aura ± visual disturbances, precipitating factors.
	Confirmed by: resolution over hours in dark room and analgesics, helped by sleep.
	Initial management: simple analgesia. Bed rest in darkened room. Plan prophylaxis.
Cluster headache	*Suggested by:* episodic, typically nightly pain in one eye for wks with nasal stuffiness on same side.
	Confirmed by: episodes resolving over hours (like migraine).
	Initial management: simple analgesia.
Cervical root headache	*Suggested by:* occipital and back of the head, temples, vertex and frontal regions, worse on neck movement or restricted neck movements.
	Confirmed by: **cervical X-ray** showing degenerative changes (or normal) and response to NSAIDs.
	Initial management: simple analgesia, NSAIDs.
Eye strain	*Suggested by:* headaches worse after reading. Refractory error.
	Confirmed by: improvement with appropriate spectacles.
	Initial management: simple analgesia, appropriate spectacles.
Drug side effect	*Suggested by:* drug history (e.g. nitrates).
	Confirmed by: improvement on drug withdrawal.
	Initial management: drug withdrawal.

Stroke

This is a sudden onset of a neurological deficit. Initial investigations (other tests in **bold** below): FBC, ESR or CRP, U&E, CT scan.

Main differential diagnoses and typical outline evidence, etc.	
Cerebral infarction	*Suggested by:* onset over minutes to hours of hemiaparesis or major neurological defect that lasts >24h.
	Confirmed by: **CT scan** apparently normal initially, ↓ attenuation after days.
	Initial management: nil by mouth and fluids IV if dysphagia. SALT assessment. DVT prophylaxis: stockings/LMW heparin (if no bleed). If infarct: stat high dose and daily regular dose aspirin. Start dipyridamole if stroke occurred whilst on aspirin.
Transient cerebral ischaemic attack due to carotid artery stenosis, etc. (see p. 598)	*Suggested by:* onset over seconds to minutes of a neurological deficit that is improving already.
	Confirmed by: deficit resolving within 24h. **CT scan** showing no area of low attenuation.
	Initial management: aspirin 75mg daily.
Cerebral embolus due to atheroma, atrial fibrillation, myocardial infarction	*Suggested by:* onset over seconds of hemiaparesis or other neurological defect that lasts >24h.
	Confirmed by: **CT scan** and **lumbar puncture** showing little change intially. Evidence of a potential source for an embolus.
	Initial management: withhold anticoagulation for weeks. Fluids IV if ability to swallow suspect. Dexamethasone if cerebral oedema. Assess for rehabilitation and plan as appropriate. Plan anticoagulation later.
Cerebral haemorrhage due to atheromatous degeneration, cerebral tumour	*Suggested by:* onset over seconds of hemiaparesis or major neurological defect that lasts >24h.
	Confirmed by: CT *showing* high attenuation ± 'low' (dark) 'oedema' area ± high density 'blood' in ventricles.
	Initial management: fluids IV if ability to swallow suspect. Dexamethasone if cerebral oedema. Assess for rehabilitation and plan as appropriate. Discuss possible evacuation of haematoma with neurosurgeons.

Subdural haemorrhage due to blunt head injury	*Suggested by:* onset over hours, days or weeks of a fluctuating hemiaparesis following history of head injury or fall especially in elderly or alcoholic.
	Confirmed by: **CT** showing low attenuation parallel to skull if chronic but high attenuation if acute.
	Initial management: plan craniotomy to remove substantial thrombus. Fluids IV if ability to swallow suspect. Dexamethasone if cerebral oedema. Assess for rehabilitation and plan as appropriate.
Extradural haemorrhage due to skull fracture lacerating middle meningeal artery	*Suggested by:* onset over minutes or hours of confusion, disturbed consciousness and hemiaparesis after 'lucid interval' of hours following head injury.
	Confirmed by: **CT head** showing high attenuation adjacent to skull ± midline shift.
	Initial management: plan craniotomy to remove thrombus. Fluids IV if ability to swallow suspect.
Subarachnoid haemorrhage from berry aneurysm	*Suggested by:* sudden onset over seconds of headache ± disturbance of consciousness (usually under 45y of age), neck stiffness.
	Confirmed by: **CT head** showing high attenuation area on surface of brain. **Lumbar puncture** showing blood.
	Initial management: fluids IV if ability to swallow suspect. Dexamethasone if cerebral oedema. Clipping of aneurysm if feasible.
Cerebellar stroke	*Suggested by:* sudden onset of ataxia.
	Confirmed by: **MRI scan** (**CT head** poorly visualizes hindbrain).
	Initial management: fluids IV if ability to swallow suspect. Dexamethasone if cerebral oedema. Assess for rehabilitation and plan as appropriate.
Pontine stroke	*Suggested by:* sudden loss of consciousness. Cheyne–Stokes breathing (speeding up and slowing down over minutes), pinpoint pupils, hemiparesis, and eyes deviated towards paresis.
	Confirmed by: above clinical findings ± **MRI scan**.
	Initial management: fluids IV if ability to swallow suspect. Assess for rehabilitation and plan as appropriate.

Dizziness

Dizziness is often non-specific (nothing significant is ever found), but one of the following will be discovered in a proportion of patients. Distinguish between dizziness and vertigo (which has a sensation of movement), the latter being more 'specific' of an identifiable lesion. Initial investigations (other tests in **bold** below): FBC, ESR or CRP, U&E, CXR.

Main differential diagnoses and typical outline evidence, etc.	
Hyperventilation due to anxiety, panic attacks	*Suggested by:* associated anxiety and claustrophobia. Finger and lip paraesthesia of hyperventilation. Resting tachypnoea, no hypoxia.
	Confirmed by: ABG: normal or ↑O2, ↓CO2; **CXR:** normal; **spirometry** normal; **VQ scan** normal. Response to anxiolytics and breathing exercises.
	Initial management: reassurance, anxiolytics, and breathing exercises.
Postural hypotension due to drugs to lower BP, loss of circulating volume, dehydration, diabetic autonomic neuropathy, old age + heavy meal, dopamine agonists, Addison's disease	*Suggested by:* associated palpitations, loss of consciousness. Supine and standing BP after 1min: >10mm drop.
	Confirmed by: response of BP changes to treatment of cause.
	Initial management: correction of underlying cause, then if necessary, fludrocortisone to raise BP.
Anaemia	*Suggested by:* subconjunctival pallor (± face, nail, and hand pallor).
	Confirmed by: **FBC:** ↓Hb.
	Initial management: treat underlying cause, e.g. recent blood loss with transfusion, iron deficiency with ferrous compound.
Hypoxic (with or without CO_2 retention)	*Suggested by:* blue hands and tongue (central cyanosis), restlessness, confused, drowsy, or unconscious.
	Confirmed by: **ABG:** ↓P_aO_2 <8kPa on blood gas analysis or **pulse oximetry** of <90% saturation (mild) or <80% (severe).
	Initial management: O_2 <28% if CO_2 retention, high flow (>28%) if no CO_2 retention.

Carotid sinus hypersensitivity	*Suggested by:* onset on head turning or shaving neck.
	Confirmed by: reproduction of symptoms while turning neck or pressure on carotid sinus.
	Initial management: advice about avoiding precipitating neck movements and/or soft collar.
Epilepsy	*Suggested by:* aura followed by other 'positive' neurological symptoms.
	Confirmed by: **EEG:** focal abnormality or 'spike and wave', etc.
	Initial management: anti-epileptic medication.
Drug effect	*Suggested by:* history of taking sedative or hypotensive drug, including alcohol.
	Confirmed by: resolution of symptom after stopping drug.
	Initial management: stopping drug.

Vertigo

Vertigo is a sensation of movement of self ± the environment, especially rotation or oscillation. Initial investigations (other tests in **bold** below): FBC, ESR or CRP, U&E, ECG.

Main differential diagnoses and typical outline evidence, etc.	
Vertebrobasilar insufficiency (brainstem ischaemia)	*Suggested by:* visual disturbances, other signs of cerebral ischaemia, e.g. dysarthria, faint. *Confirmed by:* **carotid Doppler**—evidence of arterial disease. **MR angiogram** of brain and neck vessels. *Initial management:* antiplatelet drug (e.g. aspirin), BP, cholesterol, stop smoking, control risk factors.
Benign positional vertigo	*Suggested by:* attacks with duration of minutes only. *Confirmed by:* **Hallpike head tilt test:** nystagmus after 5s, lasting a minute. Shorter duration when repeated. *Initial management:* histamine analogues (e.g betahistine) or sedatives (e.g. prochlorperazine), reassurance, positional physiotherapy. Canalith repositioning procedure.
Ménière's disease	*Suggested by:* attacks with duration of hours often incapacitating. Tinnitus ± progressive deafness in older patient. *Confirmed by:* **audiometry:** hearing loss with loudness recruitment. *Initial management:* histamine analogues (e.g betahistine) or sedatives (e.g. prochlorperazine), assessment for surgical decompression of saccus endolymphaticus.
Vestibular neuronitis (associated with viral illness)	*Suggested by:* sudden, single, prostrating attack, usually with nystagmus with resolution over weeks. *Confirmed by:* **caloric testing**. *Initial management:* histamine analogues (e.g betahistine) or sedatives (e.g. prochlorperazine), reassurance regarding resolution within days to weeks.
Middle ear disease	*Suggested by:* painful ear, recurrent attacks, or persistent vertigo and nystagmus. *Confirmed by:* **audiometry:** conductive deafness. Otoscopic appearance of otitis media or cholesteatoma. *Initial management:* histamine analogues (e.g betahistine) or sedatives (e.g. prochlorperazine), antibiotic for bacterial infection, assessment for any surgical intervention.
Reversible drug toxicity	*Suggested by:* vertigo, slurring of speech and nystagmus with suggestive drug history, e.g. alcohol, barbiturates, phenytoin. *Confirmed by:* resolution on withdrawal of drug. Drug levels if in doubt. *Initial management:* withdrawal of drug.

Wernicke's encephalopathy (due to thiamine deficiency, usually in alcoholism)	*Suggested by:* persistence of vertigo, ataxia, slurring of speech, and nystagmus despite withdrawal of alcohol.
	Confirmed by: resolution or improvement on thiamine treatment.
	Initial management: thiamine IV, then PO.

Ototoxic drugs	*Suggested by:* recurrent attacks or persistent vertigo and little nystagmus, history of streptomycin, gentamicin, kanamycin, phenytoin, quinine, or salicylates, etc.
	Confirmed by: bilateral loss of response to **caloric tests.** No signs of disease in brainstem, ears, or cerebellum.
	Initial management: stop potentially ototoxic drug.

Brainstem ischaemia or infarction	*Suggested by:* sudden onset and associated with peripheral vascular disease.
	Confirmed by: associated cranial nerve palsies, long tract signs (e.g. spastic paresis, extensor plantar response, sensory loss).
	Initial management: fluids IV if swallowing defect, antiplatelet agents after stabilization, nursing support.

Posterior fossa tumour	*Suggested by:* onset of vertigo over months, nystagmus. Bilateral papilloedema. Ipsilateral absent corneal reflex. Cranial nerve lesions V, VI, VII, X, and XI. Ipsilateral cerebellar and contralateral pyramidal signs.
	Confirmed by: **MRI scan** showing tumour.
	Initial management: histamine analogues (e.g betahistidine) or sedatives (e.g. prochlorperazine), assessment for surgical intervention.

Multiple sclerosis	*Suggested by:* sudden onset and central type nystagmus (occurs equally in both directions and sometimes vertically) in young person, other neurological disturbances, scanning speech, optic atrophy.
	Confirmed by: other similar neurological episodes 'disseminated in time and space' and multiple, enhancing lesions in various parts of nervous system on **MRI scan**.
	Initial management: histamine analogues (e.g betahistidine) or sedatives (e.g. prochlorperazine), methylprednisolone IV.

Migraine	*Suggested by:* associated headache (vertigo instead of visual aura).
	Confirmed by: resolution and recurrence consistent with natural history of migraine.
	Initial management: simple analgesia. Bed rest in darkened room. Plan prophylaxis.

(Continued)

Vertigo (continued)

Main differential diagnoses and typical outline evidence, etc. *(continued)*

Temporal lobe epilepsy	*Suggested by:* associated temporal lobe symptoms, e.g. odd taste, smells, visual hallucinations.
	Confirmed by: **EEG** findings and details of history.
	Initial management: anti-epileptic agent (e.g. carbamazepine, sodium valproate).
Ramsay Hunt syndrome due to herpes zoster	*Suggested by:* associated ear pain, lower motor neurone facial palsy.
	Confirmed by: Zoster vesicles at the external auditory meatus or fauces.
	Intial management: Histamine analogues (e.g betahistidine) or sedatives (e.g. prochlorperazine), aciclovir.

'Fit'

History of aura, loss of consciousness, tonic and clonic movements. Initial investigations (other tests in **bold** below): FBC, ESR or CRP, U&E, blood glucose, calcium, ECG.

Main differential diagnoses and typical outline evidence, etc.	
Febrile convulsion	*Suggested by:* young age, especially in childhood and associated with a febrile illness.
	Confirmed by: normal **EEG** and **CT scan**, and no subsequent recurrence without febrile illness on follow-up.
	Initial management: lower temperature with fan, oral or fluids IV, antipyretics (e.g. paracetamol).
Idiopathic epilepsy—new presentation	*Suggested by:* young age, especially in teens.
	Confirmed by: abnormal or normal **EEG**, and normal **CT scan** but subsequent recurrence.
	Initial management: if status epilepticus—benzodiazepine IV (e.g. lorazepam). If previous fit, anti-epileptic agent (e.g. carbamazepine, sodium valproate).
Known idiopathic epilepsy	*Suggested by:* history of previous fits.
	Confirmed by: past medical history of past investigations and on treatment.
	Initial management: if status epilepticus—benzodiazepine IV (e.g. lorazepam). Review ± adjust existing dose in light of drug levels.
Brain tumour	*Suggested by:* older age (but any age), headaches, papilloedema.
	Confirmed by: **CT or MRI scan** showing cerebral mass.
	Initial management: if status epilepticus—benzodiazepine IV (e.g. lorazepam). If previous fit, anti-epileptic agent (e.g. carbamazepine, sodium valproate). Assessment for possible brain surgery.
Epilepsy due to meningitis	*Suggested by:* fever, neck stiffness.
	Confirmed by: **CT scan** and lumbar puncture.
	Initial management: if status epilepticus—benzodiazepine IV (e.g. lorazepam). Benzylpenicillin IM or IV while awaiting confirmation of diagnosis, culture, and sensitivity.
Epilepsy due to old brain scar tissue	*Suggested by:* past history of serious head injury or stroke.
	Confirmed by: abnormal **EEG, CT or MRI brain scan**.
	Initial management: if status epilepticus—benzodiazepine IV (e.g. lorazepam). If previous fit, anti-epileptic agent (e.g. carbamazepine).

Alcohol withdrawal	*Suggested by:* recent heavy alcohol intake (usually superimposed on habitually high intake).
	Confirmed by: subsequent episodes in similar circumstances.
	Initial management: if status epilepticus—benzodiazepine IV (e.g. diazepam) followed by oral sedative (e.g. chlordiazepoxide 15–50mg 6-hourly).
Hypoglycaemia due to too much insulin with too little food in diabetic, or insulinoma	*Suggested by:* sweating, hunger, known diabetic on insulin or medication.
	Confirmed by: ↓blood sugar (<2mmol/L) during episode.
	Initial management: buccal glucose gel if concious (e.g. GlucoGel®) or 50% glucose IV or glucagon 1mg IV or IM if unconscious.
Sudden severe hypotension (especially cardiac arrest)	*Suggested by:* peripheral and central cyanosis, no pulse or BP.
	Confirmed by: **ECG** shows asystole or ineffectual fast or slow rhythm (or electromechanical dissociation).
	Initial management: saline IV and/or plasma expander under central venous pressure (CVP) control.
Severe electrolyte disturbance due to very high or low sodium, calcium, magnesium, etc.	*Suggested by:* abnormality on serum biochemistry.
	Confirmed by: no recurrence of fits after metabolic abnormality treated.
	Initial management: normal saline IV, then correction of hypertonicity or hypotonicity, and replacement of deficiencies.
'Functional' (pseudo-fit)	*Suggested by:* always occurring in front of audience, eyes closed during episode.
	Confirmed by: normal EEG when episode documented on video-recording. Normal **CT scan**.
	Initial management: counselling, psychotherapy.

Transient neurological deficit

Sudden dysphasia, facial or limb weakness resolving within 24h. Initial investigations (other tests in **bold** below): FBC, ESR or CRP, U&E, blood glucose, ECG, CT scan.

Main differential diagnoses and typical outline evidence, etc.	
Transient cerebral ischaemic attack (TIA) from platelet embolus? due to carotid artery stenosis or vasculitic process	*Suggested by:* onset over minutes, and then immediate improvement with prospect of complete resolution within 24h ± carotid bruit. *Confirmed by:* resolution within 24h, absence of previous fit, no throbbing migrainous headache, no chest pain, normal **ECG** and **troponin** after 12h, normal **plasma sodium**, normal **blood sugar**, no witnessed fits and normal **CT. Doppler ultrasound** of carotids (to seek operable stenosis). ↑**ESR** or ↑**CRP** (if there is a vasculitic process, e.g. cranial arteritis). *Initial management:* aspirin 75mg daily, cholesterol-lowering agent (e.g. simvastatin).
Atrial fibrillation with cerebral embolus	*Suggested by:* irregularly irregular pulse. *Confirmed by:* irregularly irregular QRS complexes, no P wave on **ECG**. *Initial management:* wait for weeks to avoid bleed into infarcted tissue, then anticoagulation (e.g. warfarin).
Intracerebral space-occuping lesion: tumour, aneurysm haematoma, arterio-venous malformation	*Suggested by:* associated headache. *Confirmed by:* **CT** or **MRI scan** appearance. *Initial management:* dexamethasone to reduce any oedema, planning for possible surgery.
Transient hypotension due to arrhythmia or myocardial infarction	*Suggested by:* history of chest pain or past medical history of ischaemic heart disease. *Confirmed by:* **ECG**: ST changes. ↑**troponin**. **24h ECG**: recurrence of arrhythmia. *Initial management:* aspirin 75mg daily, cholesterol-lowering agents (e.g. simvastatin).
Todd's paralysis (following focal epileptic fit)	*Suggested by:* witness's history of fitting. *Confirmed by:* **EEG** changes. *Initial management:* if previous fit, anti-epileptic agent (e.g. carbamazepine, sodium valproate).
Migraine	*Suggested by:* associated headache (neurological deficit instead of visual aura). *Confirmed by:* resolution consistent with other features of migraine. Normal **CT** and **MRI scan**. *Initial management:* simple analgesia for associated headache. Monitor with expectation of recovery.

Hypoglycaemic episode	*Suggested by:* a known diabetic and associated sudden hunger, sweating, confusion, loss of consciousness.
	Confirmed by: **blood sugar** <2mmol/L.
	Initial management: oral glucose gel if conscious, 50% dextrose IV bolus if unconscious.
Hyponatraemia	*Suggested by:* ↓↓sodium concentration (e.g. <120mmol/L) and ↓↓serum osmolality. Associated confusion.
	Confirmed by: resolution of deficit as **sodium concentration** and **osmolality** abnormality corrected.
	Initial management: normal saline IV, fluid restriction. Investigation and correction of underlying cause.
Multiple sclerosis (MS)	*Suggested by:* sudden onset and central type nystagmus (occurs equally in both directions and sometimes vertically) in young person, other neurological disturbances, scarring speech, optic atrophy.
	Confirmed by: other similar neurological episodes, 'disseminated in time and space' and multiple, enhancing lesions in various parts of nervous system on **MRI scan**.
	Initial management: methylprednisolone, physiotherapy, multidisciplinary (MDT) planning.
Psychological	*Suggested by:* past history of similar episodes from young (<30y) age.
	Confirmed by: absence of any objective evidence of physical cause of deficit on follow-up.
	Initial management: preliminary counselling, referral for assessment and psychotherapy.

Fatigue, 'tired all the time'

A poor lead—but consider the following possibilities during the history and examination. Initial investigations (other tests in **bold** below): FBC, U&E, fasting blood glucose, TSH, FT4.

Main differential diagnoses and typical outline evidence, etc.	
Depression	*Suggested by:* early morning wakening, fatigue worse in the morning that never goes during the day, anhedonia, poor appetite.
	Confirmed by: response to psychotherapy or antidepressants.
	Initial management: psychotherapy, antidepressants.
Anaemia—microcytic, macrocytic, or normocytic	*Suggested by:* pale palms or conjunctivae.
	Confirmed by: ↓Hb, ↓MCV (microlytic)/↑MCV (microlytic)/ normal MCV (normolytic).
	Initial management: investigate with ferritin, folate, and vitamin B12, treat underlying cause.
1° hypothyroidism	*Suggested by:* cold intolerance, tiredness, constipation, bradycardia.
	Confirmed by: ↑**TSH**, ↓**FT4**.
	Initial management: thyroxine replacement therapy.
Sleep apnoea syndrome	*Suggested by:* frequent awakening at night, snoring and breathing pauses during sleep (history from a sleeping partner), and sleepiness during the day.
	Confirmed by: multiple dips in O_2 levels whilst asleep during home or hospital monitoring.
	Initial management: home, constant pressure non-invasive ventilation.
Drug-induced	*Suggested by:* taking sedating drug, including anti-epileptic treatment.
	Confirmed by: improvement by stopping or changing drug.
	Initial management: stop or change to another drug.
Post-viral fatigue	*Suggested by:* history of recent viral illness, especially glandular fever.
	Confirmed by: resolution after weeks or months.
	Initial management: reassurance, follow-up, and investigation of new leads.
Diabetes mellitus	*Suggested by:* thirst, polyuria, polydipsia, family history (but all may be absent).
	Confirmed by: **fasting blood glucose** ≥7.0mmol/L on two occasions OR fasting, **random or GTT glucose** ≥11.1mmol/L, in combination with symptoms.
	Initial management: education on diabetes, controlled carbohydrate, and high-fibre diet.

Chronic fatigue syndrome (CFS)	*Suggested by:* (1) impaired memory/concentration unrelated to drugs or alcohol use, (2) unexplained muscle pain, (3) polyarthralgia, (4) unrefreshing sleep, (5) post-exertional malaise lasting over 24h, (6) persisting sore throat not caused by glandular fever, (7) unexplained tender cervical or axillary nodes.
	Confirmed by: 4 of 7 or more of the above present for >6mo.
	Initial management: reassurance and counselling.
Poor sleep habit	*Suggested by:* long working hours, little sleep, insomnia.
	Confirmed by: sleep diary and improvement with better sleep habits.
	Initial management: counselling.
Parasomnias	*Suggested by:* cataplexy, narcolepsy, and daytime somnolence.
	Confirmed by: response of symptoms to stimulant medication.
	Initial management: stimulant medication, e.g. methylphenidate

Examining the nervous system

If there were no symptoms at all suggestive of neurological disease, it is usual to perform a quick examination of the nervous system, and if this examination is normal, then the nervous system is not examined further. There will have been an opportunity to note the patient's posture and gait in the consulting room (or as the patient moves around the bed on the ward). If the patient's face looks normal and moves normally during speech, then there is unlikely to be a cranial nerve abnormality. The patient is then asked to hold both arms out to assess posture, to perform a 'finger-nose' test, to tap each hand on the other in turn, to 'unscrew door knobs', to tap each foot on the floor (or the examiner's hand if in bed), and then to do a 'heel-shin' test with each leg. Finally, reflexes are tested in the arms and legs. If all these are normal (and as emphasized already, there are no symptoms of neurological disorder), then the nervous system is not examined further. If there is a symptom or sign of neurological disorder, then the nervous system has to be examined carefully, perhaps beginning with the territory under suspicion.

Disturbed consciousness

Consciousness assessed using Glasgow Coma Scale (GCS) based on adding score for (a) best verbal response (see below), (b) best motor response (motor see facing page) and (c) eye opening (see facing page).

Main differential diagnoses and typical outline evidence, etc.	
Probably no current brain damage	*Suggested by:* GCS = 15 (patient complying with all requests, oriented in time and place, opening eyes spontaneously).
	Confirmed by: neurological observation.
Probable minor brain injury	*Suggested by:* GCS of 13–15.
	Confirmed by: neurological observation or **CT or MRI scan** appearance.
Probable moderate brain injury	*Suggested by:* GCS of 9–12.
	Confirmed by: neurological observation or **CT or MRI scan** appearance.
Probable severe brain injury	*Suggested by:* GCS of 3–8.
	Confirmed by: neurological observation or **CT or MRI scan** appearance.
Probable very severe brain injury	*Suggested by:* GCS = 3 (no response to pain, no verbalization, and no eye opening).
	Confirmed by: neurological observation or **CT or MRI scan** appearance.

Best verbal response

Differential diagnosis	
Oriented: score 5	*Confirmed by:* knowing own name, the place, why there, year, season and month.
Confused conversation: score 4	*Confirmed by:* conversation, but does not know name, not the place, not why there, nor year, season or month.
Inappropriate speech: score 3	*Confirmed by:* no conversation, but random speech or shouting.
Incomprehensible speech: score 2	*Confirmed by:* moaning but no words.
No speech at all: score 1	*Confirmed by:* silence.

Best motor response

Differential diagnosis	
Carrying out verbal requests: score 6	*Confirmed by:* doing simple things that you ask. (ignore grasp reflex.)
Localizing response to pain: score 5	*Confirmed by:* purposeful movement in response to pressure on fingernail, supra-orbital ridges and sternum.
Withdraws to pain: score 4	*Confirmed by:* pulling limb away from painful stimulus.
Flexor response to pain—'decorticate posture': score 3	*Confirmed by:* flexion of limbs to painful stimulus.
Extensor response to pain—'decerebrate posture': score 2	*Confirmed by:* pain causing adduction and internal rotation of shoulder, and pronation of forearm.
No response to pain: score 1	*Confirmed by:* no response to painful stimulus.

Eye opening

Comment: to be used to give GCS score.

Differential diagnosis	
Spontaneous eye opening: score 4	*Confirmed by:* eyes open and fixing on objects.
Eye opening in response to speech: score 3	*Confirmed by:* response to specific request or a shout.
Eye opening in response to pain: score 2	*Confirmed by:* response to pain.
No eye opening at all: score 1	*Confirmed by:* no response to pain.

Speech disturbance

Inability to converse can be due to disturbance in any part of the process due to deafness, poor attention, receptive dysphasia, motor dysphasia, dysarthria, dysphonia or aphonia, or combinations of these. Initial investigations (other tests in **bold** below): FBC, ESR or CRP, CT scan.

Main differential diagnoses and typical outline evidence, etc.	
Deafness due to ear disease or 8th cranial nerve lesions	*Suggested by:* no reaction to speech or noises. *Confirmed by:* conductive or nerve deafness on Rinne or Weber tests. *Initial management:* hearing aid for conductive deafness.
Inattention due to dementia, depression, etc.	*Suggested by:* normal reaction (e.g. startling) to noise or speech, but no interest in source of noise or speech. *Confirmed by:* low MMSE score ± **CT** or **MRI** of brain showing cerebral atrophy.
Sensory dysphasia due to lesion in Wernicke's area	*Suggested by:* inability to understand or comprehend speech (as if a foreign language is being spoken to patient). Worse for vocabulary or language acquired later in life. *Confirmed by:* **CT** or **MRI scan** showing lesion in Wernicke's area in dominant temporal lobe.
Motor dysphasia (or aphasia) due to lesion in dominant frontal-parietal lobe	*Suggested by:* inability to find words or names of things (nominal dysphasia). *Confirmed by:* **CT** or **MRI** scan showing lesion in Broca's area in frontal lobe. *Initial management:* speech therapy.
Dysarthria (or anarthria) due to cerebellar connections, upper or lower motor neurone lesion	*Suggested by:* inability to coordinate speech with slurring, mumbling, failure to initiate or sustain speech. *Confirmed by:* associated features of weakness or in coordination of oral muscles. *Initial management:* speech therapy.
Dysphonia (or aphonia) due to vocal cord dysfunction	*Suggested by:* hoarseness, voice loss or weakness, inability to cough properly. *Confirmed by:* indirect laryngoscopy (using mirror) to show vocal cord dysfunction or paresis. *Initial management:* treatment of underlying cause.

Dysarthria

Difficulty with articulation and incoordination of speech muscles. Initial investigations (other tests in **bold** below): FBC, ESR or CRP, U&E, CT scan.

Main differential diagnoses and typical outline evidence, etc.	
Cortical cerebral lesion (due to bleed, infarction, or tumour)	*Suggested by:* slow, stiff speech (and dysphasia if extensive lesion in dominant hemisphere, i.e. most dextrous hand is also affected) and other 'cortical' signs. *Confirmed by:* **CT** or **MRI scan** of brain. *Initial management:* speech therapy.
Internal capsule cerebral lesion (due to bleed, infarction, or tumour)	*Suggested by:* slow, stiff speech, and other internal capsule signs (e.g. spastic hemiparesis). *Confirmed by:* **CT** or **MRI scan** of brain. *Initial management:* speech therapy.
Upper motor neurone brainstem (pseudobulbar palsy due to ischaemia, motor neurone disease, MS)	*Suggested by:* slow, stiff nasal quality, slurred, and other brainstem signs (e.g. spastic hemiparesis, dysphagia). *Confirmed by:* **MRI scan** of brainstem. *Initial management:* speech therapy.
Lower motor neurone brain stem (bulbar) palsy (due to ischaemia, motor neurone disease, 'polio' syringobulbia, MS)	*Suggested by:* nasal ('Donald Duck' quality) and other brainstem signs (e.g. spastic hemiparesis, dysphagia). *Confirmed by:* **MRI scan** of brain stem. *Initial management:* speech therapy.
Extrapyramidal dysarthria (due to Parkinson's disease)	*Suggested by:* difficulty in initiating speech which is slow with other signs of parkinsonian syndrome. *Confirmed by:* response to dopaminergic drugs. *Initial management:* speech therapy.
Cerebellar lesion (due to MS, ischaemia, tumour, hereditary ataxias)	*Suggested by:* staccato, undulating, broken flow, slurred, and other cerebellar signs (e.g. ataxia). *Confirmed by:* **MRI scan** of cerebellum. *Initial management:* speech therapy.
Drug effect (e.g. alcohol, sedatives)	*Suggested by:* dysarthria (slurred) and other drug effects. *Confirmed by:* response to removal of drug. *Initial management:* await metabolism of alcohol.

Absent sense of smell

This is not tested routinely, but ask the patient if there is anything abnormal about their smell or taste. Test using bottles with familiar essences. Initial investigations (other tests in **bold** below): skull X-ray, FSH, LH.

Main differential diagnoses and typical outline evidence, etc.	
Coryza (common cold)	*Suggested by:* runny nose, fever, headache, sporadic, perhaps with contact history. *Confirmed by:* history and nasal speculum examination. *Initial management:* await resolution of infection.
Nasal allergy	*Suggested by:* runny nose, fever, headache, recurrent and recognizable precipitant. *Confirmed by:* history and nasal speculum examination. *Initial management:* nasal glucocorticoid spray.
Skull fracture	*Suggested by:* history of facial or head injury. *Confirmed by:* history or **skull X-ray** in acute phase. *Initial management:* await recovery from fracture.
Frontal lobe tumour	*Suggested by:* personality change, features of dementia, recent epilepsy. *Confirmed by:* **CT** or **MRI scan** of brain. *Initial management:* assess for feasibility of surgical removal.
Kallman's syndrome	*Suggested by:* delayed puberty or poor secondary sexual characteristics and libido, infertility. 1° amenorrhoea in females. *Confirmed by:* ↓**oestrogens** or ↓**testosterone**, and normal or ↓**FSH**, and normal or ↓**LH**. *Initial management:* as condition congenital, patient may be unaware of absent sense of smell (i.e. only detected on formal testing with scents).

Abnormal ophthalmoscopy appearance

Start with high positive (+) numbers for the eye surface and use the lowest light level possible. Look for the red reflex, and zoom into the eye until the red reflex fills the field of view. Examine the retina by rotating down to negative (−) numbers. Start with the disc, found by looking towards the patient's midline, and then follow the four main arteries out and back. Examine the macula by asking the patient to look at the light.

Main differential diagnoses and typical outline evidence, etc.	
Corneal opacity in quiet eye (old ulcer due to past trauma, trachoma—tropical countries)	*Suggested by:* grey opacity in the clear cornea without dilated blood vessels, gradual loss of vision. *Confirmed by:* absence of staining with fluorescein. *Initial management:* assess for feasibility of corneal replacement surgery.
Cataract (due to ageing (75%), diabetes, trauma, steroids, radiation, intra-uterine rubella or toxoplasmosis, or rubella, hypocalcaemia, etc.)	*Suggested by:* history of gradual onset of visual blurring, and lens opacity visible during the red reflex examination with the ophthalmoscope. Usually >65y or history of underlying condition (often already known and cataract develops later). *Confirmed by:* ophthalmoscopical appearance. *Initial management:* mydriatic eye drops, sunglasses, referral for consideration of phaco-emulsion with lens implantation.
Optic nerve swelling or (eventually) atrophy (due to papillitis from MS, or papilloedema or optic nerve infarction in temporal arteritis and retinal artery occlusion)	*Suggested by:* raised pink optic disc with blurred margins ± distended capillaries, and adjacent streak haemorrhages progressing to pale white disc with pale margins. Gradual loss of vision after initial disturbance. *Confirmed by:* visual field charting. Ophthalmoscopical appearance. *Initial management:* treat underlying cause, e.g. dexamethasone for ↑intracranial pressure, prednisolone for cranial arteritis.
Peripheral retinal damage (e.g. due to laser therapy for diabetic retinopathy)	*Suggested by:* irregular pale patches of depigmentation with central black areas of pigment clumping. *Confirmed by:* ophthalmoscopical appearance and history. *Initial management:* counsel regarding permanence.
Age-related macular degeneration (usually senile)	*Suggested by:* gradual loss of central vision, large, central, yellowish white scar or haemorrhage when patient looks at ophthalmoscope light. *Confirmed by:* ophthalmoscopical appearance. *Initial management:* referral for laser photocoagulation or photodynamic laser therapy to be considered.

Retinal vein occlusion	*Suggested by:* sudden vision loss, often in upper or lower half only.
	Confirmed by: extensive superficial retinal haemorrhages following the nerve fibre layer which may be only in the upper or lower half of the retina.
	Initial management: referral for argon laser grid photocoagulation to be considered.
Retinal artery occlusion	*Suggested by:* sudden loss of vision. May be total or partial upper or lower field.
	Confirmed by: in the first few days retinal pallor. Later, a white, thready, thin artery.
	Initial management: prevention of further episodes, e.g. aspirin, lipid-lowering drugs.
Primary optic atrophy (prior inflammation not seen—due to MS or optic nerve infarction)	*Suggested by:* gradual visual loss in a quiet eye and pale disc with sharp margins.
	Confirmed by: ophthalmoscopical appearance of pale, white, featureless disc and may have thin thready vessels.
	Initial management: prevention of further episodes, e.g. aspirin, lipid-lowering drugs.
Glaucoma	*Suggested by:* gradual loss of vision, deeply cupped disc.
	Confirmed by: ophthalmoscopical appearance of deep cupping with visible cribriform plate and nasal displacement of vessels. Loss of peripheral field. ↑intraocular pressure.
	Initial management: pilocarpine eye drops + betaxolol, or timolol.
Retinitis pigmentosa	*Suggested by:* loss of peripheral and night vision.
	Confirmed by: visual field charting. Pale disc, thin thready blood vessels, and fine star-shaped pigment without patches of depigmentation. Visual field charting.
	Initial management: counselling regarding prognosis.
Choroidoretinitis	*Suggested by:* gradual loss of vision or blurring (in acute phases), and 'patchy' visual loss—scotoma.
	Confirmed by: visual field charting showing irregular patchy areas of visual loss. Corresponding areas in the eye of irregular depigmentation with dense areas of pigment in the centre. Tests results for underlying cause: CXR, serology, sputum, lung biopsy.
	Initial management: treatment of underlying cause, e.g. for TB.

Ophthalmoscopy appearance in the diabetic

Red-free or green light of ophthalmoscope very useful for retinopathy. NB. Serial visual acuity measurements to detect early maculopathy.

Main differential diagnoses and typical outline evidence, etc.	
'Diabetic' cataract	*Suggested by:* gradual visual loss in a diabetic.
	Confirmed by: ophthalmoscopical appearance.
	Initial management: mydriatic eye drops, sunglasses, referral for consideration of phaco-emulsion with lens implantation.
'Diabetic' glaucoma	*Suggested by:* pale, deeply cupped disc with sharp margins.
	Confirmed by: ophthalmoscopical appearance and visual field test. ↑intraocular pressure.
	Initial management: pilocarpine eye drops + betaxolol, or timolol.
Diabetic micro-aneurysm and bleeding into retina	*Suggested by:* dots (micro-aneurysms or deep haemorrhages) and blots or flames (deep and superficial haemorrhages).
	Confirmed by: regular retinal photography for progress.
	Initial management: strict BP and diabetic control, referral for consideration of laser photocoagulation.
Venous irregularity preceding haemorrhage	*Suggested by:* localized widening of veins (e.g. sausage-shaped).
	Confirmed by: regular retinal photography for progress.
	Initial management: strict BP and diabetic control. Referral for consideration of laser photocoagulation.
Diabetic hard exudates	*Suggested by:* round and small pale area (after a single, serous leak), circular with central red dot (indicating a continuous leak), enlarging circle with time.
	Confirmed by: regular retinal photography for progress.
	Initial management: strict BP and diabetic control. Referral for consideration of laser photocoagulation.
Diabetic macular exudates (leading to visual loss)	*Suggested by:* star-shaped pallor (as the exudates follow the radial nerve fibre arrangement) and loss of visual acuity.
	Confirmed by: regular retinal photography for progress.
	Initial management: referral for consideration of laser photocoagulation.
Diabetic soft exudates (nerve fibre infarct pre-ceding new vessels)	*Suggested by:* pale grey area with indistinct margins.
	Confirmed by: regular retinal photography for progress.
	Initial management: strict BP and diabetic control. Referral for consideration of laser photocoagulation.

Diabetic new vessel formation (leads to haemorrhage)	*Suggested by:* 'frond' growing forwards into the vitreous (seen by adjusting focus) or like a net growing on the surface of the retina, arising from disc or larger peripheral veins.
	Confirmed by: three-dimensional clinical appearance.
	Initial management: referral for consideration of laser photocoagulation.
Retinal haemorrhage and detachment	*Suggested by:* subhyaloid haemorrhage obscuring underlying vessels, often forming 'nest shape'—flat top and round bottom.
	Confirmed by: three-dimensional clinical appearance.
	Initial management: referral for consideration of sclera silicone implants, or cryotherapy, or argon or laser coagulation.
Vitreous haemorrhage	*Suggested by:* sudden loss of vision in a diabetic and a poor red reflex on ophthalmoscopy.
	Confirmed by: retinal photography.
	Initial management: referral for consideration of vitrectomy.
Retinal vein occlusion	*Suggested by:* sudden vision loss, often in upper or lower half only.
	Confirmed by: extensive superficial retinal haemorrhages following the nerve fibre layer which may be in only the upper or lower half of the retina.
	Initial management: referral for argon laser grid photocoagulation to be considered.

Ophthalmoscopy appearances in the hypertensive

Main differential diagnoses and typical outline evidence, etc.

Grade I hypertensive retinopathy	*Suggested by:* ↑BP on three occasions typically >90mmHg diastolic or >140mmHg systolic.
	Confirmed by: segmental narrowing and tortuosity of arteries.
	Initial management: control of BP.
Grade II hypertensive retinopathy	*Suggested by:* moderately ↑BP on three occasions typically >100mmHg diastolic or >160mmHg systolic.
	Confirmed by: segmental narrowing and tortuosity of arteries, and arterio-venous nipping.
	Initial management: control of BP.
Grade III hypertensive retinopathy	*Suggested by:* severely ↑BP on three occasions typically >120mmHg diastolic or >180mmHg systolic.
	Confirmed by: segmental narrowing and tortuosity of arteries, and arterio-venous nipping, and haemorrhages and exudates.
	Initial management: control of BP.
Grade IV hypertensive retinopathy	*Suggested by:* severely ↑BP, typically >140mmHg diastolic or >200mmHg systolic.
	Confirmed by: segmental narrowing and tortuosity of arteries, and arterio-venous nipping, and haemorrhages, exudates, and papilloedema.
	Initial management: control of BP.

Sudden loss of central vision and acuity

Visual acuity is tested in each eye with a Snellen chart at 6m: 6/6 = 100% acuity and 6/60 = 10% acuity (letters normally read at 60m only readable at 6m). Fields are tested by facing patient 1m away and patient closing matching eyes. Wag your finger, moving in from the periphery horizontally and diagonally, changing hands. Test for scotoma with red marker pen top, moving horizontally, and asking for change of colour and disappearance. The rate of onset is important, sudden loss of vision is an emergency. Investgations in **bold** below.

Main differential diagnoses and typical outline evidence, etc.	
Optic nerve swelling or (eventually) atrophy (due to papillitis from MS or papilloedema or optic nerve infarction in temporal arteritis and retinal artery occlusion)	*Suggested by:* raised pink optic disc with blurred margins ± distended capillaries, and adjacent streak haemorrhages progressing to pale white disc with pale margins. Gradual loss of vision after initial disturbance. *Confirmed by:* visual field charting. Ophthalmoscopical appearance. *Initial management:* treat underlying cause, e.g. dexamethasone for ↑intracranial pressure, prednisolone for temporal arteritis.
Temporal/giant cell or cranial arteritis	*Suggested by:* scalp tenderness, jaw claudication, loss of temporal arterial pulsation, sudden loss of vision, ↑↑ESR. *Confirmed by:* **temporal artery biopsy** (may be done shortly after starting prednisolone). *Initial management:* prednisolone 40 to 60mg daily initially.
Retinal artery occlusion	*Suggested by:* sudden loss of vision. May be total or partial upper or lower field. *Confirmed by:* in the first few days, retinal pallor. Later a white, thready, thin artery. *Initial management:* prevention of further episodes, e.g. aspirin, lipid-lowering drugs.
Retinal vein occlusion	*Suggested by:* sudden vision loss, often in upper or lower half only. *Confirmed by:* extensive superficial retinal haemorrhages following the nerve fibre layer which may be in only the upper or lower half of the retina. *Initial management:* referral for argon laser grid photocoagulation to be considered.
Vitreous haemorrhage	*Suggested by:* sudden loss of vision in a diabetic and a poor red reflex on ophthalmoscopy. *Confirmed by:* retinal photography. *Initial management:* referral for consideration of vitrectomy.

Gradual onset of visual loss

Investigations in **bold** below.

Main differential diagnoses and typical outline evidence, etc.	
Cataract (due to ageing (75%), diabetes, trauma, steroids, radiation, intra-uterine rubella or toxoplasmosis, or rubella, hypocalcaemia, etc.)	*Suggested by:* gradual onset of visual blurring and lens opacity visible during the red reflex examination with the ophthalmoscope. Usually >65y or history of underlying condition (often already known and cataract develops later). *Confirmed by:* ophthalmoscopical appearance. *Initial management:* mydriatic eye drops, sunglasses, referral for consideration of phaco-emulsion with lens implantation.
Macular degeneration (age-related)	*Suggested by:* gradual loss of central vision, large, central, yellowish white scar or haemorrhage when patient looks at ophthalmoscope light. *Confirmed by:* ophthalmoscopical appearance. *Initial management:* referral for laser photocoagulation or photodynamic laser therapy to be considered.
Choroidoretinitis	*Suggested by:* gradual loss of vision, or blurring (in acute phases), and 'patchy' visual loss—scotomata. *Confirmed by:* visual field charting showing irregular patchy areas of visual loss. Corresponding areas in the eye of irregular depigmentation with dense areas of pigment in the centre. Tests results for underlying cause: **CXR, serology, sputum, lung biopsy**. *Initial management:* treatment of underlying cause, e.g. for TB.
Glaucoma	*Suggested by:* gradual loss of vision, deeply cupped disc. *Confirmed by:* ophthalmoscopical appearance of deep cupping with visible cribriform plate and nasal displacement of vessels. Loss of peripheral field. ↑intra-ocular pressure. *Initial management:* pilocarpine eye drops + betaxolol, or timolol.
Primary optic atrophy (prior inflammation not seen—due to MS or optic nerve infarction)	*Suggested by:* gradual visual loss in a quiet eye and pale disc with sharp margins. *Confirmed by:* ophthalmoscopical appearance of pale, white, featureless disc, and may have thin thready vessels. *Initial management:* treat underlying cause.

Peripheral visual field defect

An upper or lower half defect is due to ocular pathology. Lesions between eye and chiasm cause unilateral defects, but those from chiasma to brain are homonymous, i.e. affecting same area in each eye. Investigations in **bold** below.

Main differential diagnoses and typical outline evidence, etc.	
Psychogenic field defect	*Suggested by:* 'TUNNEL' vision (same diameter at all distances). Normal optic disc, visual acuity, and colour vision.
	Confirmed by: no progression on follow-up.
	Initial management: reassurance about prognosis.
Retinitis pigmentosa	*Suggested by:* funnel vision with good visual acuity in light, with inability to navigate around objects, and virtually blind in the dark.
	Confirmed by: pale atrophic disc, thin thready vessels, and asterisk or reticular type pigment in the retina without pale patches of depigmentation. Visual field charting.
	Initial management: counselling regarding prognosis.
Choroiditis (choroidoretinitis) (due to TB, sarcoid, toxoplasmosis, toxacara)	*Suggested by:* gradual loss vision or blurring (in acute phases), grey white raised patch on retina, vitreous opacities, muddiness in the anterior chamber, then white patch with pigmentation around on retina (choroidoretinal scarring).
	Confirmed by: tests results for underlying cause—**CXR, serology, sputum, lung biopsy**.
	Initial management: treatment of underlying cause, e.g. antiTB therapy.
Optic chiasm lesion (due to pituitary tumour, craniopharyngioma, aneurysm)	*Suggested by:* bitemporal hemianopia (or sometimes bitemporal upper quadrantinopia from tumour pushing up).
	Confirmed by: visual field charting. **CT or MRI scan** appearance.
	Initial management: treatment of underlying cause, e.g. surgical removal or reduction.
Optic tract lesion (due to middle cerebral artery thrombosis of contralateral side)	*Suggested by:* homonymous hemianopia.
	Confirmed by: visual field charting. **MRI scan** appearance.
	Initial management: treatment of underlying cause, prevention of recurrence, e.g. aspirin.
Visual cortex lesion (due to posterior cerebral artery occlusion, tumour)	*Suggested by:* homonymous hemianopia or occasionally quadrantanopia. May have macular sparing (visual acuity normal). Funnel vision if bilateral.
	Confirmed by: visual field charting. **CT** or **MRI scan** appearance.
	Initial management: treatment of underlying cause and prevention of recurrence, e.g. aspirin.

Ptosis

Drooping of one or both upper eyelids. Investigations in **bold** below.

Main differential diagnoses and typical outline evidence, etc.	
Oculomotor (3rd nerve) lesion due to pituitary tumour, intra-cavernous or posterior communicating artery aneurysm, meningioma, tentorial pressure cone, diabetes mellitus, syphilis, and brainstem ischaemia	*Suggested by:* ptosis, diplopia, and squint maximal on looking up and in; but therefore, in total loss, eye looks down and out. **Dilated pupil (except in diabetes mellitus, syphilis, and brainstem ischaemia when pupil not dilated)**; other cranial nerve lesions that form pattern (see p. 642). *Confirmed by:* **CT** or **MRI scan** appearance. *Initial management:* treatment of underlying cause.
Horner's syndrome due to neck trauma or tumours, cervical rib, Pancoast tumour (in lung apex), syringomyelia (in cervical spine), lateral medullary syndrome (in brainstem), hypothalamic lesion	*Suggested by:* ptosis and constricted (miotic) pupil, recessed globe of the eye, and diminished sweating on same side of face. *Confirmed by:* history of trauma or onset over week or months suggestive of tumour, or years suggestive of MS or syrinx. Other cranial nerve signs that form a pattern of cervical plexus lesion or brainstem lesion. X-ray of upper chest, ribs, or neck. **CT** of neck or upper chest or **MRI scan** of brainstem. *Initial management:* treatment of underlying cause.
Myasthenia gravis	*Suggested by:* bilateral partial ptosis worsening as day progresses. *Confirmed by:* eyes begin to droop after 15min of upgaze. +ve **Tensilon test** (edrophonium results in improvement in ptosis). *Initial management:* pyridostigmine, prednisolone, consider plasmapheresis, immunoglobulin, thymectomy.

Myopathy (dystrophia myotonica)	*Suggested by:* bilateral partial ptosis with evidence of weakness in other muscle groups. Frontal balding, inability to release hand grip.
	Confirmed by: biopsy histology of other affected muscle.
	Initial management: try mexiletine, phenytoin, acetazolamide; genetic counselling.
Congenital ptosis	*Suggested by:* unilateral or bilateral partial ptosis present since birth. Compensatory head posture.
	Confirmed by: absence of other neurological signs.
	Initial management: explanation, reassurance.

Large (mydriatic) pupil with no ptosis

Main differential diagnoses and typical outline evidence, etc.

Holmes–Adie pupil due to ciliary ganglion degeneration	*Suggested by:* dilated pupil (often widely) that only reacts slowly to light by constricting in well-lit room after 30min. Reacts to accommodation. Usually unilateral. Absent knee jerks. Usually in females.
	Confirmed by: benign outcome with no action necessary.
	Initial management: explanation, reassurance.
Traumatic iridoplegia	*Suggested by:* history of direct trauma. Dilated, fixed irregular pupil that does not accommodate nor react to light.
	Confirmed by: slit-lamp examination of anterior eye chamber.
	Initial management: explanation, reassurance.
Drug effect due to cocaine, amphetamines, tropicamide, atropine	*Suggested by:* bilateral pupil dilation.
	Confirmed by: drug history and resolution with withdrawal.
	Initial management: withdrawal of drug.
Severe brainstem dysfunction (or death)	*Suggested by:* bilateral pupil dilation with no reaction to light, comatose, long tract pyramidal signs.
	Confirmed by: absent corneal reflex response, no vestibulo-ocular reflexes, no cranial motor response to stimulation, no gag reflex, insufficient respiratory effort when P_aCO_2 >6.7kPa to prevent further ↑ of P_aCO_2 and ↓P_aO_2.
	Initial management: management of terminal illness.

Small (miotic) pupil with no ptosis

Investigations in **bold** below.

Main differential diagnoses and typical outline evidence, etc.	
Argyll Robinson pupil (due to syphilis and diabetes mellitus, rarely)	*Suggested by:* unilateral, small, irregular pupil that 'accommodates' by constricting when focusing on near finger, but does not react to light.
	Confirmed by: **syphilis serology** or **fasting blood glucose** ≥7mmol/L and random or **GTT glucose** ≥11.0mmol/L.
	Initial management: treatment of underlying cause.
Anisocoria normal variation	*Suggested by:* unilateral, small, miotic pupil that reacts normally to light and accommodation.
	Confirmed by: no change with time, benign outcome with no action necessary.
	Initial management: explanation, reassurance.
Age-related miosis due to autonomic degeneration	*Suggested by:* bilateral, small, miotic pupils that react normally to light and accommodates normally.
	Confirmed by: discovery in old age, no change with time, benign outcome with no action.
	Initial management: explanation, reassurance.
Drug effect due to opiates, pilocarpine	*Suggested by:* bilateral, small pupils. Not reacting to light.
	Confirmed by: drug history and resolution with withdrawal.
	Initial management: withdrawal of drug.
Pontine haemorrhage	*Suggested by:* bilateral, small, miotic pupils that react to light. Patient comatose, bilaterally or unilaterally, hyper-reflexic, and high or fluctuating temperature.
	Confirmed by: evolution of signs to localize to brainstem. **MRI scan.**
	Initial management: treatment of underlying cause and complications.

Squint and diplopia: ocular palsy

Elicited by asking the patient to follow the examiner's finger and asking if this results in 'seeing double', and looking for development of a convergent or divergent squint. Cover test: fix focus in the distance and alternately cover either eye in quick succession. As cover is lifted, observe the eye. If the uncovered eye now moves in, this indicates a divergent squint. If the eye moves out, this indicates a convergent squint. Initial investigations (other tests in **bold** below): FBC, ESR or CRP, CT or MRI scan.

Main differential diagnoses and typical outline evidence, etc.	
Oculomotor (3rd nerve) paresis Intra-cavernous or posterior communicating artery aneurysm, meningioma, tentorial pressure cone, diabetes mellitus, syphilis, and brainstem ischaemia	*Suggested by:* ptosis, diplopia, and squint maximal on looking up and in; but therefore, in total loss, eye looks down and out. **Dilated pupil (except in diabetes mellitus, syphilis, and brainstem ischaemia when pupil not dilated)**. *Confirmed by:* other cranial nerve lesions that form pattern (see 📖 p. 642), **skull X-ray P–A and lateral, CT or MRI scan** appearance. *Initial management:* treatment of underlying cause and complications.
Trochlear (4th cranial nerve) paresis	*Suggested by:* diplopia and squint maximal on looking down and in. Double vision for reading and walking down stairs. *Confirmed by:* other cranial nerve lesions that form pattern (see 📖 p. 642). **MRI scan** appearance. *Initial management:* treatment of underlying cause.
Abducent (6th cranial nerve) paresis	*Suggested by:* **double vision looking in direction of the affected muscle**. Head turn in direction of affected muscle. *Confirmed by:* other cranial nerve lesions that form pattern (see 📖 p. 642). **MRI scan** appearance. *Initial management:* treatment of underlying cause.
Myasthenia gravis, Graves's disease, orbital cellulitis, or tumour	*Suggested by:* diplopia and squint in all directions of gaze. *Confirmed by:* **CT or MRI scan** of orbit or +ve Tensilon test (edrophonium results in less diplopia and squint in myasthenia). *Initial management:* pyridostigmine, prednisolone, consider plasmapheresis, immunoglobulin, thymectomy.

| Internuclear ophthalmoplegia due to lesion in the medial longitudinal bundle, usually due to MS or sometimes vascular | *Suggested by:* impaired conjugate gaze (slowness of adducting eye and nystagmus in abducting eye). *Confirmed by:* other signs of brainstem lesion. *Initial management:* treatment of underlying cause. |

Loss of facial sensation

Investigations in **bold** below.

Main differential diagnoses and typical outline evidence, etc.	
Ophthalmic branch of trigeminal nerve lesion	*Suggested by:* absent corneal reflex (present corneal reflex excludes lesion) with diminished touch and pain sensation in upper face above the line of the eye.
	Confirmed by: other cranial nerve lesions that form pattern (see 📖p. 642). **MRI scan** appearance.
	Initial management: treatment of underlying cause.
Maxillary branch of trigeminal nerve lesion	*Suggested by:* diminished touch and pain sensation in midface between line of mouth and line of eye.
	Confirmed by: other cranial nerve lesions that form pattern (see 📖p. 642). **MRI scan** appearance.
	Initial management: treatment of underlying cause.
Mandibular branch of trigeminal nerve lesion	*Suggested by:* diminished touch and pain sensation in lower face below line of mouth.
	Confirmed by: other cranial nerve lesions that form pattern (see 📖p. 642). **MRI scan** appearance.
	Initial management: treatment of underlying cause.

Jaw muscle weakness

Investigations in **bold** below.

Main differential diagnoses and typical outline evidence, etc.

Motor branch of trigeminal nerve (5th cranial): lower motor neurone type on same (ipsilateral) side	*Suggested by:* weakness of jaw movement. Deviation of jaw when opening against resistance and poor contraction of masseter on clenching. Decreased jaw jerk.
	Confirmed by: other cranial nerve lesions that form pattern (see 📖p. 642). **MRI scan** appearance.
	Initial management: treatment of underlying cause.
Motor branch of trigeminal nerve (5th cranial): upper motor neurone type on other (contralateral) side.	*Suggested by:* weakness of jaw movement. Deviation of jaw when opening against resistance and poor contraction of masseter on clenching. Increased jaw jerk
	Confirmed by: other cranial nerve lesions that form pattern (see 📖p. 642). **MRI scan** appearance.
	Initial management: treatment of underlying cause.

Facial muscle weakness

Distinguish between upper (forehead muscles movement preserved) and lower (forehead movement weak) motor neurone type. Investigations in **bold** below.

Main differential diagnoses and typical outline evidence, etc.	
Facial nerve palsy (7th cranial): *upper* motor neurone type on other (contralateral) side due to internal capsule lesion—cerebrovascular accident, tumour	*Suggested by:* **able** to raise eyebrows and close eye but **unable** to grimace nor smile symmetrically; other cranial nerve lesions that form pattern (see 📖p. 642). *Confirmed by:* **MRI scan**. *Initial management:* treatment of underlying cause.
Facial nerve palsy (7th cranial): *lower* motor neurone type on same (ipsilateral) side (see below for causes)	*Suggested by:* inability to raise eyebrows nor close eye (rolls upwards to hide iris revealing the white of the eye) nor grimace nor smile symmetrically; other cranial nerve lesions that form pattern (see 📖p. 642). *Confirmed by:* **MRI scan**. *Initial management:* treatment of underlying cause.
Bell's palsy	*Suggested by:* lower motor neurone 7th nerve palsy. Prior ache behind ear. No other physical signs (NB. Corneal reflex present, and no deafness or vertigo). *Confirmed by:* above clinical features. *Initial management:* prednisolone within 5d of onset. Protective dark glasses and 'artificial tears'. Manual closure of eyelid ± tape.
Ramsay Hunt syndrome	*Suggested by:* lower motor neurone 7th nerve palsy. Taste diminished on same side. Vesicles in external auditory meatus. *Confirmed by:* above clinical features. *Initial management:* analgesia, e.g. paracetamol initially. Aciclovir.
Facial nerve palsy from parotid swelling	*Suggested by:* lower motor neurone 7th nerve palsy. Swelling in midface on same side. *Confirmed by:* above clinical features and **MRI scan**. *Initial management:* surgical decompression, release of nerve ± repair with lateral cutaneous nerve of thigh.

Cerebello-pontine lesion (e.g. tumour)	*Suggested by:* lower motor neurone 7th nerve palsy. Associated 5th (loss of corneal reflex) and 7th cranial nerve lesion.
	Confirmed by: above clinical features. **MRI scan** appearance of space-occupying lesion in or near internal auditory canal.
	Initial management: assessment for possible excision.
Cholesteatoma	*Suggested by:* lower motor neurone 7th nerve palsy. Also deafness and vertigo.
	Confirmed by: above clinical features. **MRI scan** appearance.
	Initial management: assessment for possible clearance.
Facial nerve palsy from demyelination	*Suggested by:* lower motor neurone 7th nerve palsy. Other focal neurological signs and symptoms disseminated in time and space.
	Confirmed by: above clinical features. **MRI scan** appearance.
	Initial management: methylprednisolone to hasten remission.
Facial nerve palsy from brain stem ischaemia	*Suggested by:* lower motor neurone 7th nerve palsy. Signs of adjacent dysfunction, e.g. nystagmus, long tract signs, e.g. spastic hemiparesis.
	Confirmed by: above clinical features. **MRI scan** appearance.
	Initial management: aspirin and 'statin' to prevent/reduce risk of recurrence.

Loss of hearing

Inability to hear whispering or ticking watch, and test with tuning fork held near ear (testing air and bone conduction together). Investigations in **bold** below.

Main differential diagnoses and typical outline evidence, etc.	
8th nerve conduction defect on side X due to wax, foreign body, otitis externa, recurrent otitis media, injury to tympanic membrane, otosclerosis, cholesteatoma	*Suggested by:* forehead vibration heard louder on side X than on side Y (Weber's test), and mastoid vibration on side X louder than for air (Rinne's test). *Confirmed by:* auroscope appearance, formal audiometry, and other cranial nerve lesions that form pattern (see 📖p. 642). **MRI scan** appearance. *Initial management:* treatment of underlying cause only.
Sensorineural (8th cranial) lesion on side Y due to old age, noise trauma, Paget's disease, Meniere's disease, drugs, viral infections (e.g. measles), congenital rubella, meningitis, acoustic neuroma, meningioma	*Suggested by:* forehead vibration heard louder on side X than on side Y (Weber's test), and mastoid vibration same for both sides (Rinne's test). *Confirmed by:* other cranial nerve lesions that form pattern (see 📖p. 642), formal audiometry, and **MRI scan** appearance. *Initial management:* treatment of underlying cause only.

Abnormal tongue, uvula, and pharyngeal movement

9th, 10th (not 11th), and 12th cranial nerve lesions. Investigations in **bold** below.

Main differential diagnoses and typical outline evidence, etc.	
Glossopharyngeal (9th cranial) nerve lesion	*Suggested by:* loss of gag reflex and taste on posterior one third of tongue; other cranial nerve lesions that form pattern (see 📖p. 642).
	Confirmed by: **MRI scan**.
	Initial management: treatment of underlying cause only.
Vagus (10th cranial) nerve lesion due to jugular foramen lesion, bulbar palsy	*Suggested by:* deviation of uvula away from affected side when saying 'ah'; nasal regurgitation of water. Dysarthria; other cranial nerve lesions that form pattern (see 📖p. 642).
	Confirmed by: **MRI scan**.
	Initial management: treatment of underlying cause only.
Lower motor neurone hypoglossal (12th cranial) nerve lesion on same (ipsilateral) side of deviation	*Suggested by:* deviation of tongue to side of lesion on protrusion. Fasciculation and wasting; other cranial nerve lesions that form pattern (see 📖p. 684).
	Confirmed by: **MRI scan**.
	Initial management: treatment of underlying cause only.
Upper motor neurone hypoglossal (12th cranial) nerve lesion on other (contralateral) side of deviation	*Suggested by:* deviation of tongue to one side on protrusion. Small stiff tongue and cortical or internal capsule signs.
	Confirmed by: **CT or MRI scan**.
	Initial management: treatment of underlying cause only.

Multiple cranial nerve lesions

Investigations in **bold** below.

Main differential diagnoses and typical outline evidence, etc.	
Pituitary tumour	*Suggested by:* optic tract or chiasm lesion. 3rd cranial nerve lesion.
	Confirmed by: **CT or MRI scan** appearance.
	Initial management: assessment for surgical decompression or hypophysectomy, radiotherapy or (dopamine agonist if prolactinoma).
Anterior communicating artery aneurysm cerebral artery aneurysm	*Suggested by:* optic nerve lesion, 3rd and 4th cranial nerve lesions.
	Confirmed by: **CT or MRI scan** appearance.
	Initial management: assessment for possible surgery.
Posterior carotid artery aneurysm	*Suggested by:* 4th and 5th cranial nerve lesions.
	Confirmed by: **CT** or **MRI scan** appearance.
	Initial management: assessment for possible surgery.
Gradenigo's syndrome (lesion in petrous temporal bone)	*Suggested by:* 5th and 6th cranial nerve lesions.
	Confirmed by: **MRI scan** appearance.
	Initial management: assessment for possible surgery.
Facial canal lesion, e.g. cholesteatoma	*Suggested by:* 7th and 8th cranial nerve lesions alone (no 5th or 6th).
	Confirmed by: **CT or MRI scan** appearance.
	Initial management: assessment for possible surgical clearance.
Cerebello-pontine angle lesion, e.g. tumour	*Suggested by:* 5th, 7th, and 8th ± 6th cranial nerve lesions.
	Confirmed by: **CT or MRI scan** appearance.
	Initial management: assessment for possible surgery.
Jugular foramen syndrome due to tumour, tuberculoma	*Suggested by:* 9th, 10th, and 11th cranial nerve lesions.
	Confirmed by: **MRI scan** appearance.
	Initial management: assessment for possible surgery or antitubercular antibiotic.
Lateral medullary syndrome	*Suggested by:* vertigo, nystagmus, 5th cranial nerve lesion, Horner's syndrome, contralateral spinothalamic loss on trunk.
	Confirmed by: above clinical features. **MRI scan** appearance.
	Initial management: aspirin and 'statin' to reduce risk of progression or recurrence after 1–2wk to avoid risk of bleeding into infarcted tissue.

Weber's syndrome	*Suggested by:* ipsilateral 3rd cranial nerve lesion and contralateral hemiparesis.
	Confirmed by: above clinical features. **MRI scan** appearance.
	Initial management: treatment of underlying cause only.

Odd posture of arms and hands at rest

Investigations in **bold** below:

	Main differential diagnoses and typical outline evidence, etc.
Internal capsule bleed, infarct, or tumour (or pre-central gyrus and connections, or lower pyramidal tract, i.e. upper motor neurone)	*Suggested by:* arms flexed at elbow and wrist, and weak. Increased tone and reflexes. Upper motor neurone facial weakness. *Confirmed by:* brain **CT or MRI scan** appearance. *Initial management:* assessment for treatment of any remediable underlying cause.
T1 anterior root lesion	*Suggested by:* **claw hand**, wasting of all small muscles of the hand. Loss of sensation of ulnar 1½ fingers and ulnar border of forearm. *Confirmed by:* nerve conduction study result. MRI scan appearance of neck showing root compression. *Initial management:* assessment for treatment of any remediable underlying cause.
Ulnar nerve lesion (below elbow)	*Suggested by:* **claw hand**, wasting of hypothenar eminence and dorsal guttering, especially first. Weakness of finger abduction and adduction. Loss of sensation of ulnar 1½ fingers. *Confirmed by:* nerve conduction studies. *Initial management:* assessment for treatment of any remediable underlying cause.
Radial nerve lesion (or C7 anterior root lesion)	*Suggested by:* **wrist drop**. Inability to extend wrist and grip. Loss of sensation over 1st dorsal interosseous muscle. *Confirmed by:* nerve conduction study result. *Initial management:* assessment for treatment of any remediable underlying cause.

Fine tremor of hands

Elicited by asking patient to hold arms out straight in front and placing sheet of paper to rest on them (to amplify fine tremor). Investigations in **bold** below:

Main differential diagnoses and typical outline evidence, etc.	
Thyrotoxicosis	*Suggested by:* fine tremor, anxiety, tachycardia, sweating, weight loss, goitre, increased reflexes.
	Confirmed by: ↑**FT4** or **FT3**, and ↓↓**TSH**.
	Initial management: β-blocker, e.g. propranolol to control any intolerable symptoms for few weeks, antithyroid drug, e.g carbimazole or propylthiouracil for 6–18mo (± block and replacement with thyroxine). Radio-iodine for hot nodule or recurrence.
Anxiety state	*Suggested by:* fine tremor, anxiety, tachycardia, sweating, weight loss.
	Confirmed by: normal thyroid function tests. Improvement with sedation, psychotherapy, etc.
	Initial management: β-blocker or minor tranquilizer.
Alcohol withdrawal	*Suggested by:* fine or coarse tremor, history of high alcohol intake and recent withdrawal, anxiety.
	Confirmed by: improvement with sedation, etc.
	Initial management: sedation, e.g. chlordiazepoxide in reducing dose.
Sympathomimetic drugs	*Suggested by:* fine tremor, drug history.
	Confirmed by: improvement with withdrawal of drug.
	Initial management: withdrawal of drug.
Benign essential tremor	*Suggested by:* usually coarse tremor, long history, no other symptoms or signs.
	Confirmed by: normal **thyroid test results**. Improvement with β-blocker.
	Initial management: β-blocker, e.g. propranolol.

Coarse tremor of hands

Elicited by asking patient to hold arms out straight in front and extending wrists (for asterixis or flap), then asking the patient to touch their own nose and then the examiner's finger with arm extended—repetitively (for intention tremor). Investigations in **bold** below:

Main differential diagnoses and typical outline evidence, etc.	
Hepatic failure	*Suggested by:* flapping tremor (asterixis), aggravated when wrists extended. Spider naevi. Jaundice. *Confirmed by:* abnormal **LFT** and prolonged **prothrombin time**. *Initial management:* avoid sedatives, 20° bed head uptilt, lactulose (for 2–3 stool/d).
Carbon dioxide retention	*Suggested by:* flapping tremor (asterixis), aggravated when wrists extended. Muscle twitching, bounding pulse, warm peripheries. *Confirmed by:* **ABG** show ↑P_aCO_2. *Initial management:* if on O_2, reduce %, bi-level positive airway pressure (BiPAP).
Cerebellar disease	*Suggested by:* intention tremor (past pointing) when patient attempts to touch examiner's finger. *Confirmed by:* **MRI scan**. *Initial management:* assessment for treatment of any remediable underlying cause.
Parkinsonism due to Parkinson's disease, Lewy body dementia; drug-induced (chlorpromazine, haloperidol, metoclopramide, prochlorperazine); post-encephalitis, normal pressure hydrocephalus	*Suggested by:* **resting** coarse tremor, ('pill-rolling'), 'lead-pipe rigidity', expressionless face, paucity of movement, small hand writing, rapid, shuffling ('festinant') gait with small steps. *Confirmed by:* clinical findings, e.g. persistent blinking when forehead tapped (e.g. 'glabellar tap'). Clinical improvement with appropriate treatment. *Initial management:* withdrawal of potentially causative drug or antimuscarinic, e.g. procyclidine. Counselling, explain long-term strategy, MDT planning, low dose levodopa with dopa-decarboxylase inhibitor.
Benign essential tremor	*Suggested by:* usually coarse tremor, long history, no other symptoms or signs. *Confirmed by:* normal **thyroid test** results. Improvement with β-blocker. *Initial management:* β-blocker, e.g. propranolol.

Wasting of some small muscles of hand

Inter-metacarpal grooves are prominent due to muscle wasting. Investigations in **bold** below:

Main differential diagnoses and typical outline evidence, etc.

Median nerve palsy usually due to carpal tunnel syndrome	*Suggested by:* wasting of thenar eminence. Weakness of thumb flexion, abduction, and opposition. **Unable** to lift thumb with palm upwards, but **able** to press with index finger. Loss of sensation over palmar aspect of radial 3½ fingers of hand.
	Confirmed by: **nerve conduction study** results.
	Initial management: surgery to decompress nerve.
Ulnar nerve lesion from elbow (high) to wrist (low)	*Suggested by:* wasting of hypothenar eminence. **Able** to lift thumb with palm upwards, but **unable** to press with index finger. Weakness of finger abduction and adduction. Loss of sensation in ulnar aspect 1½ fingers of hand. Claw hand (in lower lesions).
	Confirmed by: **nerve conduction study** results.
	Initial management: assessment for treatment of any remediable underlying cause, e.g. surgical decompression.
T1 lesion: anterior horn cell or root lesion	*Suggested by:* wasting of all small muscles of hand. **Unable** to lift thumb with palm upwards, but **unable** to press with index finger.
	Confirmed by: **nerve conduction study** results. **MRI scan** appearance around T1 level.
	Initial management: assessment for treatment of any remediable underlying cause, e.g. NSAID to reduce swelling around inflamed root canal, surgical decompression.
Motor neurone disease	*Suggested by:* signs of T1 lesion, prominent fasciculation, spastic paraparesis, wasted fasciculating tongue, no sensory signs.
	Confirmed by: clinical presentation and absence of structural abnormality on **MRI scan** appearance.
	Initial management: involve MDT, propantheline for drooling, analgesic ladder for pain, blend food, NG tube for dysphagia, non-invasive ventilation for early breathing difficulty.
Syringomyelia	*Suggested by:* **signs of T1 lesion**, fasciculation **not** prominent, burn scars, dissociated sensory loss, Horner's syndrome, nystagmus. History over months to years.
	Confirmed by: **MRI scan** appearances.
	Initial management: assessment for surgical decompression of foramen magnum, MDT planning.

Any prolonged systemic illness	*Suggested by:* global muscle wasting, general weight loss.
	Confirmed by: improvement in muscle wasting if primary disease treatable.
	Initial management: assessment for treatment of any remediable underlying cause
Cervical spondylosis compressing nerve root	*Suggested by:* **signs of T1 lesion**, neck pain and stiffness, and referred pain.
	Confirmed by: **MRI scan** showing root canal compression.
	Initial management: physiotherapy, NSAIDs to reduce swelling around root canal, surgical decompression if intractible pain.
Tumour compressing nerve root	*Suggested by:* **signs of T1 lesion**, referred pain. Progressing over months.
	Confirmed by: **MRI scan** showing root canal compression.
	Initial management: assessment for radiotherapy or surgical decompression.
Brachial plexus lesion	*Suggested by:* **signs of T1 lesion**, and history of trauma to shoulder area or birth injury.
	Confirmed by: **nerve conduction study** results.
	Initial management: treatment of underlying cause.
Cervical rib	*Suggested by:* **signs of T1 lesion** aggravated by movement or posture.
	Confirmed by: **neck and chest X-ray**—presence of cervical rib.
	Initial management: physiotherapy, assessment for possible rib removal, or band division.
Pancoast tumour	*Suggested by:* **signs of T1 lesion**, Horner's syndrome, features of lung cancer (clubbing, chest signs, etc.).
	Confirmed by: **CXR** and **CT scan** appearances.
	Initial management: assessment for radiotherapy.

Wasting of arm and shoulder

Loss of rounded contour of deltoid and biceps muscle. Fasciculation is localized twitching of muscle. Note facial expression. Investigations in **bold** below:

Main differential diagnoses and typical outline evidence, etc.	
Progressive muscular atrophy	*Suggested by:* bilateral wasting of hand, arm, and shoulder girdle with fasciculation.
	Confirmed by: **EMG** results.
	Initial management: MDT planning, especially occupational and physiotherapy.
Motor neurone disease (amyotrophic lateral sclerosis) with anterior horn cell degeneration	*Suggested by:* initially unilateral wasting of shoulder abductor and biceps. Weakness of speech, swallowing. No sensory signs.
	Confirmed by: **EMG** results.
	Initial management: MDT planning, propantheline for drooling, analgesic ladder for pain, blend food, NG tube for dysphagia, non-invasive ventilation for early breathing difficulty.
1° muscle disease	*Suggested by:* bilateral wasting of shoulder abductor, and biceps.
	Confirmed by: **EMG** findings or **muscle biopsy**.
	Initial management: MDT planning, especially occupational and physiotherapy.

Abnormalities of arm tone

Elicited by supporting elbow in one hand, and asking patient to allow you to flex and extend arm at the elbow without assistance. Investigations in **bold** below:

Main differential diagnoses and typical outline evidence, etc.	
Cerebellar lesion	*Suggested by:* **tone diminished**, no wasting. diminished reflexes. Past pointing, truncal ataxia, nystagmus.
	Confirmed by: **CT or MRI scan** appearance of cerebellum.
	Initial management: assessment for treatment of any remediable underlying cause. MDT planning, especially occupational and physiotherapy.
1° muscle disease	*Suggested by:* **tone diminished** with wasting ± fasciculation.
	Confirmed by: **EMG** findings or **muscle biopsy**.
	Initial management: MDT planning, especially occupational and physiotherapy.
Upper motor neurone	*Suggested by:* **tone increased**. Brisk reflexes below lesion.
	Confirmed by: **CT or MRI scan** of brain or spinal cord.
	Initial management: MDT planning, especially occupational and physiotherapy.
Parkinson's disease	*Suggested by:* **tone increased** with cogwheel effect (superimposed tremor). Poor facial movement, shuffling, hesitant, 'festinant' gait, coarse tremor.
	Confirmed by: response to drug therapy.
	Initial management: withdrawal of potentially causative drug or antimuscarinic, e.g. procyclidine. Counselling, MDT planning, low dose levodopa initially with dopa-decarboxylase inhibitor.

Weakness around the shoulder and arm without pain

Elicited by asking the patient to flex and extend wrist and elbow against resistance, and to abduct, adduct, flex and extend shoulder against resistance, comparing both sides. Investigations in **bold** below:

Main differential diagnoses and typical outline evidence, etc.	
C4–5 root lesion	*Suggested by:* weakness of abduction at the shoulder only (**not elbow or wrist**).
	Confirmed by: **nerve conduction studies** and **MRI scan** of neck.
	Initial management: physiotherapy, assessment for treatment of any remediable underlying cause.
C5–6 root lesion Erb's palsy	*Suggested by:* weakness of flexion at the shoulder and lbow, but not wrist. Arm externally rotated and adducted behind back (note porter's tip position). History of birth trauma.
	Confirmed by: **nerve conduction studies** and **MRI scan** of neck.
	Initial management: physiotherapy.
C7 root lesion	*Suggested by:* wrist drop or weakness of grip, and extension at the **elbow and wrist**.
	Confirmed by: **nerve conduction studies** and **MRI scan** of neck.
	Initial management: physiotherapy.
Radial nerve lesion	*Suggested by:* wrist drop or weakness of grip and extension at the wrist but **not** at the elbow.
	Confirmed by: **nerve conduction studies** and history of trauma.
	Initial management: physiotherapy, assessment for possible surgical repair.
C8–T1 root lesion (Klumpke's paralysis)	*Suggested by:* arm held in adduction, paralysis/paresis of the small muscles of the hand, loss of sensation over ulnar border of the hand. History of birth trauma.
	Confirmed by: **nerve conduction studies** and **MRI scan** of neck.
	Initial management: physiotherapy.

Incoordination (on rapid wrist rotation or hand tapping)

Comment: this is often used as a 'screening' test (i.e. if normal, you can discount any significant neuromuscular condition of the upper limbs in the absence of other symptoms or signs. Investigations in **bold** below:

Main differential diagnoses and typical outline evidence, etc.	
Upper motor neurone paresis	*Suggested by:* spastic weakness (i.e. with increased tone) in upper limb.
	Confirmed by: **CT scan** of brain or **MRI scan** of neck.
	Initial management: physiotherapy.
Lower motor neurone paresis	*Suggested by:* flaccid weakness (i.e. with decreased tone) in upper limb.
	Confirmed by: **nerve conduction studies** and **MRI scan** of neck.
	Initial management: physiotherapy.
Ipsilateral cerebellar lesion	*Suggested by:* decreased tone, past pointing, diminished reflexes.
	Confirmed by: **CT or MRI scan** of cerebellum.
	Initial management: physiotherapy, assessment for treatment of any remediable underlying cause.
Loss of proprioception	*Suggested by:* loss of joint position sense and vibration sense.
	Confirmed by: **nerve conduction studies**.
	Initial management: physiotherapy, assessment for treatment of any remediable underlying cause.

Muscle wasting

Comment: has to be assessed in context of the bulk of other muscles. Investigations in **bold** below:

Main differential diagnoses and typical outline evidence, etc.
Adjacent bone, joint or muscle disease *Suggested by:* wasting with pain and limitation of movement. Visible swelling or deformity of bone or joint. *Confirmed by:* **X-ray of affected part. EMG.** *Initial management:* physiotherapy, assessment for treatment of any remediable underlying cause.
Lower motor neurone lesion *Suggested by:* wasting and fasciculation. Tone decreased. Weakness and diminished reflexes. *Confirmed by:* **nerve conduction studies**. *Initial management:* physiotherapy, assessment for treatment of any remediable underlying cause.
Muscle disease *Suggested by:* wasting. Tone decreased. Weakness and diminished reflex. *Confirmed by:* **EMG**. *Initial management:* physiotherapy, assessment for treatment of any remediable underlying cause.

Weakness around one lower limb joint

These weaknesses may point strongly to one nerve root lesion. Test by asking the patient to perform the movement against your resistance. Initial investigations (other tests in **bold** below):

Main differential diagnoses and typical outline evidence, etc.	
L1/2 root lesion or femoral nerve	*Suggested by:* weakness of hip flexion alone. *Confirmed by:* **X-ray of lumbar spine and sacrum. Nerve conduction studies. MRI scan** if lesion can be localized clinically. *Initial management:* physiotherapy, assessment for treatment of any remediable underlying cause.
L2/3 root lesion or obturator nerve	*Suggested by:* weakness of hip adduction alone. *Confirmed by:* **X-ray of lumbar spine and sacrum. Nerve conduction studies. MRI scan** if lesion can be localized clinically. *Initial management:* physiotherapy, assessment for treatment of any remediable underlying cause.
L3/4 root lesion or femoral nerve	*Suggested by:* weakness of knee extension alone. *Confirmed by:* **X-ray of lumbar spine and sacrum. Nerve conduction studies. MRI scan** if lesion can be localized clinically. *Initial management:* physiotherapy, assessment for treatment of any remediable underlying cause.
L4/5 root lesion or tibial nerve	*Suggested by:* weakness of foot dorsiflexion and inversion at the ankle. *Confirmed by:* **X-ray of lumbar spine and sacrum. Nerve conduction studies. MRI scan** if lesion can be localized clinically. *Initial management:* physiotherapy, assessment for treatment of any remediable underlying cause.
L5/S1 root lesion or common peroneal nerve	*Suggested by:* weakness of knee flexion alone. *Confirmed by:* **X-ray of lumbar spine and sacrum. Nerve conduction studies. MRI scan** if lesion can be localized clinically. *Initial management:* physiotherapy, assessment for treatment of any remediable underlying cause.
S1/2 root lesion or sciatic nerve	*Suggested by:* weakness of toe flexion alone. *Confirmed by:* **X-ray of lumbar spine and sacrum. Nerve conduction studies. MRI scan** if lesion can be localized clinically. *Initial management:* physiotherapy, assessment for treatment of any remediable underlying cause.

Lateral popliteal nerve palsy (usually traumatic)	*Suggested by:* flaccid 'foot drop with weakness of eversion and dorsiflexion of the foot, and a sensory loss over lateral aspect of leg.
	Confirmed by: **nerve conduction study** result.
	Initial management: physiotherapy, assessment for possible surgical repair.

Bilateral weakness of all foot movements

Initial investigations (other tests in **bold** below): FBC, ESR or CRP, U&E, CT scan.

Main differential diagnoses and typical outline evidence, etc.	
Guillain–Barré syndrome.	*Suggested by:* onset over days, preceding viral illness.
	Confirmed by: ↑**CSF protein**. Progressive course then variable recovery.
	Initial management: monitor breathing and make arrangements for possible ventilation in ITU.
Lead poisoning	*Suggested by:* gradual onset over weeks to months.
	Confirmed by: **nerve conduction studies**, and history of exposure. **Serum lead** levels.
	Initial management: identify and remove source of poisoning, assess need for EDTA (e.g. if levels >45mcg/dL).
Porphyria	*Suggested by:* onset over months to years. Usually known to have porphyria.
	Confirmed by: **EMG** and ↑urine or **faecal porphobilinogens**.
	Initial management: stop potentially precipitating drug, fluids IV, ↑carbohydrate intake, haematin IV.
Charcot–Marie–Tooth disease	*Suggested by:* onset over years. Associated with foot drop and peroneal atrophy upper limbs affected later.
	Confirmed by: **EMG**.
	Initial management: MDT planning, especially occupational and physiotherapy. Assessment for possible nerve release.

Spastic paraparesis

Bilateral lower limb paresis with increased tone. This is a **medical emergency**, if acute. Initial investigations (other tests in **bold** below): FBC, ESR or CRP, U&E, MRI scan.

Main differential diagnoses and typical outline evidence, etc.	
Prolapsed disc (anteriorly thus compressing spinal cord)	*Suggested by:* sudden onset often associated with change in spinal posture. *Confirmed by:* **MRI scan** appearance. *Initial management:* urgent referral for possible spinal cord decompression surgery.
Traumatic vertebral displacement or fracture	*Suggested by:* sudden onset associated with violent injury. *Confirmed by:* **MRI scan** appearance. *Initial management:* urgent referral for possible spinal cord decompression surgery.
Collapsed vertebra (due to 2° carcinoma or myeloma)	*Suggested by:* sudden onset over minutes or hours. Other symptoms suggestive of neoplasia over months. *Confirmed by:* **nerve conduction studies**. **MRI scan** appearance. *Initial management:* urgent referral for possible spinal cord decompression surgery.
Spondylitic bone formation compressing spinal cord	*Suggested by:* onset over months to years. Often past history of spondylitic back pain. *Confirmed by:* **MRI scan** appearance. *Initial management:* referral for possible spinal cord decompression surgery.
MS affecting spinal cord	*Suggested by:* this and other intermittent neurological symptoms disseminated in site and time. *Confirmed by:* **MRI scan** appearance. *Initial management:* methylprednisolone, physiotherapy, MDT planning.
Infective space-occupying lesion, e.g. TB or abscess	*Suggested by:* onset over days or weeks with fever from low grade to spiking. *Confirmed by:* **MRI scan** and findings at surgery, **histology**, and **microbiology**. *Initial management:* urgent assessment for surgery.
Glioma or ependymoma in spinal cord	*Suggested by:* gradual onset over months. *Confirmed by:* **MRI scan** and findings at surgery, **histology**. *Initial management:* assessment for surgery.
Parasagittal cerebral meningioma or other tumour	*Suggested by:* gradual onset over months. *Confirmed by:* **MRI scan** and findings at surgery, **histology**. *Initial management:* assessment for surgery.

Hemiparesis (weakness of arm and leg)

During the history and examination, other leads may appear, e.g. dysphagia, cough and breathlessness, limited or no support at home, ipsilateral facial weakness, cognitive impairment, raised urea and creatinine, opacification on the CXR. Some of these may lead to additional diagnoses which are causes and complications of one of those below. Initial investigations (other tests in **bold** below): FBC, ESR or CRP, U&E, CT scan.

Main differential diagnoses and typical outline evidence, etc.	
Occlusion of upper branch of middle cerebral artery with infarction, including Broca's area	*Suggested by:* expressive dysphasia and contralateral lower face and arm weakness. *Confirmed by:* **MRI or CT scan** appearance. *Initial management:* nil by mouth, fluids IV until swallowing assessed, attention to pressure areas, MDT planning for physiotherapy and occupational therapy and social services.
Occlusion of perforating branch of middle cerebral artery with lacunar infarction	*Suggested by:* hemiparesis alone with subsequent spasticity (or receptive dysphasia alone or hemi-anaesthesia alone). *Confirmed by:* **MRI or CT scan** appearance. *Initial management:* nil by mouth, fluids IV until swallowing assessed, attention to pressure areas, MDT planning for physiotherapy and occupational therapy and social services.
Total middle cerebral artery territory infarction (usually embolic)	*Suggested by:* contralateral flaccid hemiplegia (with little subsequent spasticity) and hemi-anaesthesia with deviation of head to side of lesion. Also homonymous hemianopia with aphasia if dominant hemisphere affected or 'neglect' if non-dominant hemisphere affected. *Confirmed by:* **MRI or CT scan** appearance. *Initial management:* nil by mouth, fluids IV until swallowing assessed, attention to pressure areas, MDT planning for physiotherapy and occupational therapy and social services.
Posterior cerebral artery infarction	*Suggested by:* contralateral homonymous hemianopia or upper quadrantinopia, mild contralateral hemiparesis and sensory loss, ataxia and involuntary movement, memory loss, dyslexia, and ipsilateral 3rd nerve palsy. *Confirmed by:* **MRI or CT scan** appearance. *Initial management:* nil by mouth, fluids IV until swallowing assessed, attention to pressure areas, MDT planning for physiotherapy and occupational therapy and social services.

Anterior cerebral artery infarction	*Suggested by:* paresis of contralateral leg, rigidity, perseveration, grasp reflex in opposite hand, urinary incontinence, and dysphasia if in dominant hemisphere.
	Confirmed by: **MRI or CT scan** appearance.
	Initial management: nil by mouth, fluids IV until swallowing assessed, attention to pressure areas, MDT planning for physiotherapy and occupational therapy and social services.

Disturbed sensation in upper limb

Elicit by testing touch (a piece of cotton wool), heat (a cold metal object), and pain (pinprick with a sterile needle) in each dermatome distribution. Note any discrepancy between these modalities of sensation. In the palm, examine the radial 3½ fingers and the ulnar 1½ fingers. Test joint position sense (by holding digits at their sides) and vibration with a tuning fork over bony prominences. Then use a two-pointed device (2-point discrimination), placing objects into the patients hand and asking to guess what they are with eyes closed, e.g. a 20-pence piece (stereognosis) and drawing figures on the palm (graphaesthesia). Consider if you have discovered any of the patterns described below. Investigations in **bold** below.

Main differential diagnoses and typical outline evidence, etc.	
Contralateral cortical (pre-central gyrus) lesion	*Suggested by:* asterognosis, diminished 2-point discrimination, and graphaesthesia. *Confirmed by:* **CT or MRI scan** of brain. *Initial management:* treatment of any remediable underlying cause, e.g. surgical removal of tumour.
Peripheral neuropathy	*Suggested by:* loss of touch and pinprick sensation worse in hand, progressing upwards. *Confirmed by:* **nerve conduction studies**. *Initial management:* treatment of any remediable underlying cause, e.g. stop drug, better control of diabetes.
Spinothalamic tract damage (no dorsal column loss) due to syringomyelia in cervical cord	*Suggested by:* loss of pinprick and temperature sensation, normal or disturbed touch, but normal joint position and vibration sense in hand. *Confirmed by:* **nerve conduction studies**. **MRI** of cervical cord. *Initial management:* treatment of underlying cause, e.g. assessment for surgical decompression of foramen magnum, MDT planning.
Cervical or thoracic nerve root lesion	*Suggested by:* loss of sensation in dermatome distribution in hand or forearm or upper arm. *Confirmed by:* **nerve conduction studies**. **X-ray** and **MRI scan** of neck. *Initial management:* assessment for treatment of any remediable underlying cause, e.g. NSAIDs to reduce swelling around inflamed root canal, surgical decompression.
Peripheral nerve lesions in arm	*Suggested by:* loss of sensation localized to the forearm, upper arm or radial 3½ fingers or ulnar 1½ fingers in the palm. *Confirmed by:* **nerve conduction studies**. *Initial management:* assessment for treatment of any remediable underlying cause by surgical decompression.

Diminished sensation in arm dermatome

Investigations in **bold** below:

Main differential diagnoses and typical outline evidence, etc.	
C5 posterior root lesion	*Suggested by:* loss of sensation of **lateral aspect of upper arm**.
	Confirmed by: **nerve conduction studies. MRI scan** appearance.
	Initial management: assessment for treatment of any remediable underlying cause, e.g. NSAIDs to reduce swelling around inflamed root canal, surgical decompression.
C6 posterior root lesion	*Suggested by:* loss of sensation of **lateral forearm and thumb**.
	Confirmed by: **nerve conduction studies. MRI scan** appearance.
	Initial management: assessment for treatment of any remediable underlying cause, e.g. NSAIDs to reduce swelling around inflamed root canal, surgical decompression.
C8 posterior root lesion	*Suggested by:* loss of sensation of **palmar and dorsal aspect of ulnar 1½ fingers** and the ulnar border of the wrist.
	Confirmed by: **nerve conduction studies. MRI scan** appearance.
	Initial management: assessment for treatment of any remediable underlying cause, e.g. NSAIDs to reduce swelling around inflamed root canal, surgical decompression.
T1 posterior root lesion	*Suggested by:* loss of sensation of **ulnar border of the forearm**.
	Confirmed by: **nerve conduction studies. MRI scan** appearance.
	Initial management: assessment for treatment of any remediable underlying cause, e.g. NSAIDs to reduce swelling around inflamed root canal, surgical decompression.
T2 posterior root lesion	*Suggested by:* loss of sensation of **inner aspect of upper arm and breast**.
	Confirmed by: **nerve conduction studies. MRI scan** appearance.
	Initial management: assessment for treatment of any remediable underlying cause, e.g. NSAIDs to reduce swelling around inflamed root canal, surgical decompression.

Diminished sensation in the hand

Investigation in **bold** below.

Main differential diagnoses and typical outline evidence, etc.	
Median nerve lesion due to carpal tunnel syndrome, 'pill', pregnancy, hypothyroidism, acromegaly, rheumatoid arthritis, or nerve trauma	*Suggested by:* loss of sensation of **palmar aspect of radial 3½ fingers** (in carpal tunnel syndrome, also discomfort in forearm and tingling if front of wrist tapped). If nerve severed, wasting of thenar eminence and thumb opposition. *Confirmed by:* **X-ray wrist and elbow. Nerve conduction studies** and **thyroid function tests, rheumatoid factor**, etc. *Initial management:* assessment for treatment of any remediable underlying cause, e.g. thyroid hormone replacement, surgical decompression of carpal tunnel.
Ulnar nerve lesion due to compression of deep palmar branch from trauma or ulnar groove at elbow from trauma or osteoarthritis	*Suggested by:* loss of sensation of **palmar and dorsal aspect of ulnar 1½ fingers** but *not* the ulnar border of the wrist. *Confirmed by:* **nerve conduction studies.** *X-ray wrist and elbow*. *Initial management:* assessment for surgical decompression.
Radial nerve lesion due to local compression (e.g. arm left hanging over chair)	*Suggested by:* loss of sensation of **dorsal aspect of radial 3½ fingers**. *Confirmed by:* **nerve conduction studies**. *Initial management:* physiotherapy if cause self-limiting.
C7 posterior root lesion due to cervical osteophytes	*Suggested by:* loss of sensation of **middle finger alone**. *Confirmed by:* **nerve conduction studies. MRI scan** appearances. *Initial management:* NSAIDs to reduce swelling around inflamed root canal, physiotherapy, surgical decompression.
C8 posterior root lesion due to cervical osteophytes	*Suggested by:* loss of sensation of **palmar and dorsal aspect of ulnar 1½ fingers** and the ulnar border of the wrist. *Confirmed by:* **nerve conduction studies. MRI scan** appearances. *Initial management:* NSAIDs to reduce swelling around inflamed root canal, physiotherapy, surgical decompression.

Disturbed sensation in lower limb

Look for specific patterns as indicated below. Investigations in **bold** below:

Main differential diagnoses and typical outline evidence, etc.	
Contralateral cortical (pre-central gyrus) lesion	*Suggested by:* graphaesthesia. *Confirmed by:* **CT or MRI scan** of brain. *Initial management:* treatment of any remediable underlying, e.g. surgical removal of tumour.
Peripheral neuropathy (due to diabetes mellitus, carcinoma, vitamin B$_{12}$ deficiency, drugs therapy, heavy metal, or chemical exposure	*Suggested by:* loss of touch and pinprick sensation worse in foot (e.g. stocking distribution), progressing upwards. *Confirmed by:* **nerve conduction studies. MRI scan** appearance. *Initial management:* treatment of any remediable underlying cause, e.g. stop drug, better control of diabetes.
Spinothalamic tract damage (no dorsal column loss) due to contralateral hemisection of the cord	*Suggested by:* loss of pinprick and temperature sensation, normal or disturbed touch, but normal joint position and vibration sense in foot. *Confirmed by:* **nerve conduction studies. MRI** of cervical cord. *Initial management:* treatment of any remediable underlying cause.
Dorsal column loss due to vitamin B$_{12}$ deficiency, ipsilateral hemisection of the cord, rarely tabes dorsalis	*Suggested by:* loss of joint position and vibration sense in foot. Pinprick and temperature sensation normal. *Confirmed by:* **nerve conduction studies.** Vitamin B12 levels. *Initial management:* treatment of any remediable underlying cause, e.g. vitamin B12 injections.
L1 posterior root lesion	*Suggested by:* loss of sensation in **inguinal region**. *Confirmed by:* **nerve conduction studies.** X-ray of lumbar spine and sacrum. *Initial management:* NSAIDs to reduce swelling around inflamed root canal, physiotherapy.
L2/3 posterior root lesion	*Suggested by:* loss of sensation in **anterior thigh**. *Confirmed by:* **nerve conduction studies.** X-ray of lumbar spine and sacrum. *Initial management:* NSAIDs to reduce swelling around inflamed root canal, physiotherapy.

L4/5 posterior root lesion	*Suggested by:* loss of sensation in ***anterior shin***.
	Confirmed by: **nerve conduction studies**. X-ray of lumbar spine and sacrum.
	Initial management: NSAIDs to reduce swelling around inflamed root canal, physiotherapy.
S1 posterior root lesion	*Suggested by:* loss of sensation in ***lateral border of foot***.
	Confirmed by: **nerve conduction studies**. X-ray of lumbar spine and sacrum.
	Initial management: NSAIDs to reduce swelling around inflamed root canal, physiotherapy.

Brisk reflexes

Investigations in **bold** below:

Main differential diagnoses and typical outline evidence, etc.	
Thyrotoxicosis	*Suggested by:* brisk reflexes in all limbs with normal flexor plantar responses.
	Confirmed by: ↑**FT4** and ↓↓**TSH** levels.
	Initial management: β-blocker, e.g. propranolol to control distressing symptoms, carbimazole or propylthiouracil to block thyroid hormone production.
High level pyramidal tract lesion (cervical cord, brainstem, bilateral internal capsule, or diffuse bilateral cortical lesion)	*Suggested by:* brisk reflexes in all limbs with **extensor** plantar responses.
	Confirmed by: normal **FT4** and **TSH** levels. **MRI scan** appearances.
	Initial management: physiotherapy, identification of any underlying treatable cause, e.g. tumour or removable haematoma.
Contralateral pyramidal tract lesion in internal capsule, primary cortex, brainstem, or cervical cord	*Suggested by:* unilateral brisk reflexes in upper and lower limb.
	Confirmed by: **MRI** of brain or cervical cord.
	Initial management: physiotherapy, identification of any underlying treatable cause, e.g. tumour or removable haematoma.

Diminished reflexes

Investigations in **bold** below:

Main differential diagnoses and typical outline evidence, etc.	
Sensory neuropathy	*Suggested by:* diminished reflexes, most marked peripherally. Normal muscle power. Normal bplantar responses.
	Confirmed by: **nerve conduction studies**.
	Initial management: protection of vulnerable areas, e.g. feet from neuropathic trauma.
Motor neuropathy	*Suggested by:* diminished reflexes, muscle wasting, fasciculation and weakness.
	Confirmed by: **nerve conduction studies** and normal EMG.
	Initial management: physiotherapy to optimize function.
1° muscle disease	*Suggested by:* diminished reflexes, muscle wasting and weakness. No fasciculation.
	Confirmed by: **nerve conduction studies** and abnormal EMG and muscle biopsy.
	Initial management: physiotherapy to optimize function.
Cerebellar disease	*Suggested by:* unilateral brisk reflexes in upper and lower limb.
	Confirmed by: **CT** and **MRI** of brain posterior fossa.
	Initial management: identification of any underlying treatable cause, e.g. tumour or removable haematoma.
Posterior root lesion in C7/C8	*Suggested by:* loss of **triceps** jerk.
	Confirmed by: **MRI** of disc space.
	Initial management: NSAIDs to reduce swelling around inflamed root canal, physiotherapy.
Posterior root lesion in C5/C6	*Suggested by:* loss of **biceps** jerk.
	Confirmed by: **MRI** of disc space.
	Initial management: NSAIDs and physiotherapy.
Posterior root lesion in L3/L4	*Suggested by:* loss of **knee** jerk.
	Confirmed by: **MRI** of disc space.
	Initial management: NSAIDs and physiotherapy.
Posterior root lesion in S1/S2	*Suggested by:* loss of **ankle** jerk.
	Confirmed by: **MRI** of disc space.
	Initial management: NSAIDs and physiotherapy.

Gait abnormality

Initial investigations (other tests in **bold** below):

Main differential diagnoses and typical outline evidence, etc.	
Somatomization 'functional' cause	*Suggested by:* **bizarre gait with exaggerated delay on affected limb**. No other physical signs of a le sion.
	Confirmed by: careful follow-up.
	Initial management: reassurance.
Contralateral pyramidal tract lesion (in cerebral hemisphere, internal capsule, brainstem or spinal cord)	*Suggested by:* **stiff leg swung in arc**. Other motor (± sensory) localizing signs indicating level of lesion.
	Confirmed by: **CT scan** or **MRI** of probable site.
	Initial management: identification of any underlying treatable cause, e.g. tumour or removable haematoma.
Parkinsonism	*Suggested by:* **shuffling festinant gait**, paucity of facial expression and movement, stiffness, tremor, etc.
	Confirmed by: response to treatment by dopamine agonist drugs, etc.
	Initial management: counselling, explain long-term strategy, MDT planning, low dose levodopa with dopa-decarboxylase inhibitor.
Cerebellar lesion (tumour, ischaemia, etc.)	*Suggested by:* **wide-based gait**, inability to stand with feet together, falling to one side (truncal ataxia). Loss of tone and reflexes on same side as lesion.
	Confirmed by: **MRI** of posterior fossa of brain.
	Initial management: identification of any underlying treatable cause, e.g. tumour or removable haematoma.
Dorsal column loss or peripheral neuropathy (due to vitamin B12 deficiency, etc.)	*Suggested by:* **bilateral stamping, high-stepping gait**, unsteadiness made worse by closing eyes (positive Rombergism).
	Confirmed by: **nerve conduction studies** and response to treatment of cause (if found).
	Initial management: identification of any underlying treatable cause, e.g. tumour or removable haematoma.
Bilateral upper motor neurone lesion (usually in spinal cord)	*Suggested by:* **'scissors'** or **'wading through mud' gait**. Bilateral leg weakness and brisk reflexes.
	Confirmed by: **MRI** of clinically probable site of lesion.
	Initial management: identification of any underlying treatable cause, e.g. tumour or removable haematoma.

Pelvic girdle and proximal muscle weakness (e.g. due to hereditary muscular dystrophy	*Suggested by:* **waddling gait (hip tilts down when leg lifted)**. Hypotonic limb weakness and poor reflexes.
	Confirmed by: EMG.
	Initial management: identification of any underlying treatable cause, e.g. tumour or removable haematoma.
Joint, bone, or muscle lesion	*Suggested by:* **hobbling with minimal time spent on affected limb**. Tenderness and limited range of movement.
	Confirmed by: X-rays and response to treatment or resolution of cause.
	Initial management: identification of any underlying treatable cause.
Lateral popliteal nerve palsy	*Suggested by:* **unilateral stamping, high-stepping gait with foot drop**. Flaccid weakness around ankle. Loss of sensation of lateral lower leg.
	Confirmed by: **nerve conduction studies**.
	Initial management: identification of any underlying treatable cause.
Drug effect	*Suggested by:* wide-based gait, nystagmus, past pointing. History of alcohol intake or other drug.
	Confirmed by: ↑alcohol or other drug level, improvement with withdrawal.
	Initial management: stopping drug.

Difficulty in rising from chair or squatting position

Investigations in **bold** below:

Main differential diagnoses and typical outline evidence, etc.	
Polymyositis	*Suggested by:* muscle wasting, weakness, and poor reflexes. *Confirmed by:* **EMG** and **muscle biopsy**. *Initial management:* physiotherapy to optimize function.
Carcinomatous neuromyopathy	*Suggested by:* muscle wasting, weakness, and poor reflexes. Evidence of cancer (usually late stage). *Confirmed by:* **EMG** and evidence of carcinomatosis. *Initial management:* physiotherapy to optimize function.
Thyrotoxicosis	*Suggested by:* weight loss, tremor, sweating, anxiety, loose bowels. ↑T3 or T4 and ↓↓TSH. *Confirmed by:* response to treatment of thyrotoxicosis. *Initial management:* non-selective β-blocker, e.g. propranolol followed by carbimazole or propylthiouracil.
Diabetic amyotrophy	*Suggested by:* long history of diabetes mellitus. *Confirmed by:* **nerve conduction studies** and muscle biopsy. *Initial management:* physiotherapy to optimize function.
Cushing's syndrome	*Suggested by:* facial and truncal obesity with limb wasting, ↑**midnight cortisol**, ↑**24h urinary free cortisol**. *Confirmed by:* failure of 9 a.m cortisol and failure of 24h urinary cortisol to suppress in **dexamethasone test**. Bilateral adrenal hyperplasia or unilateral adenoma on **CT scan**. *Initial management:* stopping or reducing glucocorticoid therapy or assessment for surgical removal of cortisol secreting adrenal adenoma or ACTH secreting pituitary adenoma. Metyrapone preoperatively to reduce cortisol.
Osteomalacia	*Suggested by:* ↓**serum calcium** and ↑**alkaline phosphatase**. *Confirmed by:* response to treatment with calcium and vitamin D. *Initial management:* treatment with calcium and vitamin D.
Hereditary dystrophy	*Suggested by:* evidence of 1° muscle disease and family history. *Confirmed by:* **muscle biopsy**. *Initial management:* physiotherapy to optimize function.

Chapter 11

Laboratory tests

Microscopic haematuria

This is detected on routine urine 'dipstick' testing. Initial investigations (other tests in **bold** below): MSU, FBC.

Main differential diagnoses and typical outline evidence, etc.	
Menstruation	*Suggested by:* history of current, recent or imminent periods, and no urinary symptoms.
	Confirmed by: 'dipstick' –ve on repeating in mid-cycle.
	Initial management: reassurance.
Urinary tract infection	*Suggested by:* fever, frequency, or dysuria. ↑nitrites, ↑leucocytes on 'dipstick'.
	Confirmed by: **MSU microscopy and culture**, response to antibiotics. **US scan** for possible anatomical abnormality.
	Initial management: increased fluid intake, cranberry juice, and regular bladder emptying. Provisional 1st line antibiotic pending MSU result, e.g. trimethoprim, cefalexin for 5d; 2nd line, e.g. ciprofloxacin bd for 5d.
Recent urethral trauma	*Suggested by:* recent urethral catheterization.
	Confirmed by: history, no infection in **MSU**.
	Initial management: explanation, reassurance.
Bleeding diathesis	*Suggested by:* bruising, anticoagulant therapy.
	Confirmed by: abnormal **platelet and clotting screen**.
	Initial management: treatment of underlying cause, e.g. vitamin K, platelet transfusion.
Kidney calculus	*Suggested by:* excruciating pain that fluctuates in the back below ribs, cloudy dark urine with a foul smell, recurrent dysuria, gout, persistent x3 microscopic haematuria.
	Confirmed by: **renal ultrasound, intravenous urography (IVU), cystoscopy** by urologist.
	Initial management: immediate analgesia, e.g. diclofenac IM or suppository, or pethidine IM with metoclopramide IM, and antibiotics. Emergency surgery if renal tract obstruction proved on imaging.
Glomerulonephritis 1° or 2° to SLE, SBE, etc.	*Suggested by:* persistent x3 microscopic haematuria, associated proteinuria, hypertension.
	Confirmed by: **urine microscopy, renal ultrasound, immunoglobulins, complement, ANA, ANCA** positive **blood cultures**/response to antibiotics.
	Initial management: corticosteroids and/or immunosuppression with cyclophosphamide. Plasmapharesis to remove auto-antibodies in rapidly progressive glomerulonephritis.

Nephritis 2° to NSAIDs, etc.	*Suggested by:* persistent ×3 microscopic haematuria, taking NSAIDs or other suspicious drug.
	Confirmed by: **urine microscopy, renal ultrasound**, improvement on stopping suspected drug, IVU, etc.
	Initial management: eliminate possible causes; treat infection with antibiotics, treat renal failure.
Tumour of kidney	*Suggested by:* flank pain and abdominal mass, dark urine, weight loss, varicocoele (forms blockage of testicular vein), persistent ×3 microscopic haematuria.
	Confirmed by: **renal ultrasound, IVU, then cystoscopy** by urologist.
	Initial management: treat infection. Stenting, surgical resection, radio- or chemotherapy as single or combined treatments.

Asymptomatic proteinuria

Total protein excretion is usually <50mg/24h, of which albumin alone is normally <30mg/24h. Abnormal proteinuria is regarded as >150mg/24h. Initial investigations (other tests in **bold** below): urine 'dipstick' ± MSU, FBC, U&E.

Main differential diagnoses and typical outline evidence, etc.	
Postural or orthostatic proteinuria	*Suggested by:* specimen from ambulant person <40y.
	Confirmed by: protein testing –ve on early morning urine specimen.
	Initial management: explanation to patient and reassurance.
Non-specific febrile illness	*Suggested by:* known febrile illness.
	Confirmed by: normal when illness resolved.
	Initial management: monitor progress.
Urinary tract infection	*Suggested by:* strong urge to pass urine, dysuria, increased frequency and fever. ↑nitrites, ↑leucocytes on 'dipstick'.
	Confirmed by: **MSU microscopy and culture,** response to antibiotics. **US scan** for possible anatomical abnormality.
	Initial management: increased fluid intake, cranberry juice, and regular bladder emptying. Provisional 1st line antibiotic pending MSU result, e.g. trimethoprim, cefalexin for 5d; 2nd line, e.g. ciprofloxacin bd for 5d.
Glomerulonephritis 1° or 2° to SLE, etc.	*Suggested by:* proteinuria >1g/24h, persistent x3 microscopic haematuria, hypertension.
	Confirmed by: **urine microscopy, renal ultrasound, immunoglobulins, complement, ANA, ANCA, etc.**
	Initial management: corticosteroids and/or immunosuppression with cyclophosphamide. Plasmapharesis to remove auto-antibodies in rapidly progressive glomerulonephritis.
Nephritis 2° to NSAIDs, etc.	*Suggested by:* proteinuria >1g/24h, taking NSAIDs or other suspicious drug.
	Confirmed by: **urine microscopy, renal ultrasound,** improvement on stopping suspected drug, IVU, etc.
	Initial management: eliminate possible causes; treat renal failure.
Nephrotic syndrome due to minimal change glomerulonephritis, diabetes mellitus, etc.	*Suggested by:* frothy urine, oedema of legs, and swelling around the eyes, reduced quantity of urine, high blood pressure, and blood in urine.
	Confirmed by: **proteinuria** >3g/24h. **Serum albumin** low (<30g/L), and ↑cholesterol and ↑triglycerides.
	Initial management: treat specific disease. Monitor U&E, BP, fluid balance, and weight. Lifestyle advice: no smoking, exercise, and low fat diet. Restricted salt and normal protein intake ± diuretics and ACE Inhibitors.

Glycosuria

Almost always indicates diabetes and blood sugar has to be tested, but consider other possibilities. Initial investigations (other tests in **bold** below): urine 'dipstick' ± MSU, FBC, fasting glucose, U&E.

Main differential diagnoses and typical outline evidence, etc.	
Diabetes mellitus	*Suggested by:* fatigue or other unexplained symptoms, thirst, polydipsia, polyuria.
	Confirmed by: **fasting blood glucose** ≥7.0mmol/L OR random or **2h glucose tolerance test (GTT)** glucose ≥11.1mmol/L once only with symptoms or on two occasions if no symptoms.
	Initial management: lifestyle advice—stop smoking, exercise, and weight reduction. Dietary advice, ↓saturated fat, ↓glucose and ↑carbohydrate. When dietary measures are not enough in type 2 diabetes, oral treatment, e.g. metformin or sulphonylurea. Insulin for all type 1 diabetics, and if ↑HbA1c despite oral treatment in type 2 diabetics.
Renal glycosuria	*Suggested by:* patient well or renal disease or pregnant.
	Confirmed by: glycosuria when blood sugar shown to be normal on **glucose tolerance test**.
	Initial management: explanation and reassurance.

Raised urine or serum bilirubin

Initial investigations (other tests in **bold** below): US scan of liver.

Main differential diagnoses and typical outline evidence, etc.	
Hepatocellular jaundice (due to hepatitis or very severe liver failure) (see 📖p.694)	*Suggested by:* jaundice with dark stools and dark urine. Also ↑urine urobilinogen (you can check this immediately).
	Confirmed by: ↑**serum bilirubin** and ↑**urine urobilinogen**. Highly abnormal **LFT**. Normal bile ducts but abnormal liver parenchyma on **US scan**.
	Initial management: depends on cause (see 📖p.694.)
Obstructive jaundice due to intrahepatic causes (drugs, hepatitis, etc.) or extrahepatic (stones, tumours, etc.) (see 📖p.696)	*Suggested by:* jaundice with pale stools and dark urine. Also NO ↑urine urobilinogen.
	Confirmed by: ↑plasma bilirubin but ↑↑alkaline phosphatase, otherwise slightly abnormal LFT. Dilated bile ducts on US scan.
	Initial managemewnt: depends on cause (see 📖p.649.)

Hepatocellular jaundice

Suggested by: jaundice with pale or normal stools and dark urine.

Confirmed by: ↑serum bilirubin and ↑urine urobilinogen. Highly abnormal LFT. Normal bile ducts on US scan.

Main differential diagnoses and typical outline evidence, etc.	
Acute (viral) hepatitis A	*Suggested by:* flu-like illness, pruritis, loss of appetite, jaundice, and tender hepatomegaly. *Confirmed by:* presence of **hepatitis A IgM antibody** suggests acute infection. *Initial management:* conservative, advise rest, nutritious diet, and no alcohol. General hygiene. Alfa-interferon for fulminant hepatitis. Immunize contacts with hepatitis A vaccine.
Acute hepatitis B	*Suggested by:* history of IV drug use, transfusion, needle punctures, tattoos, tender hepatomegaly. *Confirmed by:* presence of **HBsAg** in serum. *Initial management:* conservative advice—no alcohol. Chronic despite antiviral treatment: alfa-interferon. Immunize sexual contacts.
Acute hepatitis C	*Suggested by:* history of transfusion or other blood products. Tender hepatomegaly. *Confirmed by:* presence of **anti-HCV antibody and antigen**. *Initial management:* combination of ribavirin + peg-interferon-alfa for moderate and severe chronic hepatitis (response depends on ethnic group, age, viral load, and HCV genotype).
Alcoholic hepatitis	*Suggested by:* history of drinking, presence of spider naevi, and other signs of chronic liver disease. *Confirmed by:* **raised GGT, raised ALT, liver biopsy**. *Initial management:* stop alcohol, treatment of alcohol withdrawal, high dose vitamin B, low protein intake, steroids in severe disease if no infection.
Drug-induced hepatitis, e.g. paracetamol (dose-dependent), halothane (independent)	*Suggested by:* drug history, recent surgery. *Confirmed by:* improvement after stopping the offending drug. *Initial management:* stop causative agent, conservative treatment.

1° hepatoma	*Suggested by:* weight loss, abdominal pain, heaviness feeling in right upper abdomen, excessive alcohol intake, right upper quadrant (RUQ) mass.
	Confirmed by: **US scan/CT liver, liver biopsy,** ↑**alpha-fetoprotein**.
	Initial management: resection for solitary tumour <3cm diameter. Liver transplantation, chemotherapy, percutaneous ablation, tumour embolizations.
Right heart failure (due to pulmonary hypertension, COPD, tricuspid incompetence, worsened by anaemia, infection	*Suggested by:* shortness of breath, tiredness, racing heart, rapid weight gain, ↑JVP, hepatomegaly, ankle oedema.
	Confirmed by: **CXR, ECG, echocardiogram, radionuclide ventriculography**.
	Initial management: diuretics, β-blockers, and digoxin. Treatment of cause. Lifestyle advice on weight reduction, diet, and smoking cessation.

Obstructive jaundice

Suggested by: jaundice with pale stools and dark urine.

Confirmed by: ↑urine and serum bilirubin but NO ↑urobilinogen in urine. ↑↑alkaline phosphatase, otherwise slightly abnormal **LFT**. Dilated bile ducts on **US liver scan**.

Main differential diagnoses and typical outline evidence, etc.	
Common bile duct stones	*Suggested by:* pain in RUQ ± Murphy's sign.
	Confirmed by: **US scan liver/biliary ducts**.
	Initial management: analgesics, anti-emetics, and antibiotics. Emergency or elective cholecystectomy.
Cancer of head of pancreas	*Suggested by:* painless jaundice, itching, appetite and weight loss, development of diabetes mellitus, palpable gallbladder (Courvoisier's law).
	Confirmed by: **CT pancreas, ERCP or MRCP**.
	Initial management: relief of symptoms caused by jaundice with an endoscopic or percutaneous stent insertion. Pain control with opiates. Surgery if patient fit with no metastases and tumour is <3cm.
Sclerosing cholangitis	*Suggested by:* progressive fatigue, pruritus, dark urine, right upper abdominal pain, and jaundice.
	Confirmed by: ↑**serum alkaline phosphatase**, no gallstones on **US scan**, normal **antimitochondrial antibodies**, **ERCP** (beading of the intra- and extra-hepatic biliary ducts).
	Initial management: colestyramine for pruritis. Ursodeoxycholic acid to improve LFT and jaundice. Antibiotics for infection, endoscopic stenting for strictures, yearly follow-up, and liver transplantation for end-stage disease.
1° biliary cirrhosis	*Suggested by:* scratch marks, non-tender hepatomegaly ± splenomegaly, xanthelasmata and xanthomas, arthralgia.
	Confirmed by: +ve **anti-mitochondrial antibody**, ↑↑serum **IgM, liver biopsy**.
	Initial management: colestyramine for pruritis. Codeine for diarrhoea. Vitamins D and K if clotting abnormal. Ursodeoxycholic acid to improve LFT, jaundice, and ascites.
Drug-induced, e.g. oral contraceptive pill, phenothiazines, anabolic steroids, erythromycin	*Suggested by:* drug history.
	Confirmed by: symptoms recede when offending drug is discontinued.
	Initial management: eliminate the cause, conservative treatment.

Pregnancy (last trimester)	*Suggested by:* jaundice during pregnancy and severe itching.
	Confirmed by: resolution following delivery.
	Initial management: explanation and reassurance.
Alcoholic hepatitis/ cirrhosis	*Suggested by:* history of drinking, presence of spider naevi, and other signs of chronic liver disease.
	Confirmed by: **liver biopsy**.
	Initial management: stop alcohol. Treat withdrawal symptoms. High dose vitamin B, thiamine low protein intake, and steroid in severe disease if no infection.
Dubin–Johnson syndrome (see 📖p.381)	*Suggested by:* intermittent jaundice and associated pain in the right hypochondrium. No hepatomegaly.
	Confirmed by: normal **alkaline phosphatase**, normal **LFT**. ↑**urinary bilirubin**. Pigment granules on **liver biopsy**.

Hypernatraemia

Initial investigations (other tests in **bold** below): repeat U&E, blood glucose, urine and simultaneous serum osmolality.

Main differential diagnoses and typical outline evidence, etc.	
Hypertonic plasma with hypervolaemia (e.g. excess IV saline) or hypovolaemia (e.g. diabetic polyuria or diabetes insipidus)	*Suggested by:* little hypotonic fluid orally or intra-venously and thirsty, high volume of urine with low sodium content (e.g. in diabetic polyuria). *Confirmed by:* ↑**plasma osmolality** and **urine osmolality** higher (unless diabetes insipidus). *Initial management:* replace fluids. Avoid rapid changes. Give water PO or IV in form of 5% dextrose. Monitor serum electrolytes regularly.
Diabetes inspidus with hypovolaemia	*Suggested by:* drinking excessively and passing large volumes of urine (polydipsia and polyuria). Thirsty. *Confirmed by:* ↑plasma osmolality and ↓urine osmolality. *Initial management:* replace fluids. Avoid rapid changes. The aim is to reduce sodium at a rate of <10mmol/L per day. Normal saline may be used initially if serum sodium was >170mmol/L. Desmopressin 100-200mcg tid orally IM might be used.
Primary aldosteronism due to adrenal hyperplasia or Conn's sydrome with adrenal tumour	*Suggested by:* normal fluid intake, ↑BP. ↓serum potassium. *Confirmed by:* ↓**plasma renin** activity and ↑**aldosterone** levels. **CT or MRI scan** appearance. *Initial management:* spironolactone, amiloride, or eplerenone for cases of bilateral adrenal hyperplasia. Adrenalectomy for aldosterone-producing adenoma.

Hyponatraemia

Also usually indicates hypotonicity—low plasma osmolality. Initial investigations (other tests in **bold** below): U&E, blood glucose, urine and simultaneous serum osmolality

Main differential diagnoses and typical outline evidence, etc.	
Hypotonic with hypovolaemia due to excess renal or non-renal loss (excessive diuretic therapy, history of renal tubular disease, diarrhoea, vomit, fistula, burns, small bowel obstruction, blood loss)	*Suggested by:* ↓**serum sodium** and ↓**osmolality**. Loss of skin turgor, tachycardia, ↓BP. History of possible cause. *Confirmed by:* response to removal or treating of cause. *Initial management:* treat the cause. If symptomatic, saline water. In chronic conditions, fluid restriction. Avoid rapid changes, e.g. maximum change of sodium of 12–15mmol/L/d.
Hypotonic with normovolaemia, including pseudohyponatraemia (severe hypothyroidism or glucocorticoid deficiency). Symptoms of severe diabetes mellitus	*Suggested by:* ↓**serum sodium** and ↓**osmolality**. Normal skin turgor, normal pulse and BP. *Confirmed by:* response to treating cause, balancing fluid intake. **Blood glucose** of >20mmol/L in pseudohyponatraemia. *Initial management:* treatment of the cause, e.g. hypothyroidism, Addison's disease, or diabetes mellitus.
Hypotonic with hypervolaemia (water overload, cardiac failure, cirrhosis, renal failure, nephrotic syndrome, inappropriate antidiuretic hormone (**ADH**) secretion)	*Suggested by:* ↓**serum sodium** and ↓**osmolality**. Oedema, basal lung crackles. *Confirmed by:* response to treating cause, reducing fluid intake. *Initial management:* treatment of the underlying condition.
Syndrome of inappropriate ADH secretion (malignancy, CNS disorders, chest infections, metabolic problems, drugs)	*Suggested by:* **serum sodium** usually <120mmol/L. Confusion, progressing to coma, mild oedema. *Confirmed by:* **urine osmolality** > **serum osmolality** despite ↓serum osmolality (<270mmol/L). **Urine sodium** >20mmol/L. *Initial management:* fluid restriction. Treat the underlying cause. If not possible, demeclocycline for long-term control.

Hyperkalaemia

Initial investigations (other tests in **bold** below): U&E, blood glucose

Main differential diagnoses and typical outline evidence, etc.	
Drug effect: potassium administration or other drug effect	*Suggested by:* potassium supplements, blood transfusion, ACE inhibitor, spironolactone, amiloride, triamterene, etc.
	Confirmed by: normal potassium when drug reduced or stopped.
	Initial management: stop suspect drug.
Metabolic acidosis, renal failure, diabetic ketoacidosis	*Suggested by:* usually obvious illness and severe metabolic disturbance, ↓pH and ↓plasma **HCO₃**.
	Confirmed by: response to treatment of metabolic disturbance.
	Initial management: If K⁺ >6.5 and not falling, calcium gluconate IV, glucose + insulin, calcium resonium. Treatment of cause.
Addison's disease	*Suggested by:* fatigue, ↓BP, pigmented buccal mucosa and palmar creases, ↓Na, ↑K.
	Confirmed by: ↓random and **9 a.m cortisol**, ↑**ACTH**, and poor response to **Synacthen® stimulation**. Response to hydrocortisone IV and normal saline.
	Initial management: hydrocortisone, e.g. 10–20mg mane and 5–10mg evening. Fludrocortisone, e.g. 50–100mcg daily.
Recent blood transfusion	*Suggested by:* history.
	Confirmed by: fall of potassium after few hours.
	Initial management: monitor potassium. If K⁺ >6.5 and not falling, calcium gluconate IV, glucose + insulin, calcium resonium.
Spurious result due to haemolysis in specimen bottle	*Suggested by:* laboratory reporting haemolysis in specimen bottle.
	Confirmed by: normal potassium when repeated with no delay in delivery to lab.
	Initial management: repeat potassium.

Hypokalaemia

Initial investigations (other tests in bold below): U&E, plasma glucose

Main differential diagnoses and typical outline evidence, etc.	
Diuretic therapy	*Suggested by:* taking thiazide or loop diuretic (fondness of liquorice of Pernod drink). *Confirmed by:* normal potassium after stopping diuretic. *Initial management:* stop suspected cause ± oral potassium supplements.
β-agonist treatment	*Suggested by:* taking high doses of β-agonist, usually in nebulizer for acute asthmatic attack in hospital. *Confirmed by:* normal potassium after stopping drug. *Initial management:* stop β-agonist.
Vomiting, e.g. pyloric stenosis	*Suggested by:* history of severe vomiting with poor fluid intake. *Confirmed by:* normal potassium without subsequent need for replacement when cause of vomiting treated. *Initial management:* depending on severity, replacement of fluids and electrolytes, correction of acid-base imbalance, and dealing with specific underlying causes.
Chronic diarrhoea, purgative abuse, intestinal fistula, villous adenoma of rectum	*Suggested by:* history of severe diarrhoea or mucous loss. *Confirmed by:* normal potassium without need for further replacement when cause treated subsequently. *Initial management:* oral potassium supplements if not dehydrated, potassium IV with IV fluid replacement, treatment of cause.
1° hyperaldosteronism due to adrenal hyperplasia or Conn's syndrome with adrenal tumour	*Suggested by:* normal fluid intake, ↑BP, ↓serum potassium. *Confirmed by:* ↓**plasma renin activity** and ↑**aldosterone. CT or MRI scan** appearance. *Initial management:* spironolactone, amiloride, or eplerenone for bilateral adrenal hyperplasia. Adrenalectomy for 'Conn's syndrome' (aldosterone-producing adenoma).
Renal tubular defect (due to recovery phase from renal failure, recent pyelonephritis, associated myeloma, heavy metal poisoning, congenital renal tubular defects)	*Suggested by:* hypokalaemia and history of possible cause. *Confirmed by:* **test for renal concentrating ability**. *Initial management:* treatment of underlying cause. If serum K^+ <3mmol/L, potassium PO or IV not exceeding 20mmol/L/h. Serum U&E and ECG monitoring during treatment.

Hypercalcaemia

Present when specimen taken without a venous cuff, and calcium result was corrected for albumin concentration. Initial investigations (other tests in **bold** below): U&E, calcium, alkaline phosphatase.

Main differential diagnoses and typical outline evidence, etc.	
Severe hypercalcaemia	*Confirmed by:* calcium <3.5 mmol/L.
	Initial management: saline infusion ± furosemide to maintain fluid balance and prevent overload. Correct hypokalaemia and hypomagnesaemia. If calcium remains high, pamidronate to lower over 2–3d.
Thiazide diuretics	*Suggested by:* mild hypercalcaemia, drug history, normal phosphate and alkaline phosphatase.
	Confirmed by: normal calcium when drug stopped.
	Initial management: stop thiazide.
Bone metastases from breast, bronchus, kidney, thyroid, ovary, colon	*Suggested by:* normal phosphate and ↑alkaline phosphatase.
	Confirmed by: 2°s on **bone scan**.
	Initial management: pamidronate to lower calcium over 2–3d. Appropriate treatment of neoplastic process.
Thyrotoxicosis	*Suggested by:* weight loss with good appetite, tremor, palpitation and agitation, goitre, mild ↑calcium.
	Confirmed by: ↑**T4** or ↑**T3** and ↓↓**TSH**. Normal phosphate and alkaline phosphatase. Response to treatment of thyrotoxicosis.
	Initial management: propranolol 40 to 80mg 8mg hourly to control symptoms (avoid in asthmatics). Carbimazole, e.g. 40mg reduced to 10 ± 5mg for 18mo according to test results. Written warning about agranulocytosis.
1° (or tertiary) hyperparathyroidism	*Suggested by:* fatigue, constipation, depression, impaired memory, renal colic and kidney stones, stomach ulcer, ↑BP, pancreatitis, low phosphate, and ↑alkaline phosphatase.
	Confirmed by: ↑**plasma parathyroid levels** with ↑calcium.
	Initial management: correct very high calcium. Surgical removal of parathyroid adenoma.

Myeloma	*Suggested by:* low back pain, polyuria and polydypsia, spinal fracture, normal serum phosphate and alkaline phosphatase.
	Confirmed by: paraprotein with immunoparesis on **electrophoresis, ↓Hb, Bence–Jones protein in urine**, spinal X-ray showing fracture with an osteolytic lesion.
	Initial management: correct very high calcium. Analgesics for bone pain. Oral bisphosphonate to keep calcium down. Local radiotherapy in progressive disease. Prompt treatment of infections. Transfusions for anaemia. Chemotherapy using melphalan or cyclophosphamide in conjunction with steroids. More aggressive treatment for fitter patients.
Sarcoidosis	*Suggested by:* cough, weight loss, night sweats, shortness of breath, erythema nodosum, ↑phosphate and alkaline phosphatase. Bilateral hilar shadows on CXR.
	Confirmed by: **lung function tests, Kveim test, biopsy** from a granuloma, ↑vitamin D levels and ↑ACE levels.
	Initial management: correct very high calcium. Long-term prednisolone to control calcium. If severe cases, methylprednisolone IV or immunosuppression, e.g. methotrexate and cyclophosphamide.
Vitamin D excess	*Suggested by:* drug history and ↑phosphate.
	Confirmed by: normal calcium when drug stopped.
	Initial management: stop suspected rug.
Ectopic parathyroid hormone due to lung cancer usually	*Suggested by:* ↓phosphate and ↑alkaline phosphatase.
	Confirmed by: ↑plasma parathyroid levels with high calcium presence of underlying neoplasm.
	Initial management: correct very high calcium. Surgical resection of cancer in appropriate cases.

Hypocalcaemia

Present when specimen taken without a venous cuff and corrected for albumin concentration. Investigations in **bold** below:

Main differential diagnoses and typical outline evidence, etc.	
Vitamin D deficiency—due to dietary deficiency or 1,25 (OH)$_2$D abnormality	*Suggested by*: diet history, ↓phosphate and ↑alkaline phosphatase. *Confirmed by*: **↓1, 25(OH)2 vitamin D**, normal calcium after adequate treatment with vitamin D. *Initial management*: calcium + vitamin D, 1–2 tablets daily.
Hypoparathyroidism (transient or permanent after thyroid surgery, autoimmune disease, radiations)	*Suggested by*: neck surgery, ↑phosphate. *Confirmed by*: **↓parathyroid hormone** or normal in presence of ↓calcium. *Initial management*: alfacalcidol with careful monitoring of calcium levels.
Chronic renal failure	*Suggested by*: **↑phosphate, ↑↑creatinine, ↑alkaline phosphatase, ↓Hb**. *Confirmed by*: improvement with control of renal failure and phosphate levels. *Initial management*: stop nephrotoxic drugs, relieve obstruction; prompt treatment of infections; treat ↑BP with ACE inhibitors or angiotensin receptor blockers (ARBs); hyperlipidaemia with statins. Restriction of fluids and furosemide for oedema. Erythropoietin for severe anaemia. Alfacalcidol for renal bone disease. Dialysis.
Pseudohypo-parathyroidism	*Suggested by*: short stature, obesity, round face, short metacarpals, ↑phosphate. *Confirmed by*: **↑plasma parathyroid levels** with ↓ or normal calcium. *Initial management*: alfacalcidol with careful monitoring of calcium levels.
Pancreatitis	*Suggested by*: abdominal pain and tenderness, ↓phosphate, normal alkaline phosphatase. *Confirmed by*: **↑↑serum amylase** and **US scan** of abdomen. *Initial management*: nil by mouth, nasogastric (NG) tube, saline infusion to correct dehydration, strong analgesics (e.g. pethidine IM), regular monitoring.
Fluid overload	*Suggested by*: history and ↓phosphate and normal alkaline phosphatase. *Confirmed by*: normalization with correction of fluid balance. *Initial management*: reduced fluid intake to allow correction ± diuretic.

Rhabdomyolysis

Suggested by: severe muscle pains, weakness, dark or cola-coloured urine, racing heart, history of extreme muscle activity, ↑phosphate.

Confirmed by: ↑↑**CPK**, ↑**creatinine**, ↑urinary **myoglobin**, **CT and MRI scans** of the muscles and **muscle biopsy**.

Initial management: correct electrolyte disturbances, e.g. hyperkalaemia. Rehydration to maintain a urine output of 300 mL/h until myoglobinuria disappears. Sodium bicarbonate IV ± dialysis.

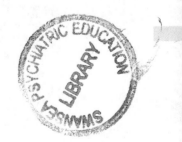

Raised alkaline phosphatase

Investigations in **bold** below:

Main differential diagnoses and typical outline evidence, etc.	
Paget's disease	*Suggested by:* deformity of skull or tibia typically, ↑↑alkaline phosphatase.
	Confirmed by: bone deformity, especially on **skull and tibia X-ray** and **↑urinary hydroxyproline**.
	Initial management: analgesics for bone pain. If not enough, try alendronic acid.
Vitamin D deficiency due to dietary deficiency	*Suggested by:* diet history, ↓phosphate and ↑alkaline phosphatase.
	Confirmed by: **↓1,25 (OH)2 vitamin D level**, and normal calcium after oral vitamin D and calcium supplement.
	Initial management: dietary treatment and calcium supplement with vitamin D.
Bone metastases from breast, bronchus, kidney, thyroid, ovary, colon	*Suggested by:* normal phosphate, ↑calcium and ↑alkaline phosphatase.
	Confirmed by: 2°s on **bone scan**.
	Initial management: appropriate management of malignancy.
1° or tertiary hyperparathyroidism	*Suggested by:* ↓phosphate and ↑alkaline phosphatase after years of 2° hyperparathyroidism.
	Confirmed by: **↑plasma parathyroid** levels with ↑calcium.
	Initial management: correct very high calcium. Surgical removal of parathyroid adenoma.
Cholestasis	*Suggested by:* jaundice with pale stools and dark urine. Bilirubin (i.e. conjugated and thus soluble) in urine.
	Confirmed by: **↑urine and serum bilirubin** but NO ↑urobilinogen in urine. ↑↑alkaline phosphatase, otherwise slightly **abnormal LFT**.
	Initial management: colestyramine for pruritis. Treat infections. Relieve obstruction by stenting or surgery.

Raised serum urea and creatinine

Investigations in **bold** below:

Main differential diagnoses and typical outline evidence, etc.	
High protein load due to gastrointestinal (GI) bleed, catabolism, sepsis, etc.	*Suggested by:* ↑blood urea and normal creatinine or urea/creatinine ratio strongly in favour of urea. *Confirmed by:* recovery when catabolism or GI bleeding stops. *Initial management:* IV line—IV fluids and then blood transfusion, regular monitoring. Reduce acidity e.g. with PPI.
Pre-renal failure due to hypovolaemia (due to low fluid intake, or high fluid loss of any cause)	*Suggested by:* ↑blood urea and ↑creatinine. History of fluid imbalance with fluid loss exceeding intake. Urea/creatinine ratio in favour of urea. *Confirmed by:* improvement (↓**creatinine**) with restoration of fluid volume. *Initial management:* correction of fluid and electrolyte imbalance. Antibiotics for infection. Stop nephrotoxic drugs. Rehydration orally, via NG tube or IV infusion. Monitor urine output ± central venous pressure (CVP) monitoring.
Chronic renal failure due to pyelonephritis, glomerulonephritis, interstitial nephritis, diabetes mellitus, renovascular disease, analgesic nephropathy, hypertension, etc.	*Suggested by:* ↑**blood urea** and ↑creatinine and not rising rapidly over days. ↓Hb, small renal size on **US scan**. *Confirmed by:* **renal biopsy** appearance. *Initial management:* Treat infections, stop nephrotoxic drugs, relieve obstruction: treat ↑BP with ACE inhibitors or ARBs, and hyperlipidaemia with statins. Restriction of fluids and furosemide for oedema. Erythropoietin for severe anaemia. Alfacalcidol for renal bone disease. Dialysis.
Acute tubular necrosis, severe hypotension, nephrotoxins (NSAIDs, aminoglycosides, amphotericin B, etc.)	*Suggested by:* ↑blood urea and ↑creatinine and rising rapidly over days. Hb normal. Recent acute illness with hypotension and oliguria (fall in urine output <1mL/kg/h). **US scan**: normal kidney size and no obstructive uropathy. *Confirmed by:* no improvement when normovolaemic and **renal biopsy**. *Initial management:* eliminate any causes. Maintain fluid balance with careful monitoring of output and input + insensible loss (± CVP). Temporary dialysis.
Obstructive post-renal failure	*Suggested by:* ↑blood urea and ↑creatinine and rising. Hb normal. ↓urine output. *Confirmed by:* **US scan** showing dilatation of renal calyces or ureters. *Initial management:* catheterization for acute retention of urine. Ureteric stenting or nephrostomy.

Low haemoglobin

Investigations in **bold** below:

Main differential diagnoses and typical outline evidence, etc.	
Microcytic anaemia (see 📖p.716)	*Suggested by:* history of blood loss or familial microcytic anaemias (especially in Mediterranean origin). *Confirmed by:* ↓Hb and ↓MCV.
Macrocytic anaemia (see 📖p.718)	*Suggested by:* sore tongue, diarrhoea. Family history of pernicious anaemia (PA), medication or alcohol. *Confirmed by:* ↓Hb and ↑MCV.
Normocytic anaemia (see 📖p.720)	*Suggested by:* history of chronic intercurrent illness, e.g. pancytopaenia, chronic renal failure. *Confirmed by:* ↓Hb and MCV normal.

Microcytic anaemia

Usually accompanied by low mean corpuscular Hb concentration. Investigations in **bold** below:

Main differential diagnoses and typical outline evidence, etc.	
Iron deficiency anaemia	*Suggested by:* history of blood loss (e.g. history of heavy periods, passing blood rectally), or poor diet.
	Confirmed by: ↓**serum iron, ↓ferritin,** and ↑**total iron binding capacity**.
	Initial management: treat the cause. Iron replacement therapy.
Thalassaemia: α, β, intermedia, and variants	*Suggested by:* persistent mild anaemia, failure to thrive, family history, Mediterranean origin. Hepatosplenomegaly, ↓↓MCV for degree of anaemia.
	Confirmed by: **blood film:** target and nucleated cells. **Hb electrophoresis** shows ↑HbF or ↑HbA2, ↑serum iron and iron binding capacity
	Initial management: regular blood transfusions to keep Hb above 9g/dL. Iron-chelating agents, eg desferrioxamine infusion 8–10h per day. Splenectomy when increased frequency of transfusions; treat complications such as 2° diabetes mellitus. Bone marrow transplantation.
Sideroblastic anaemia rarely congenital or acquired due to alcohol lead poisoning, etc.	*Suggested by:* history of chronic intercurrent illness, e.g. chronic renal failure.
	Confirmed by: ↑**serum iron, ↑ferritin** and **total iron binding capacity** normal.
	Initial management: eliminate cause. Pyridoxine. Blood transfusion in severe anaemia.

Macrocytic anaemia

Investigations in **bold** below:

Main differential diagnoses and typical outline evidence, etc.

B$_{12}$ deficiency: pernicious anaemia, intestinal malabsorption	*Suggested by:* associated autoimmune disease, e.g. primary hypothyroidism, vitiligo, etc. ↓Hb, ↓WCC, and ↓platelets. *Confirmed by:* ↑**serum B$_{12}$** (± ↓**folate** too due to anorexia) + pernicious anaemia diagnosed in absence of general malabsorption. *Initial management:* treat any malabsorption. In pernicious anaemia, hydroxocobalamin 1mg IM every 3–4mo after loading doses (e.g. 6x 1mg IM over 2wk).
Folate deficiency	*Suggested by:* poor diet, pregnancy, lactation, general malabsorption. *Confirmed by:* ↓**folate** but **serum B$_{12}$** normal. *Initial management:* eliminate cause + folic acid, e.g. 5mg daily for 4mo. Correct any B$_{12}$ deficiency before starting folic acid.
Antifolate drugs	*Suggested by:* phenytoin typically, barbiturates and similar, methotrexate and similar. *Confirmed by:* response to high dose folic acid treatment or stopping drug (**serum folate** may be normal). *Initial management:* stopping antifolate drug.
Alcohol abuse	*Suggested by:* history of abuse and poor diet. *Confirmed by:* response to abstinence (**serum folate** may be normal). *Initial management:* stop alcohol; treat withdrawal symptoms—high dose vitamin B and low protein intake in the presence of advanced liver disease.
Hepatitis and liver disease	*Suggested by:* abnormal liver enzymes. *Confirmed by:* normal (or ↑) **serum B$_{12}$** and poor response to folic acid. *Initial management:* conservative treatment. Advise no alcohol. If chronic, trial of alfa–interferon or antiviral treatment.
Hypothyroidism	*Suggested by:* ↓**FT4** and ↑**TSH**. *Confirmed by:* **normal B$_{12}$** and response to treatment with thyroxine. *Initial management:* levothyroxine replacement, e.g. 25–50mcg per day and adjust, based on TSH.
Haemolysis	*Suggested by:* **urobilinogen in urine**. *Confirmed by:* ↑reticulocytes on **blood film**. *Initial management:* avoid precipitating factors. Blood transfusion if anaemia is severe. Treatment depends on cause, e.g. steroid and immunosuppressants in autoimmune haemolytic anaemia.

Myelodysplasia

Suggested by: hepato- or splenomegaly.

Confirmed by: **bone marrow examination**, normal B_{12} and folate.

Initial management: intensive combination or single-agent chemotherapy. Frequent transfusion of RBC and platelets. Stem cell transfusions if young patient.

Normocytic anaemia

Investigations in **bold** below:

Main differential diagnoses and typical outline evidence, etc.	
Anaemia of chronic disease (e.g. rheumatoid arthritis, hypogonadism, etc.)	*Suggested by:* associated chronic disease.
	Confirmed by: **iron**, **B₁₂** normal. ↓**folate** or normal. Normal or ↑ferritin from inflammation.
	Initial management: treatment of underlying cause.
Chronic renal failure	*Suggested by:* high **creatinine** and **urea**.
	Confirmed by: response to erythropoietin treatment only.
	Initial management: erythropoietin.
'Anaemia of pregnancy'	*Suggested by:* pregnant state.
	Confirmed by: persistence despite folic acid and iron supplements, resolution after birth.
	Initial management: explanation, reassurance.
Hypothyroidism	*Suggested by:* ↓**FT4** and ↑**TSH**.
	Confirmed by: **normal B₁₂** and response to treatment with thyroxine.
	Initial management: thyroxine replacement, e.g. 25–50mcg per day and adjust based on TSH.
Haemolysis (e.g. due to reticulosis)	*Suggested by:* urobilinogen in urine.
	Confirmed by: ↑reticulocytes on **blood film**.
	Initial management: avoid precipitating factors. Blood transfusion if severe haemolysis. Treat infection depending on the cause, e.g. steroids, immunosuppressants, splenectomy, anticoagulation, and stem cell transplantation.
Bone marrow failure	*Suggested by:* pancytopaenia.
	Confirmed by: **bone marrow examination**.
	Initial management: blood cell transfusion to support blood count. Immunosuppression (e.g. ciclosporin) may be effective but not curative. Allogeneic marrow transplantation for younger patients who are severely affected.

Very high ESR, CRP, or plasma viscosity

An ESR or CRP or plasma viscosity which is just above normal is non-specific as it is associated with any cause of inflammation, including infection—but an ESR near 100 or above is a good lead. Initial investigations (other tests in **bold** below): FBC

Main differential diagnoses and typical outline evidence, etc.	
Severe bacterial infection, e.g. osteomyelitis empyema, peritonitis	*Suggested by:* high fever, ↑leucocytes.
	Confirmed by: positive **bacterial culture** from blood and/or site of infection and response to antibiotics and/or **surgical drainage**.
	Initial management: antibiotics according to culture and sensitivity. Clearance of pus.
Giant cell arteritis	*Suggested by:* localized headache, especially over temple, late loss of vision ± muscle pain and stiffness in shoulder area.
	Confirmed by: vessel wall inflammation on **biopsy**.
	Initial management: prednisolone 40–60mg per day and reduce the dose gradually after a week. Bisphosphonates as a prophylaxis for osteoporosis.
Bacterial endocarditis	*Suggested by:* fever, changing heart murmurs, nail splinter haemorrhages.
	Confirmed by: bacterial growth from several **blood cultures**, **echocardiogram** may show vegetations.
	Initial management: aggressive antibiotic treatment, e.g. benzylpenicillin 1.2g/4h IV + gentamicin 1mg/kg/8h IV for 4wk. To add flucloxacillin 2g qds IV in acute causes. Surgical treatment, e.g if unstable infected prosthetic valve.
Myeloma	*Suggested by:* bone pain or fractures. **Bence–Jones protein** in urine and monoclonal protein band on **electrophoresis**.
	Confirmed by: myeloma cells on **bone marrow examination**.
	Initial management: treat severe hypercalcaemia (🔲see p.706). Analgesics for bone pain. Bisphosphonates to reduce fracture rates. Local radiotherapy in rapidly progressive disease. Prompt treatment of infection. Transfusions for anaemia, chemotherapy using melphalan or cyclophosphamide in conjunction with steroids. More aggressive treatment for fitter patients.
Prostatic carcinoma	*Suggested by:* bone pain, few urinary symptoms.
	Confirmed by: sclerotic changes in **pelvic bones X-ray** and ↑**prostatic-specific antigen (PSA)** and prostatic biopsy.
	Initial management: for localized disease, radical prostatectomy or radiotherapy with hormonal therapy. For metastatic disease, hormonal therapy.

Radiology

The general approach

- Use good viewing conditions—preferably a light box in a dark area. Many systems are now electronic, but monitors (especially on wards) can be of variable quality, so don't look at screens with any electronic interference!
- Check the patient's name, gender, age, and address to ensure correct identity.
- Check if the film is marked P–A (X-rays passing from posterior to anterior in a standard way) or A–P (X-rays passing from anterior to posterior). A–P views are done when the patient is ill, using a portable X-ray tube—these will often be semi-erect films with suboptimal exposure factors. This projection magnifies the mediastinum so A–P films should not be used to assess cardiac size or hilar configuration.
- Check which sides are marked left and right, and whether the cardiac apex is on the left (if not, the patient may have dextrocardia).
- Check the patient's positioning. Are the sternoclavicular joints equidistant from the spinous processes of the vertebral column? If not, then the patient was rotated. Rotation causes asymmetry of shoulder girdle muscles projected over the lung fields. The side which has the less space between the end of the clavicle and spinous process has more muscle projected over the lung fields and should be whiter than the other side. Be cautious in the interpretation of a rotated chest radiograph.
- Can you see the vertebral column through the heart shadow? If not, then it is 'under-penetrated' (the X-ray beam was too weak). This means that normal lung tissue will look abnormally opaque (white).
- If the lungs appear dark, the vertebral column can be seen very clearly and the heart shadow is vague, it was over-penetrated and abnormalities may be missed.
- Is the diaphragm between the 5th/6th anterior rib ends? If it is higher, then the patient did/could not take a deep breath, and interpretation of the appearance of the lungs and mediastinum will be suboptimal. If the diaphragm is flattened, then emphysematous changes are likely.
- Having considered the technical issues, is there anything that strikes you immediately? Check for foreign bodies, e.g. endotracheal tubes, chest drains, etc. A striking radio-opaque (white) or lucent (dark) area is likely to be a good lead.
- After noting the obvious finding or if there is nothing dramatic, assess the X-ray systematically as there could well be more subtle abnormalities.
- Compare the lung fields in the lower zones, mid-zones, and upper zones, and check 'behind' the heart.
- Look at the superior mediastinum, the hilum, the heart, the cardiophrenic angles, the diaphragms, and the costophrenic angles.
- Lastly, look at the ribs, the shoulders, the overlying soft tissue from the neck down to the upper abdomen. Note artefacts from skin folds, electrodes, hair and clothing, especially braids, piercings, and buttons.
- Initially, try to look at the film without considering the clinical setting (otherwise, there is a tendency to miss obvious things which do not

fit in with your differential diagnosis), then look again with the clinical setting in mind.
- Remember to compare any chest film with an abnormality with any previous X-rays. Progression over time will often hold the key to the correct diagnosis.

This brief account only includes some common X-ray features of some common diagnoses. Get the X-rays formally reported by a radiologist urgently if you do not recognize a sign and the patient is unwell. Remember that all radiation exposures have to be justified by clinical benefit to comply with IR(ME)R (Ionising Radiation (Medical Exposure) Regulations).

Abnormal chest X-ray (CXR) appearances

Many CXR appearances may be recognizable immediately as indicating a specific diagnosis but if not, classify an appearance into one of the leads on the following pages, and then approach the lead systematically.

X-rays cannot be used to decide management alone. Their appearances can be used as diagnostic leads—the symptoms, signs, and other test results being differentiators between the diagnoses. The X-ray appearance can also be used to differentiate between differential diagnoses provided by symptoms and signs. Some patients with highly abnormal CXR may be relatively well and have self-limiting conditions, and monitoring only is needed. In immunocompromised patients, the findings are altered so that diagnostic leads may have wider (or longer) differential diagnoses that include many other infections (think also of mycobacterial disease such as TB-MAI (mycobacterium avium Intracellulare), fungal, lymphoma, and Kaposi's sarcoma, etc). Do not treat X-rays but patients!

Area of uniform lung opacification (whiteness) with a well-defined border

This typically occurs when there is abnormal substance (liquid, cells, pus, blood) in the alveolar spaces next to an anatomical border (e.g. a fissure), causing a sharp border definition. The silhouette sign consists of loss of normal demarcation between white tissue and darker lung due to latter's abnormal opacification. The position of this sign can help localize an affected lobe as follows: loss of a diaphragm silhouette ⇒ (implies) lower lobe consolidation same side; loss of right (R) heart border silhouette ⇒ (R) middle lobe consolidation; loss of left heart border silhouette ⇒ lingular segment consolidation; loss of upper (R) mediastinal border silhouette ⇒ (R) upper lobe consolidation. A veil-like shadow over the whole left hemithorax ⇒ left upper lobe opacification. Investigations in **bold** below.

Main differential diagnoses and typical outline evidence, etc.	
Consolidation (usually due to lobar pneumonia)	*Suggested by:* well-demarcated uniform whiteness, with a straight border (due to containment by fissural pleura) **with no volume loss** ± air bronchograms. History of productive cough, chest pain, breathlessness, bronchial breathing, fever, ↑neutrophils.
	Confirmed by: clinical resolution on antibiotics and clearing of opacification; repeat **CXR after 8wk**.
	Initial management: analgesia and provisional antibiotic, e.g. amoxicillin/clarithromycin PO for 5d. If >2 features of Confusion, Resp rate >30/min, BP <90/60, age >65y), then antibiotic IV, e.g. amoxicillin/augmentin or cefuroxime + controlled O_2 and fluids. If suspected aspiration, then anaerobic antibiotic, e.g. cefuroxime/metronidazole IV. If hospital/nursing home acquired, cefuroxime or piperacillin with tazobactam IV.
Collapsed lobe due to bronchial obstruction from carcinoma, mucus plugs, foreign body, misplacement of endobronchial tube	*Suggested by:* dense, well-demarcated whiteness with straight borders (due to containment by fissures **with volume loss**). Background clinical picture suggestive of cause (e.g. cachexia, monophonic wheeze, and central soft tissue opacity in carcinoma or inhalation of foreign body, recent endotracheal intubation, etc).
	Confirmed by: **CT thorax** and/or **bronchoscopy** or CXR resolution following appropriate treatment for intraluminal blockage, e.g. clearing of foreign body, mucus impaction.
	Initial management: If suspected aspiration, then anaerobic antibiotic, e.g. cefuroxime/metronidazole IV.
Pulmonary infarction/embolus	*Suggested by:* wedge-shaped regions of opacification peripherally ± atelectasis and pleural effusion. History of pleuritic chest pain, breathlessness, haemoptysis. May have hypoxia, tachycardia, signs of deep vein thrombosis (DVT).
	Confirmed by: **CT pulmonary angiogram** (**V/Q** is only helpful when CXR is completely normal).
	Initial management: LMW heparin, then warfarin for >3mo. Thrombolysis if ↓βP, large bilateral clots, or acutely dilated right ventricle on echocardiogram.

Dense pulmonary fibrosis	*Suggested by:* bilateral parenchymal opacification (i.e. reticulonodular shadowing), usually with volume loss, often shrunken against apical pleura. Often idiopathic, but may have history of previous TB exposure, radiation, extrinsic allergic alveolitis, chronic sarcoid, ankylosing spondylitis, pneumoconiosis, etc. *Confirmed by:* **high resolution CT thorax**. *Initial management:* address cause. Consider immunosuppression. Controlled O_2 if hypoxic.
Pleural effusion: transudate due to heart failure or exudate due to tumour/ pneumonia, etc.	*Suggested by:* homogeneous dense area of opacification, obscuring the hemidiaphragm in erect position, less dense superiorly with concave meniscus. No air bronchogram. Shift with change of position ± interfissural or subpulmonary loculation. Stony dullness to percussion. *Confirmed by:* aspiration of fluid in diagnostic tap ± **US scan** to differentiate from consolidation. *Initial management:* controlled O_2 if breathless/hypoxic. If heart failure: diuretics, β-blockers, and ACE inhibitors; if pneumonia/TB: antibiotics; if cancer, pleural drainage and pleurodesis by a specialist; if autoimmune disease, immunosuppression.
Empyema	*Suggested by:* large, lentiform pleural opacification. Recent chest infection, spiking temperature. *Confirmed by:* **pleural tap** (pus cells, ↓pH, bacteria present). *Initial management:* drainage with intercostal (IC) drain. High dose antibiotics IV according to cultures/setting. If slow/poor drainage and loculated effusion, intrapleural thrombolytics or surgical decortication.
Pneumonectomy	*Suggested by:* dense white area over entire lung with ispilateral displacement of mediastinal structures and trachea towards side of surgery. *Confirmed by:* history of pneumonectomy. *Initial management:* observation.
Complete lung collapse	*Suggested by:* dense white area over entire lung, trachea and heart (mediastinum) shifted towards affected side, dullness to percussion, ↑tactile vocal fremitus, absent breath sounds. *Confirmed by:* **CT thorax** and complete obstruction of main bronchus at **bronchoscopy**. *Initial management:* controlled O_2, analgesia. Management of underlying cause, e.g. carcinoma.
Drugs	Amiodarone, nitrofurantoin, etc.

Round opacity (or opacities) >5mm in diameter

Beware skin/rib lesions or artefact from hair, braids, or clothing, which can mimic intrathoracic pathology. Positron Emission Tomography (PET) scans are being increasingly used in assessing solitary pulmonary nodules to help distinguish between malignant (increased metabolic uptake in, for example, lung cancer) and benign (low/no metabolic activity) causes. Investigations in **bold** below.

Main differential diagnoses and typical outline evidence, etc.	
Carcinoma of bronchus	*Suggested by:* solitary opacity with irregular or lobulated or spiculated border ± other features of metastases (hilar enlargement, destructive bone changes in ribs, etc.). Often smoker, symptoms of cough, chest pain, haemoptysis, weight loss.
	Confirmed by: tissue diagnosis via **sputum cytology, bronchoscopy** or **CT guided biopsy**.
	Initial management: controlled O_2 if breathless/hypoxic. Analgesia. Refer to chest physician for staging and other therapies.
Pulmonary metastasis	*Suggested by:* multiple rounded opacities ± background history of neoplasia or lymphoma.
	Confirmed by: **CT scan appearance ± biopsy**.
	Initial management: controlled O_2 if breathless/hypoxic. Analgesia. Refer to chest physician for staging and other therapies.
'Rounded pneumonia' or lung abscess	*Suggested by:* round opacity in child, cavitating thick-rimmed lesion in adult. Background of raised inflammatory markers, neutrophilia and cough, pyrexia, spiking (in abscess).
	Confirmed by: **sputum microscopy**, culture and sensitivity resolution following appropriate antibiotic therapy.
	Initial management: antibiotics IV according to cultures/setting. Analgesia.
TB granuloma	*Suggested by:* coin lesion ± cavitation in upper lobe. History of TB exposure, weight loss, lymphadenopathy.
	Confirmed by: **CT scan** appearance. Acid-fast bacilli (AFB) on Ziehl-Neelsen (ZN) **smear** or **culture**.
	Initial management: refer to chest physician. Keep in isolation if hospitalized until smear status is known. Rifampicin, pyrazinamide, isoniazid, ethambutol PO ± pyridoxine if malnourished.
Rheumatoid nodule	*Suggested by:* peripherally positioned, multiple soft tissue nodules ± cavitation. History/signs of rheumatoid arthritis.
	Confirmed by: **CT scan** appearance and +ve **rheumatoid serology**. Consider **PET scan** in equivocal cases.
	Initial management: no action, keep under observation.

Histoplasmosis	*Suggested by:* coin lesion ± cavitation, mainly in upper lobe. Patient from USA, Africa, or HIV +ve.
	Confirmed by: **CT scan** appearance. Yeast-like organisms in sputum. +ve complement fixation test.
	Initial management: itraconazole/ketoconazole PO. Amphotericin B if very ill/immunosuppressed.
Wegener's granuloma	*Suggested by:* multiple rounded opacities ± cavitation with background of proteinuria, nasal/skin lesions, etc.
	Confirmed by: **biopsy of lung lesion or kidney**.
	Initial management: immunosuppression with cyclophosphamide, steroids, azathioprine.
Klebsiella pneumonia	*Suggested by:* multiple cavitating opacities, especially in the upper lobes in an elderly person. History of aspiration/hospitalization/institutionalization.
	Confirmed by: growth of *klebsiella* on **blood culture** and response to antibiotics.
	Initial management: cefuroxime IV ± metronidazole.
Hydatid cyst (echinococcus)	*Suggested by:* opacity in a lower lobe with dark cavity ± daughter cysts within large cyst. Water lily sign may be seen. Patient from endemic area in contact with working sheep dogs.
	Confirmed by: **CT scan** appearance. +ve **complement fixation test** or **ELISA**.
	Initial management: albendazole and refer for surgery if symptomatic/enlarging.
Pulmonary A-V malformation	*Suggested by:* other symptoms or signs ± occasional haemoptysis.
	Confirmed by: **CT thorax** showing feeding blood vessel on contrast-enhanced scan.
	Initial management: refer for embolization (significant risk of right-to-left systemic emboli causing cerebrovascular accident).
Benign tumours	*Suggested by:* no other symptoms and no change over 6mo.
	Confirmed by: **excision and histology**.
	Initial management: excision if symptomatic.
Also	Thymoma, Kaposi's sarcoma, carcinoid, drugs (including amiodarone)

Multiple 'nodular' shadows and 'miliary mottling'

These are round lesions 2–5mm in diameter of variable density, from small and soft in miliary (<2mm) mottling to larger and calcified in old chickenpox. Investigations in **bold** below.

Main differential diagnoses and typical outline evidence, etc.	
Metastases	*Suggested by:* low density nodules more profuse in the lower lung zones ± mediastinal widening and other manifestations of malignancy, e.g. lytic lesions in ribs. History of malignancy, e.g. thyroid or renal cell carcinoma. Anorexia and weight loss.
	Confirmed by: **histological** diagnosis.
	Initial management: controlled O_2 if breathless/hypoxic, analgesia. Refer to oncologist for consideration of chemotherapy.
Miliary TB	*Suggested by:* innumerable, grain-like, low density, discrete nodules with background history of TB contact. Weight loss.
	Confirmed by: AFB in **sputum, culture of bone marrow or biopsy** specimens from pleura, lung, liver, or lymph nodes.
	Initial management: isolate if in hospital until sputum smear results known. Refer to chest physician to start quadruple therapy (rifampicin, pyrazinamide, isoniazid, and ethambutol), notification, and contact tracing.
Sarcoidosis	*Suggested by:* low density nodules more profuse in the perihilar and mid-lung zones. Bilateral hilar ± paratracheal lymph node enlargement. Background of rash, uveitis, etc.
	Confirmed by: **histology** showing non-caseating granuloma with no AFB, ↑serum angiotensin-converting enzyme (ACE).
	Initial management: refer to chest physician; consider (long-term) steroids if evidence of end-organ damage, e.g. low transfer factor.
Past chickenpox	*Suggested by:* very dense opacities suggesting calcification. No current symptoms. Past history of chickenpox.
	Confirmed by: no change over months on **serial X-rays**.
	Initial management: explanation and reassurance.
Mitral stenosis with pulmonary hypertension	*Suggested by:* dense opacities due to calcification. Background of tapping left ventricular impulse (palpable 1st heart sound), ECG findings—M-shaped P wave,
	Confirmed by: **echocardiogram** and **cardiac catheterization**.
	Initial management: aspirin, diuretics ± ACE inhibitors. Anticoagulate if atrial fibrillation. Refer to cardiologist for advice on valvotomy/replacement.

Pneumoconiosis	*Suggested by:* discrete (worsening) opacities mainly in upper lobe. Employment history of >10y (coal mining, metal mining, quarrying).
	Confirmed by: comparison with previous CXR. **High resolution CT scan**.
	Initial management: controlled home O_2 if breathless/ hypoxic. Refer for industrial compensation.

Diffuse poorly defined hazy opacification

Invetigations in **bold** below.

Main differential diagnoses and typical outline evidence, etc.	
Pulmonary oedema: (cardiogenic or fluid overload or both)	*Suggested by:* symmetrical haziness more florid in a perihilar distribution, fluffy alveolar opacities ± confluence, (if fluid is in air spaces), Kerley B lines or peri-bronchial cuffing (if in interstitium), or effusion (if in pleural space). Cardiomegaly if cardiogenic. Background history of fluid overload ± heart disease ± abnormal ECG, S3, fine bibasal crackles in lungs.
	Confirmed by: ventricular dysfunction on **echocardiogram** if cardiogenic, and response to diuretics or vasodilators.
	Initial management: stop any IV fluids. Controlled O_2 if breathless/hypoxic, diuretics IV, nitrates IV. Long-term diuretics, ACE-inhibitors, β-blockers according to BP and renal function.
Acute respiratory distress syndrome (ARDS)	*Suggested by:* symmetrical, diffuse, poorly defined opacies which become confluent. Normal heart size. Acutely ill patient with severe hypoxia. History of precipitating cause (e.g. smoke inhalation, aspiration, drug exposure, fat/amniotic fluid emboli, viral infection, disseminated intravascular coagulation (DIC)), no clinical signs of left ventricular failure.
	Confirmed by: (1) acute onset, (2) bilateral infiltrates, (3) **pulmonary capillary wedge pressure** <19mmHg or no congestive cardiac failure, (4) P_aO_2:FiO_2 <200 in the presence of good left ventricular function. Around 40% fatality.
	Initial management: intubation; ventilation with small volumes and consider prone ventilation/steroids. Treatment of underlying cause.
Infective infiltration: due to viral pneumonia, Gram −ve organisms	*Suggested by:* region of patchy pulmonary infiltrate ± air bronchogram ± pleural effusion. History of cough, increased sputum; fever, ↑inflammatory markers, neutropaenia (viral) or neutrophilia (bacterial).
	Confirmed by: +ve **cultures** or resolution following appropriate antibiotics.
	Initial management: antibiotics or antivirals; route and type according to setting and cultures.
Alveolar cell carcinoma	*Suggested by:* region of poorly defined opacification which may contain air bronchogram. Background of progressive breathlessness, copious watery productive cough, weight loss. No resolution with antibiotic therapy.
	Confirmed by: **sputum cytology, lung biopsy**.
	Initial management: analgesia. Surgical referral/radiotherapy ± chemotherapy.

Lung haemorrhage	*Suggested by:* region of poorly defined opacification ± air bronchogram. Background history of trauma/contusion, clotting abnormality, necrotizing pneumonia or rarer causes such as Hamman–Rich/Goodpasture's syndrome.
	Confirmed by: haemoptysis or profuse bleeding through endotracheal tube. Resolution if trauma/clotting corrected; **CT appearances** + **renal/lung biopsy** (for Goodpasture's syndrome, Hamman–Rich).
	Initial management: correct reversible causes and clotting disorders; steroids.

Increased linear markings

Indicates thickening of the interstitial tissues. Investigations in **bold** below.

Main differential diagnoses and typical outline evidence, etc.	
Pulmonary fibrosis: idiopathic or 2° to, extrinsic allergic alveolitis, asbestosis, sarcoidosis, collagen vascular disease, pneumoconiosis, etc.	*Suggested by:* increased interstitial markings with relevant exposure history and clinical/X-ray features of above conditions. *Confirmed by:* typical appearances on **high resolution CT scan. Lung biopsy**. *Initial management:* treat cause, e.g. remove birds, immunosuppression if autoimmune disease, etc. Controlled home O_2 if breathless/hypoxic.
Interstitial fluid = pulmonary oedema	*Suggested by:* smooth thickening of the interlobular septa (Kerley B lines) with background lung crackles. *Confirmed by:* rapid resolution following diuretic therapy or correct fluid balance or dialysis. *Initial management:* controlled O_2 if breathless/hypoxic, diuretics IV, nitrates IV. Long-term diuretics, ACE-inhibitors, β-blockers according to BP and renal function.
Metastatic cells = lymphangitis carcinomatosis	*Suggested by:* irregular thickening of the interlobular septa (Kerley B lines) with background of other features of malignancy. Usually no crackles. *Confirmed by:* **high resolution CT**, **lung biopsy**, or progressive malignant disease. *Initial management:* consider steroids and palliation.
Bronchiectasis (congenital, e.g. Young's, Kartagener's; post-infective, e.g. post-whooping cough; obstruction, etc. e.g. hypogammag-lobulinaemia	*Suggested by:* tram lines and rings with background of cough with high volume of sputum (± foul and purulent (if super-added infection). *Confirmed by:* **High resolution CT** (bronchiole bigger than its accompanying artery). *Initial management:* sputum cultures and antibiotics according to results when symptomatic. Chest physiotherapy. Bronchodilator and mucolytics if wheeze/airways obstruction.

Symmetrically dark lungs

CXR film exposure is correct. Another clue to presence of pathology is abnormal lung size. Investigations in **bold** below.

Main differential diagnoses and typical outline evidence, etc.	
Chronic obstructive pulmonary disease (COPD) (emphysema)	*Suggested by:* long, narrow heart and chest, flat diaphragms, ribs horizontal, 7th rib visible anteriorly and 11th rib visible posteriorly. Prominent pulmonary arteries with paucity of interstitial markings, peripheral pruning (in pulmonary hypertension). Large, thin-rimmed, dark areas with no lung markings are bullae. History of smoking at least 10 pack years.
	Confirmed by: **High resolution CT** and lung function tests showing fixed obstructive deficit **FEV$_1$**<80%, FEV$_1$/FVC <70%.
	Initial management: stop smoking, bronchodilators (short-acting prn, then regular long-acting bronchodilators), inhaled steroids if FEV$_1$ <50–60% predicted and recurrent exacerbations. Refer for specialist opinion if rapid decline in FEV$_1$, atypical features, respiratory failure, or recurrent exacerbations.
Asthma	*Suggested by:* hyperexpanded lungs. No loss of lung markings. Background history of variable wheeze, cough, and breathlessness.
	Confirmed by: **peak flow/FEV$_1$** improvement following appropriate treatment.
	Initial management: remove allergen if possible (e.g. occupation, stop NSAIDs, stop smoking, etc).
	Acute: controlled O$_2$ if breathless/hypoxic, nebulized/high dose repeated inhaled bronchodilators, systemic steroids. Treat infection, dehydration, and closely monitor clinical response, ABG, and K$^+$. Long term: stepwise increase in treatment starting with inhaled bronchodilators prn, then regular inhaled steroids, then combination inhaler: long-acting β-agonist and inhaled steroids. Specialist follow-up.

Single dark lung

Investigations in **bold** below.

Main differential diagnoses and typical outline evidence, etc.	
Pneumothorax	*Suggested by:* visible lung edge with absence of lung markings peripheral to this. Central mediastinum. Beware skin folds, which may mimic a lung edge. History of sudden onset of breathlessness and/or pleuritic chest pain. Hyper-resonance and reduced breath sounds.
	Confirmed by: convincing appearances on CXR. Hint—best seen in an expiration film.
	Initial management: controlled O_2 if breathless/hypoxic, analgesia. Aspirate if symptomatic, >15% collapse or co-existing lung disease. If aspiration fails, insert intercostal (IC) drain through the 'triangle of safety'. If <15%, monitor for 12–24h and repeat CXR.
Tension pneumothorax (medical emergency: this should have been diagnosed clinically before doing the CXR)	*Suggested by:* visible lung edge with absence of lung markings peripheral to this, mediastinal shift away from the black lung. Background of acute progressive dyspnoea, tachycardia, ↓BP. Shifted mediastinum away from collapsed lung.
	Confirmed by: relief when needle or catheter inserted and re-expansion of lung when chest tube inserted later.
	Initial management: insert large Venflon into 2nd IC space, mid-clavicular line (on side with absent breath sounds). Then insert IC chest drain before requesting CXR.
Bulla	*Suggested by:* loss of lung markings inside lucent, thin-rimmed, circular region ± background history of COPD.
	Confirmed by: comparison with previous CXR, **CT thorax**.
	Initial management: observation, bullectomy if very large or symptomatic (e.g. recurrent pneumothorax).
Mastectomy	*Suggested by:* no breast shadow.
	Confirmed by: history of mastectomy.
	Initial management: explain and reassure.
Large pulmonary embolus (area of oligaemia on affected side)	*Suggested by:* wedge-shaped regions of opacification peripherally ± atelectasis and pleural effusion. History of pleuritic chest pain, breathlessness, haemoptysis. May have hypoxia, tachycardia, signs of DVT.
	Confirmed by: **CT pulmonary angiogram** (**V/Q** is only helpful when the CXR is completely normal).
	Initial management: LMW heparin, then warfarin for >3mo. Thrombolysis if ↓BP, large bilateral clots, or acutely dilated right ventricle on echocardiogram.
Lobar collapse	*Suggested by:* usually not whole lung looks dark. Signs of volume loss, e.g. 'sail' sign, raised diaphragm, etc.
	Confirmed by: CXR appearance. **CT chest** and/or **bronchoscopy** to establish cause.
	Initial management: treatment of underlying cause.

Abnormal hilar shadowing— homogeneous

Check that the film is not rotated—this can give a false positive diagnosis.
Compare with old films, if possible, for duration of abnormality.
Investigations in **bold** below.

Main differential diagnoses and typical outline evidence, etc.	
Metastatic lymphadenopathy, bronchial carcinoma	*Suggested by:* unilateral hilar opacity ± lung opacity or bilateral hilar opacity ± evidence of metastatic deposits, e.g. lytic rib lesions. Background history of neoplasia.
	Confirmed by: **bronchoscopy ± CT staging. Sputum cytology/biopsy** showing cancer cells.
	Initial management: controlled O₂ if breathless/hypoxic, analgesia. Refer for chest opinion for possible surgery, radiotherapy ± chemotherapy.
Hodgkin's or non-Hodgkin's lymphoma	*Suggested by:* bilateral hilar shadows ± parenchymal opacification. Anaemia, lymph node enlargement elsewhere, hepatosplenomegaly.
	Confirmed by: **histology** (Reed–Sternberg cells in Hodgkin's or without in non-Hodgkin's).
	Initial management: chemotherapy ± radiotherapy.
Primary TB with hilar node (primary complex)	*Suggested by:* unilateral hilar mass (lymphadenopathy) and poorly defined opacification in peripheral lung field, often with paratracheal nodal enlargement. Clinical features of TB.
	Confirmed by: **CT scan** showing no tumour. AFB on **ZN stain** and **culture growth from sputum**. Resolution on specific antiTB therapy.
	Initial management: isolate if in hospital until sputum smear results known. Refer to chest physician to start quadruple therapy (rifampicin, pyrazinamide, isoniazid, and ethambutol), notification, and contact tracing.
Prominent pulmonary artery due to embolus	*Suggested by:* smooth, non-lobular appearance tapering off peripherally with dark peripheral lung fields.
	Confirmed by: **CT pulmonary angiogram**.
	Initial management: LMW heparin, then warfarin for >3mo. Thrombolysis, e.g. if ↓BP, large bilateral clots, or acutely dilated right ventricle on echocardiogram.
Prominent pulmonary arteries due to pulmonary hypertension	*Suggested by:* bulky, bilateral hila with outline suggestive of prominent pulmonary arteries, tapering off peripherally with dark peripheral lung fields ± widening of upper mediastinum (superior vena cava) ± bulging right heart border.
	Confirmed by: **echocardiogram** and **CT pulmonary angiogram**.
	Initial management: treat cause; controlled O₂ if breathless/hypoxic. Specialist management.

Sarcoidosis

Suggested by: bilateral, hilar, convex shadows, possibly with other lung changes of sarcoid. Erythema nodosum, arthralgia, uveitis, etc.

Confirmed by: **histology** showing non-caseating granuloma with no AFB.

Initial management: refer to chest physician; long-term steroids if end-organ damage, e.g. low transfer factor.

Abnormal hilar shadowing—streaky

Investigations in **bold** below.

Main differential diagnoses and typical outline evidence, etc.	
Left ventricular failure (due to myocardial infarction, arrhythmia, fluid overload)	*Suggested by:* smooth thickening of the interlobular septa (Kerley B lines), cardiomegaly, bilateral fine lung crackles.
	Confirmed by: rapid resolution following diuretic therapy or correct fluid balance or dialysis.
	Initial management: controlled O_2 if breathless/hypoxic, diuretics IV, nitrates IV. Treat cause. Long-term diuretics, ACE inhibitors, β-blockers according to BP and renal function.
Bronchopneumonia (bilateral)	*Suggested by:* breathlessness, chest pain, productive cough.
	Confirmed by: +ve **sputum/blood cultures**, atypical serology.
	Initial management: controlled O_2 if breathless/hypoxic, antibiotics to cover *Streptococcus pneumoniae* (penicillins) and other organisms (clarithromycin).
Pneumocystis carinii pneumonia	*Suggested by:* breathlessness, chest pain, dry cough, known immunosuppression (or risk factors), and lymphopaenia.
	Confirmed by: +ve sputum/bronchial washings, cultures, immunostaining.
	Initial management: controlled O_2 if breathless/hypoxic, co-trimoxazole.
Also	Histioplasmosis, pulmonary alveolar proteinosis.

Upper mediastinal widening

Investigations in **bold** below.

Main differential diagnoses and typical outline evidence, etc.	
Retrosternal goitre	*Suggested by:* superior mediastinal mass shadow extending from the neck. *Confirmed by:* clinical examination, **US or radioisotope scan**. *Initial management:* surgery if local symptoms of compression. Correct thyroid function if hypothyroid (↑TSH, ↓FT4) or thyrotoxic (↓TSH, ↑FT4 or ↑FT3).
Hodgkin's or non-Hodgkin's lymphoma or metastatic lymphadeno-pathy	*Suggested by:* dense, often multinodular masses, causing mediastinal widening. CT scan appearances. *Confirmed by:* **mediastinoscopy** or surgical removal showing **histology**. *Initial management:* referral to oncologist for chemotherapy ± radiotherapy.
Thymoma	*Suggested by:* clearly outlined opacity (calcification in 20%). Background features of myasthenia gravis (in 30%). *Confirmed by:* **CT scan** appearance and **histology** from **mediastinoscopy** or surgical removal. *Initial management:* surgical removal ± chemo-radiotherapy according to histological subtype and staging. Check for associated myasthenia gravis (30%).
Teratoma: benign or malignant	*Suggested by:* anterior mediastinal opacification, rarely with calcification, e.g. in teeth. *Confirmed by:* **CT scan** appearance ± fat, hair, teeth, and histology from **mediastinoscopy** or surgical removal. *Initial management:* surgical removal, consider chemoradiotherapy according to histological subtype and staging.
Kinked or aneurysmal aorta	*Suggested by:* opacification continuous with descending aorta shadow. Risk factors for aneurysms (↑BP, smoker, trauma, syphilis, collagen disease, etc). Signs of aortic regurgitation. *Confirmed by:* **CT scan** appearance. *Initial management:* reassure if kinked. Refer to vascular surgeon if aneurysmal. Modify risk factors.

Abnormal cardiac shadow

Investigations in **bold** below.

Main differential diagnoses and typical outline evidence, etc.	
Left ventricular failure due to ischaemic heart disease, recent myocardial infarction, arrhythmia (e.g. atrial fibrillation)	*Suggested by:* large heart, mainly to left of midline (with central trachea), linear upper lobe opacities, and fluffy lung opacities—centrally more than peripherally. *Confirmed by:* **echocardiogram** showing poor contraction of left ventricle. *Initial management:* controlled O_2 if breathless/hypoxic, diuretics IV, nitrates IV. Long-term diuretics, ACE inhibitors, β-blockers according to BP and renal function. Treat cause.
Pulmonary hypertension	*Suggested by:* prominent right heart border (of right ventricle), upwardly rounded apex and bilateral prominence of hila. Loud S2 (pulmonary valve closure), ↑JVP ± history of pulmonary embolus, tall R waves in V1 to V3 and right axis deviation on ECG. *Confirmed by:* **echocardiogram** (estimated pulmonary pressure >25 mmHg at rest). *Initial management:* controlled O_2 if breathless/hypoxic, treat reversible causes, e.g. pulmonary emboli, vasculitis. Diuretics if swollen legs. Specialist centre follow-up.
Cardiomyopathy	*Suggested by:* generally large heart with clear borders (indicating poor contraction). Predisposing condition, e.g. ischaemia, chronic alcohol abuse, amyloid, leukaemia, rheumatoid arthritis, etc. *Confirmed by:* **echocardiogram** showing poor contraction of left ventricle. *Initial management:* controlled O_2 if breathless/hypoxic, diuretics IV, nitrates IV. Long-term diuretics, ACE inhibitors, β-blockers according to BP and renal function.
Pericardial effusion	*Suggested by:* large globular cardiac outline and clear borders (indicating little or no contraction). Quiet hear sounds, impalpable apex. Low voltage **ECG** complexes. *Confirmed by:* echocardiogram. *Initial management:* if distressed, emergency pericardiocentesis. If stable, refer for echocardiogram-guided drainage and pericardial window.
Atrial septal defect	*Suggested by:* unusually convex right heart border, upwardly rounded cardiac apex, and bilateral prominence of hila. *Confirmed by:* **echocardiogram**. *Initial management:* refer to cardiology to consider surgical correction.

Mitral stenosis	*Suggested by:* large heart, enlarged left atrium (rounded opacity behind the heart which 'splays' the carinal angle) ± calcification in position of mitral valve and dense nodules due to haemosiderosis. History of rheumatic heart disease.
	Confirmed by: **echocardiogram** and **cardiac catheterization**.
	Initial management: aspirin, diuretics, and ACE inhibitors. Warfarin if AF. Refer to cardiology to consider valvotomy/ valve replacement.
Left ventricular aneurysm	*Suggested by:* bulge in left ventricular border ± calcification. Background history of ischaemic heart disease ± myocardial infarction. Persistent ST elevation on ECG.
	Confirmed by: **echocardiogram**.
	Initial management: refer to cardiology to consider surgery. Warfarin if associated thrombus.
Mediastinal emphysema	*Suggested by:* gas around the mediastinal contour ± surgical emphysema. Background history of acute asthma, OGD, oesophageal rupture, etc., signs of surgical emphysema.
	Confirmed by: **CT thorax**.
	Initial management: nil by mouth, prophylactic cefuroxime IV and metronidazole if oesophageal rupture. Surgical repair if no spontaneous healing after 2–3d.
Hiatus hernia	*Suggested by:* circular shadow behind the heart ± air/fluid level, absent gastric bubble. Intermittent appearance on previous CXR.
	Confirmed by: **barium swallow, endoscopy**.
	Initial management: lifestyle modification. Antacids, e.g. PPI if symptoms continue.
Also	Diaphragmatic hernia, atrial myxoma, radiation pneumonitis.

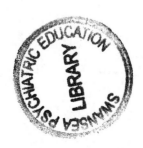

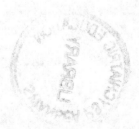

Making the diagnostic process evidence-based

Evidence-based diagnoses and decisions

The purpose of this chapter is to explain how the differential diagnostic process can be made 'evidence-based'. The first chapter explained how a diagnostic lead can be used to provide a differential diagnosis; examples of such diagnostic leads and their differential diagnoses are shown throughout this book. These pages also show how other findings can be used to differentiate between the differential diagnoses so that some become more probable and others less probable. One of the differential diagnoses can be 'confirmed' by showing that some findings occur by definition only in patients with that single diagnosis and not in others. By specifying the individual patient's 'particular evidence', we make this process 'partially' evidence-based.

In order to make the diagnostic process completely evidence-based, it is necessary to show that the differential diagnoses of a diagnostic lead actually account for a high proportion of patients with that diagnostic lead in an appropriate study. In order to show that other findings can actually differentiate between the lead's differential diagnoses, we also have to show in a study that they actually occur more commonly in some diagnoses than in others. The greater this difference, the better the differentiation. The problem is that this information has not been collected yet, and so completely evidence-based differential diagnosis is in its infancy. All we can do at present is to describe the patient's particular evidence in the form of particular symptoms, signs and test results, making the process 'partially' evidence-based.

Before the evidence about diagnostic leads and diagnostic differentiators can be collected, it is also necessary to provide evidence that the findings used to confirm diagnoses can justify their use in that way. These confirmatory findings are also called diagnostic or 'gold standard' criteria. These criteria identify groups of patients within which there are further subgroups defined by different treatment indication criteria and other subgroups with different prognoses and different risks of complications. Therefore, the diagnostic criterion can be thought of as an 'envelope' that encloses other various treatment and prognostic groups. The current approach is to choose these criteria in a non-evidence-based way because experts or expert committees consider them to be the most theoretically suitable.

Epidemiologists provide evidence that a test result is useful for screening a population by describing its 'sensitivity' and 'specificity'. Thus, the frequency with which a test is positive in those with the diagnostic criterion is a measure of its 'sensitivity' in detecting the diagnosis. A negative test is supposed ideally to predict the absence of the diagnosis; the frequency of a negative result in those without the diagnosis is called its 'specificity'. Both these proportions should be as high as possible. However, these indices are also used to assess the usefulness of tests in the clinical setting. When a number of symptoms, signs, and test results have to be taken into account, their individual 'sensitivities' are multiplied together. The same is done with 'one minus each specificity'. The probability of the diagnosis is then found by using a simple formula called Bayes theorem (named after an 18th century clergyman who is said to have described it in a paper published after his death). This simple arithmetical process (see p.757) has been proposed as a representation of the 'intuitive', non-explicit diagnostic process. However, it does not represent the explicit, transparent, differential diagnostic process described in this book.

The remainder of this chapter will explain the logical and mathematical basis of the differential diagnostic process described in this book. The explanation only requires a basic understanding of set and probability theory to follow it. However, this may require patience and perseverance from those whose memory of these subjects has faded. It will provide statisticians and those students and doctors who wish to conduct research in this area to in order to make it 'evidence-based' with a detailed understanding of the mathematics of the differential diagnostic process.

Before considering the type of general scientific evidence required to support the use of findings during the differential diagnostic process, it is important to understand what general scientific evidence is required to support the use of findings as criteria to confirm diagnoses and to begin treatment or to provide some other advice.

The logic of diagnostic criteria

A diagnostic term, e.g. 'diabetes mellitus', is the title to what we imagine is wrong with a patient. There will be considerable variation between what medical professionals imagine when a diagnosis is discussed. This depends on what they have read, their personal experience, and research experience. What is imagined will also vary when a diagnosis is applied to different patients. It will be governed by the patient's general appearance and demeanour, symptoms, signs and test results. This is the imaginative meaning of diagnosis. However, when we communicate our thoughts to others, we have to use descriptive terms with shared meanings. This gives rise to another parallel meaning of diagnosis, which is connected with diagnostic terms, classifications, and set theory.

A diagnostic term is also the label that we would apply to the group or set of patients, e.g. 'those with diabetes mellitus'. This label is usually chosen for historical reasons (e.g. 'sweet-tasting urine' or 'diabetes mellitus'). The rule for when or when not to use the label is chosen because it is close to the 'essence' of the disease as generally understood. Formal definitions for general use are usually drawn up by experts in the field. For example, in the case of diabetes mellitus, we might state that all those patients with two fasting blood glucose results of at least 7.0mmol/L have diabetes. A single rule based on fasting glucose would not define diabetes properly because it does not specify that all such patients and only such patients have diabetes. In other words, it is a 'sufficient' criterion that confirms the diagnosis, but its absence does not exclude the diagnosis. This means that it is not a 'necessary' criterion because some other rule can also be used. For example, patients with two random blood glucose results of at least 11.1mmol/L also have diabetes. If there are many rules, then we have to say patients with rule A or B or C or D have diabetes. In order to complete the definition, we say 'all those and only those' with A or B or C or D have diabetes.

If we say that a patient does not have diabetes (i.e. is not a member of the set of diabetics), then we are also implying that there is no significant prospect of that patient benefiting from the treatments directed at diabetes. Therefore, it is important that the 'envelope' that encloses and excludes those with and without diabetic patients does not 'rule out' those who might benefit from its treatments. This is why the World Health Organization and the American Diabetes Association widened the definition by lowering the blood sugars to include those who needed treatment for diabetic retinopathy who had blood sugars that lay outside the criteria for diabetes. The diagnostic label is helpful because it implies that 'diabetic' patients should be assessed to see if they would benefit from a range of treatments (which include preventative treatments as well as those that relieve existing symptoms).

One approach to defining diagnostic 'envelopes' would be to identify all the treatment indication criteria that can be explained by the theories of that diagnosis, and then defining diagnostic envelopes in terms of these treatment indication criteria. The different treatment indication criteria for diabetes might be (A) the indication for a diabetic diet alone, (B) the indication for metformin, etc. up to (Z) the indication for an insulin pump. Those with diabetes mellitus could then be defined as all those and only those with one or more of the treatment indication criteria A or B up to Z. This would ensure that the 'envelope' would not omit any patient who required treatment. The approach of basing diagnostic definitions on individual treatment indication criteria might depend on demonstrating the presence of a large amount of information, especially for broad diagnostic categories such as diabetes. Therefore, it is more practical to use a simple test if possible, e.g. based on fasting or random blood sugars, and to adjust the criteria when required. The approach of basing definitions on treatment indications might be more practical for diagnostic groups connected to few treatments or a single treatment such as 'diabetic microalbuminuria'.

Using a diagnosis to make predictions

Having confirmed a diagnosis by showing the presence of at least one of its 'sufficient criteria', the next step is to consider the different subgroups of patients requiring different treatments within the diagnostic 'envelope'. In some cases, all the patients within the 'envelope' may need some action, e.g. all diabetic patients need dietary and lifestyle advice, and regular follow-up. Some of the subgroups may have their own diagnostic labels, e.g. 'diabetic microalbuminuria' (see figure 13.1). The treatment may be to reduce symptoms or to prevent future problems such as nephropathy. Ideally, the diagnosis of 'diabetic microalbuminuria' should be based on the test whose results identify all those who might benefit and exclude all those who do not. Some candidate tests would be an overnight microalbumin excretion rate, a 24-h microalbumin excretion rate, or an albumin/creatinine ratio based on an early morning urine specimen.

The perfect test for use as a treatment criterion for diabetic microalbuminuria would have a cut-off point below which no patients develop nephropathy so that there is no point to treat them and above which, all patients get nephropathy so that they all need treatment. In practice, only a proportion (e.g. 25%) of patients with microalbuminuria would develop nephropathy (see figure 13.1). The cut-off point is currently set at an albumin excretion rate (AER) of 20mcg/min because this happens to be two standard deviations above the mean of the log of AERs in healthy volunteers. It is also assumed that patients with an AER below 20mcg/min have a negligible risk of developing nephropathy; above this level, it is assumed that about 25% develop nephropathy irrespective of the value of the AER (see figure 13.2). In reality, it is an oversimplification to think that there is a sharp difference between those with an AER above or below 20mcg/min.

In one study, it was discovered that the proportion of patients with an AER between 20 and 40mcg/min who developed nephropathy within 2 years was less than 1%, suggesting that the cut-off point of 20mcg/min is incorrect. The same study showed that the proportion developing nephropathy within 2 years was higher for those with an AER between 40 and 80 mcg/min, higher again in patients with an AER between 80 and 120 and higher still in those with an AER between 120 and 160 mcg/min (see figure 13.3). This rise in risk is quite shallow. A better test ('X') might show a steeper rise in risk of nephropathy as in figure 13.4. Nevertheless, distinct sets and subsets such as those in figure 13.1 are helpful simplifications. If data are plotted as shown in figures 13.2 to 13.4, then their cut-offs points can be placed more accurately so that less than 1% are excluded from the diagnosis, e.g. an AER of 40mcg/min.

Therefore, it is possible to choose a cut-off point for a test's results, below which a low proportion of patients (e.g. <1%) get a complication such as nephropathy. The best test would then be the one which has the greatest proportion of patients developing nephropathy above such a cut-off point (e.g. test X in figure 13.4 would be better than the AER in figure 13.2). If this cut-off point was used to initiate treatment, this would mean that a higher proportion of those treated would benefit and fewer would be treated unnecessarily who had little prospect of benefiting.

This is an example of how 'gold standard' tests can be chosen so that they provide the best predictions and help the decision of when and when not to treat. However, even if some cut-off point suggests that there might be some benefit in treatment, a decision still has to be made as to whether the probability of benefit would outweigh the risk of adverse events in the individual patient, and in many countries, the cost. For example, if a test result was just above the cut-off point and at that particular result, there was a 2% chance of response to treatment compared to 1% chance of response to placebo, then the probability of benefit would be 2% − 1% = 1%, and the number needed to treat (NNT) for one to benefit would be 100. The cost and risk of side effects might lead to a decision not to accept treatment. However, if the test result was much higher with a 76% − 1% = 75% chance of benefit, then the treatment might be accepted.

The diagnostic envelope would include patients 'inside' the diagnostic cut-off point when its treatment should be considered and exclude those with no prospect of benefit. It is important to note that the upper or lower 'limit of normal' (the upper or lower two standard deviations) acts only as a guide to the region where this cut-off point might be. Therefore, the purpose of the diagnostic process is to identify those patients who need specific treatments and advice. Even the best treatments will be ineffective if given to the wrong patients. For example, if a placebo-controlled trial of thyroxine was conducted on patients with 'hypothyroidism' who were diagnosed by using faulty hormone assays that merely generated random numbers, then there would be little difference between treatment and placebo as most of those selected would be normal.

The same principles apply to surgical treatment. However, the diagnostic process continues during the surgical procedure. For example, during a laparotomy for suspected appendicitis, the patient may be found to have an appendix abscess or a retrocaecal appendix or one wrapped in adherent loops of bowel. Therefore, the 'diagnostic envelope' of those with appendicitis would contain a number of subgroups with different surgical treatment requirements. Nevertheless, the surgeon would prefer to have a clear picture of what will probably be found from preoperative imaging methods so that surprises are minimized.

Evidence-based differential diagnosis

If a finding (e.g. right lower quadrant (RLQ) abdominal pain) has been shown in a study to have a small number of differential diagnoses, and these diagnoses account for a very high proportion of patients with that finding, then this will be evidence of its ability to act as a good lead during the differential diagnostic process. This is one type of general evidence of a finding's ability to perform well during the differential diagnostic process.

If a finding (e.g. 'guarding') occurs commonly in one of the differential diagnoses of a lead (e.g. appendicitis) and less commonly in another of the differential diagnoses (e.g. non-specific abdominal pain—NSAP), then this will be another type of general evidence of a finding's ability to perform well during a differential diagnostic process. If 'guarding' is 'likely' to occur in appendicitis but 'less likely' to occur in NSAP, thus giving a strong 'differential likelihood ratio', such a strong ratio provides general evidence of a finding's ability to perform well as a 'differentiator' during a diagnostic process.

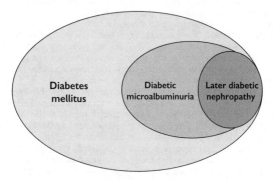

Fig.13.1 Diagnostic 'envelopes' and distinct proportions with subgroups

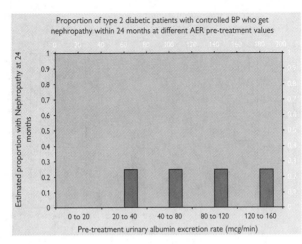

Fig.13.2 Abrupt change in proportions

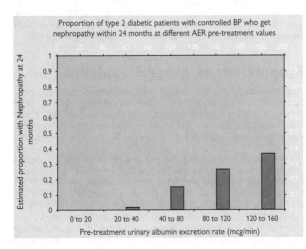

Fig.13.3 Gradual and shallow change in proportions

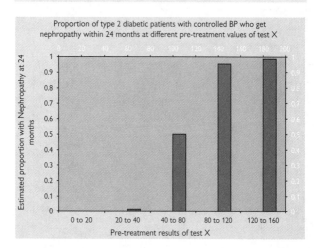

Fig.13.4 Steep change in proportions

The lead of 'abdominal pain in the right lower quadrant' could be due to appendicitis, salpingitis, an ectopic pregnancy, or 'NSAP'. If the patient is male, the pain cannot be due to an ectopic pregnancy or salpingitis (because being female is a necessary criterion for these gynaecological conditions). However, being male is obviously frequent in those with appendicitis, giving a differential likelihood ratio of zero. If the patient has 'guarding', this occurs less often in NSAP and more often in appendicitis, making appendicitis more probable and NSAP less probable.

Proportions as 'general' evidence

Most patients arriving in a surgical admission unit with RLQ abdominal pain would have appendicitis (e.g. 75/200) or NSAP (e.g. 123/200) with a few (e.g. 2/200) having something else. If the proportion with RLQ pain in the studied population was 200/300, then the proportion with 'something else' in those with RLQ pain and any other finding could be no more than $2/200 \times 200/300 = 2/300$.

If the patient had 'guarding' and this only occurred in 6/150 patients with NSAP, then the combination of 'guarding' with RLQ pain can be no more than 6/150 of those with NSAP. If the proportion with NSAP in the surgical admission unit was 150/300, then the proportion with NSAP and guarding and RLQ pain could be no more than $6/150 \times 150/300 = 6/300$.

If 'guarding' occurred in 80/100 of those with appendicitis and RLQ pain occurred in 75/100, then both must occur together in at least $80/100 + 75/100 - 100/100 = 55/100$ even if they occur together as infrequently as possible. If the proportion with appendicitis in the surgical admission population was 100/300, then the proportion with appendicitis and guarding and RLQ pain would be at least $100/300 \times 55/100 = 55/100$.

If the proportion with RLQ pain and guarding and appendicitis in the study population was exactly 55/300, the proportion with RLQ pain and guarding and NSAP was exactly 6/300, and the proportion with RLQ pain and guarding and 'something else' was exactly 2/300, the proportion of patients with RLQ pain and guarding who had appendicitis would be 55/300 / (55/300+6/300 + 2/300) = 55/63 = 0.873. But as 55/300 was a minimum value and as 6/300 and 2/300 were maximum values, then at least 87.3% must have appendicitis. (The actual proportion in this example data set is 76/80 = 0.95 = 95%)

Simplifying the arithmetic

The proportion of patients with RLQ pain and guarding who have appendicitis was shown to be at least 87.3% in the above reasoning process. The arithmetic used can be put together in one calculation as follows, providing the minimum probability of appendicitis given the presence of RLQ pain and guarding:

$$1/\left\{1+\frac{[150/300 \times 6/150]+[200/300 \times 2/200]}{100/300 \times [75/100 + 80/100 - 100/100]}\right\} = 55/63 = 0.873 \quad (A)$$

$$1/\left\{1+\frac{[0.5 \times 0.04]+[0.67 \times 0.01]}{0.33 \times [0.75 + 0.80 - 1]}\right\} = 0.873 \quad (B)$$

The calculation can be simplified by making an assumption of statistical 'depvendence' (see 📖p.766) to give approximations which tend to slightly underestimate the actual proportion of appendicitis in those with RLQ pain and guarding. These approximations use the ratio of incidences (e.g. 0.5/0.33 below), differential odds (e.g. 0.01/0.375 below) and differential likelihood ratios (e.g. 0.04/0.8 below). The differential likelihood ratio (DLR) is the frequency of a finding in one diagnosis (e.g. guarding in NSAP = 0.04) divided by the frequency in another (e.g. guarding in appendicitis = 0.80). The differential odds (DO) are the proportion of patients with one diagnosis category in those with a 'lead' finding (e.g. the proportion with unspecified diagnoses in those with RLQ pain = 0.01) divided by the proportion of patients with a different diagnosis in patients with the same 'lead' finding (e.g. the proportion with appendicitis in those with RLQ pain = 0.375). The probability of appendicitis given RLQ pain and guarding is thus approximately:

$$1/\left\{1+\frac{0.5 \times 0.04}{0.33 \times 0.80}+\frac{0.01}{0.375}\right\} = 0.908 \quad (C)$$

A simple rearrangement of the above equation (for details see 📖pp.768–769) uses differential odds alone (i.e. 0.05/0.67 and 0.01/0.375). The probability of appendicitis given RLQ pain and guarding is thus approximately:

$$1/\left\{1+\frac{0.05}{0.67}+\frac{0.01}{0.375}\right\} = 0.908 \quad (D)$$

The above expressions provide a mathematical explanation as to why leads with small number of differential diagnoses perform well in the differential diagnostic process. They also explain why differential likelihood ratios are important in 'evidence-based' differential diagnosis. The reasoning in the above two pages is repeated in great detail on 📖pp.766–769 below for those who wish to reflect more deeply.

Evidence-based 'active' diagnosis

Diagnoses can be pursued actively by looking for findings that are 'likely' to occur in patients with the diagnosis that you are trying to confirm, and 'unlikely' to occur in those with diagnoses that you are trying to discount. The process starts by first looking at the patient's findings and choosing the best lead. This is the finding with the shortest list of differential diagnoses that can explain 99% say of patients with the lead.

RLQ abdominal pain is such a lead, its differential diagnosis being appendicitis (in 37.5% of patients) or NSAP (in 61.5% of patients), these accounting for 99% of patients with RLQ pain. The 'unlisted' 1% is all other possible diagnoses. In order to differentiate between these diagnostic categories, the diagnostician has to choose one to 'chase' (the postulated diagnosis). This should be the most probable diagnosis (to be correct first time as often as possible) or dangerous diagnosis (to avoid delay).

If it was decided to pursue appendicitis first, then a finding is sought that occurs commonly in appendicitis but less commonly in NSAP. Guarding is such a finding because it occurs in 80% of those with appendicitis (the 'likelihood' is 0.8) but in only 4% of those with NSAP (the 'likelihood' is 0.04). The ratio is thus 0.04/0.80 = 0.05.

The differential ratio (i.e. 0.04/0.8) is multiplied by the incidence of NSAP (i.e. 150/300 = 0.5) divided by the incidence of appendicitis in the same population (i.e. 100/300 = 0.33) to give the differential odds. This also has to be done for the other differential diagnoses (but there was only one here, NSAP). The differential odds of the 'unlisted' diagnoses (0.01/0.375) then have to be added. The frequency with which appendicitis will be found in RLQ pain and guarding is estimated by using equation (C) on page 757:

$$1/\left\{1+\frac{0.5 \times 0.04}{0.33 \times 0.80}+\frac{0.01}{0.375}\right\}=0.908$$

This equation uses <u>differential</u> likelihood ratios: the frequency of a finding in patients with a diagnosis divided by its frequency in patients with another diagnosis. This has to be distinguished from the 'overall likelihood ratio' which is the frequency of a finding in patients with a diagnosis divided by its frequency in all patients <u>without that diagnosis</u>.

The 'overall likelihood ratio' is difficult to measure because it is affected by patients with other diagnoses or healthy individuals in the study population. The absolute incidence and prevalence are affected in the same way. However, in the expressions used here, all is required is the ratio of two incidences or prevalences. This ratio of 0.5/0.333 = 1.5 can also be calculated indirectly from the probability of NSAP given RLQ pain (0.615) divided by the likelihood of RLQ pain given NSAP (0.82) multiplied by the likelihood of appendicitis given RLQ pain (0.75) divided by the probability of appendicitis given RLQ pain (0.375): $0.615/0.82 \times 0.75/0.375 = 1.5$.

Evidence-based 'passive' diagnosis

Diagnoses can be pursued actively by looking for findings that are 'likely' to occur in patients with the diagnosis that you are trying to confirm, and 'unlikely' to occur in those with diagnoses that you are trying to discount. However, the 'passive' approach is to think of each the patient's findings in turn (e.g. RLQ pain, guarding, etc), and to consider if there is only one diagnosis that is common to each list of differential diagnoses. This passive approach does not depend on 'likelihoods' or 'likelihood ratios'.

If there is only a single diagnosis (e.g. appendicitis) common to a number of findings (e.g. RLQ pain and guarding), it follows that the diagnosis will be probable, i.e. it will occur very frequently in a group of patients with those findings (e.g. appendicitis will occur frequently in those with RLQ pain and guarding). The frequency with which the diagnosis will be found can be estimated by using equation (D) on page 757.

In order to estimate the frequency given a combination of findings by using observed frequencies given single findings, choose the finding associated with the 'common' diagnosis that has the best lead (i.e. the finding with shortest list of differential diagnoses). Thus the differential diagnosis of RLQ pain is appendicitis (in 37.5%) or NSAP (in 61.5%), these accounting for 99% of patients with RLQ pain, the other 1% not being in the list. For each other diagnosis in the list (i.e. NSAP alone in this case), choose another finding which provides the best (i.e. the lowest) 'differential odds'. For example, guarding is associated with NSAP in only $6/120 = 5\%$ of cases and appendicitis occurs in $80/120 = 75\%$ of cases, so the differential odds is $5/75 = 0.067$.

The best (i.e. lowest) DO for each of the differential diagnoses to be discounted can be used to estimate the probability of the diagnosis to be confirmed (e.g. appendicitis). This is done by adding the lowest DOs for each differential diagnosis to give the sum of the lowest DOs. The probability of the suspected diagnosis (e.g. appendicitis) is thus:

$1/[1 + \text{sum of all the lowest DOs}]$.

If the sum of all the lowest DOs is zero, then the probability of the diagnosis will be one, of course.

The lowest DO for NSAP is 0.067 (provided by guarding) and the lowest DO for the 'unlisted' diagnoses is provided by RLQ pain is $1/37.5 = 0.027$. Therefore, the estimated probability of appendicitis give RLQ pain and guarding is $1/(1 + 0.067 + 0.027) = 0.908$ (see equation (D) on p.757). Note that this does not use incidence or prevalence.

In order to practice evidence-based differential diagnosis (and thus evidence-based medicine) properly, research is needed to find the frequency with which patients with each differential diagnosis occur in those with a diagnostic lead in different clinical settings (i.e. to calculate the various DOs) and the DLRs. There will be differences between general practices, hospitals, parts of the country, etc.

Likelihood ratios as diagnostic evidence

The 'likelihood ratio' is a term usually used for the frequency of a finding occurring in a diagnosis (e.g. 'guarding' in appendicitis) divided by the frequency of that finding <u>in all those without</u> the diagnosis (e.g. 'guarding' in those without appendicitis). The 'likelihood' is the probability of a finding occurring in a diagnosis (also known as the 'sensitivity'); the term 'probability' is used when predicting a diagnosis from a finding.

In 300 patients admitted to a surgical department, 120 had 'guarding' and 100 patients turned out to have appendicitis. Eighty patients had both appendicitis and 'guarding'. This meant that of those 100 patients with appendicitis, 80/100 = 80% had 'guarding'. Also, of the 120 patients with 'guarding', 80/120 = 66.67% also had appendicitis.

The frequency of 'guarding in those <u>without appendicitis</u> was 40/200 = 20% or 0.20 (because many patients had other conditions that can cause guarding). Therefore, the 'overall' likelihood ratio would be 0.80/0.20 = 4. This 'overall likelihood ratio' is widely regarded as a measure of a finding's diagnostic usefulness.

If the 300 patients had been admitted to the surgical ward in a month and 100 of these had appendicitis, then the incidence per month would be 100/300 = 0.33. If 120 of these 300 patients had 'guarding', then its incidence would be 120/300 = 0.40%. However, if <u>all patients with appendicitis and all patients with 'guarding'</u> during the same month had been sent to hospital from a catchment area of 300,000, then the incidence of appendicitis in the catchment population would be 100/300,000 = 0.00033 and the incidence of guarding would be 0.00040 per month.

In the catchment area, the proportion of those with appendicitis who had guarding would also be 80/100 = 80%. The proportion of those <u>without</u> appendicitis who had 'guarding' would be 40/299,900 = 0.00013. Therefore, the likelihood ratio would be 0.8/0.00013 = 5998 (five thousand nine hundred and ninety eight!)—compared to four inside the surgical department. Despite this, the probability of any patient in the catchment area having appendicitis who is known to have guarding would still be 80/120 = 66.67%, which is exactly the same as for patients in the hospital. If the frequency of guarding in those with NSAP is also 4% in the community, the DLR, DO and probability of the diagnosis will also be same.

So, the overall likelihood ratio (OLR) becomes inflated if the population contains large numbers of patients <u>without the diagnosis or the finding</u> (e.g. healthy people). Therefore, it is very important only to use an OLR with an incidence or prevalence measured in exactly that same population used to obtain the OLR. However, if the spectrum of illness is similar (e.g. in terms of severity) in different populations, then the sensitivities or likelihoods will also be similar and so will the DLRs. Therefore, the DLR is better a measure of test performance than the OLR.

Diagnosis and statistical dependency

If guarding occurs in 6/150 (0.04 or 4%) of patients with NSAP and if RLQ pain occurs in 123/150 (0.82 or 82%) of patients with NSAP, then both occur together in 6/150 = 0.04 = 4% or less. If both findings do actually occur as often as possible together, then they will occur in 0.04 of cases. In this case, there would be positive statistical dependence between these two findings. However, if there was statistical independence, they would occur together in $0.82 \times 0.04 = 0.0328$ or 3.28% of cases. If there was negative statistical dependence, they would never occur together.

If guarding occurred in 80/100 = 0.8 = 80% of patients with appendicitis and if RLQ pain occurred in 75/100 = 0.75 = 75% of patients with appendicitis, then both must occur together in $0.75 + 0.8 - 1 = 0.55 = 55\%$ of cases. If they did occur together in 55% of cases, then this would represent negative statistical dependence. If there was statistical independence, then both would occur together in $0.75 \times 0.8 = 0.6$ or 60% of cases. If there was positive statistical dependence, they would occur together in 0.75 or 75% of cases (i.e. equal to the lowest frequency).

If there was statistical independence between RLQ pain and guarding in NSAP, then both would occur in 0.0328 of cases of NSAP. If there was statistical independence between RLQ pain and guarding in appendicitis, then both would occur in $0.8 \times 0.75 = 0.6$ of cases of appendicitis. The estimated DLR for appendicitis over NSAP for the combination of RLQ pain and guarding based on assuming statistical dependence would be 0.6/0.0328 = 18.28. The same estimated DLR based on statistical independence can also be found by multiplying the DLR for guarding (0.8/0.04 = 20) by the DLR for RLQ pain (0.75/0.82 = 0.914). This gives ($20 \times 0.914 = 18.28$).

If there was statistical dependence between RLQ pain and guarding in appendicitis and NSAP, then the DLR of the combination can be assumed to be equal to the highest of the individual DLRs. The DLRs for appendicitis over NSAP was 20 for guarding and 0.914 for RLQ pain, so the highest would be 20. Therefore, the estimated DLR for the combination would be estimated to be 20. This is similar to the estimation, assuming statistical independence in this case, which was 18.28. However, the estimate based on the dependence assumption is the simpler of the two.

No assumption can be guaranteed to be accurate of course. The dependence assumption may be more accurate if there are strong individual likelihood ratios whereas the independence assumption may work better for weaker individual DLRs. It is also possible that errors in the assumption may be similar (e.g. both degrees of dependence may be overestimated) so that the errors cancel out. The answer is to 'audit' the accuracy of estimated probabilities, e.g. by checking whether predictions with estimated probabilities between 0.85 and 0.90 actually turn out to be correct in 85% to 90% of cases when making these assumptions.

The detailed arithmetic of differential diagnosis

The purpose of this section is to show how it is possible to work out the frequency with which a diagnosis such as appendicitis occurs in combinations of findings such as RLQ pain and guarding without having to know the frequency of every diagnosis in every combination of findings. It is based on the familiar reasoning process that states: 'RLQ pain is usually due to appendicitis or NSAP. Guarding occurs often in appendicitis but it occurs infrequently in NSAP. Therefore, when there is RLQ pain and guarding, the diagnosis will usually be appendicitis.' The basis of this diagnostic reasoning, which is fundamental to the differential diagnostic process, and to making it evidence-based, will be described here in detail; it is also described elsewhere.[1, 2, 3]

The formulae or equations that summarize this reasoning were described on 🕮p.757. When:

- 150/300 is the proportion with NSAP in the studied population
- 6/150 is the proportion with guarding in those with NSAP
- 200/300 is the proportion with RLQ pain in the studied population
- 2/200 is the proportion with unlisted diagnoses in those with RLQ pain
- 100/300 is the proportion with appendicitis in the studied population
- 75/100 is the proportion with RLQ pain in those with appendicitis
- 80/100 is the proportion with guarding in those with appendicitis
  then the proportion of patients with appendicitis in those with RLQ pain and guarding is at least:

$$1/\left\{1+\frac{[150/300\times6/150]+[200/300\times2/200]}{100/300\times[75/100+80/100-1]}\right\}=55/63=0.873$$

This expression is rigorous—it always gives a correct answer. However, it gives a minimum value for the actual proportion. In other words, the actual proportion will be between 0.873 and 1. The following expression (when 75/200 is the proportion with appendicitis in those with RLQ pain) gives an approximate answer instead and is simpler and easier to apply:

$$1/\left\{1+\frac{150/300\times6/150}{100/300\times80/100}+\frac{2/200}{75/200}\right\}=0.908$$

A simple rearrangement of the above equation (when 6/20 is the proportion of patients with NSAP in those with guarding and 80/120 is the proportion of those with appendicitis in those with guarding) also gives an approximate answer to the proportion of those with appendicitis in those RLQ pain and guarding:

$$1/\left\{1+\frac{6/120}{80/120}+\frac{2/200}{75/200}\right\}=0.908$$

This section will show how these equations were derived.

Reasoning with proportions

The reasoning behind the equations is based on simple proportions and assumptions. However, the mathematical reasoning is intricate and following it requires patience. It cannot be read quickly or 'skimmed'. It is central to evidence-based differential diagnosis.

Most patients arriving in a hypothetical general surgical admission unit with RLQ pain had appendicitis or NSAP, with a low proportion (perhaps 2/200) having something not in the list of two possibilities. If the proportion with RLQ pain in the surgical admission population was 200/300, then the proportion with 'an unlisted diagnosis' in combination with RLQ pain in that population is $2/200 \times 200/300 = 2/300$. This also means that the proportion of patients with 'an unlisted diagnosis' in combination with RLQ pain and guarding is equal to or less than 2/300.

This can also be stated in another way, which is the converse of the reasoning in the above paragraph. If the proportion with an 'unlisted' diagnosis (i.e. other than appendicitis or NSAP) in the population of the surgical unit was 50/300 and 2 of these 50 had RLQ pain, then the proportion with an 'unlisted' diagnosis in the studied population would be $2/50 \times 50/300 = 2/300$. This means that the proportion of patients with RLQ pain AND guarding AND the unlisted group of diagnoses in the studied population can be no more than 2/300. But this $2/300 = 2/50 \times 50/300$ is the same as the converse reasoning of $2/300 = 2/200 \times 200/300$ in the previous paragraph.

As an aside, the simple arithmetic relationship of $2/200 \times 200/300 = 2/300 = 2/50 \times 50/300$ is the basis of 'Bayes theorem' named after an 18th century clergyman who wrote a celebrated paper (published post humously) on the way observed events could be used predict future events. 'Bayes theorem' is used often when reasoning about diagnosis. If the above equation of $2/200 \times 200/300 = 2/300 = 2/50 \times 50/300$ is rearranged, it gives 'Bayes theorem':

$$2/200 = \frac{2/50 \times 50/300}{200/300}$$

'Bayes theorem' in words is that 'the proportion with a diagnostic category in those with a finding (2/200) is equal to the proportion with the finding in those with the diagnostic category (2/50), multiplied by the proportion of those with the diagnostic category in the studied population (50/200), divided by the proportion with the finding in the studied population (200/300).

However, we have reasoned already that in differential diagnosis, the proportion of patients with RLQ pain AND guarding AND the unlisted group of diagnoses in the studied population can be no more than the proportion with RLQ pain in the surgical admission population, multiplied by the proportion with 'an unlisted diagnosis' in the studied surgical admission population, which is $2/200 \times 200/300 = 2/300$.

If the patient had 'guarding' and this only occurred in 6/150 = of patients with NSAP, then the combination of 'guarding' with RLQ pain can occur in no more than 6/150 of those with NSAP. If the proportion with NSAP in the surgical admission population was 150/300, then the proportion with

NSAP and guarding and RLQ pain in the surgical admission population could be no more than $6/150 \times 150/300 = 6/300$.

If 'guarding' occurred in 80/100 of those with appendicitis and RLQ pain occurred in 75/100, then both must occur together in at least $80/100 + 75/100 - 100/100 = 55/100$ even if they occur together as infrequently as possible. If the proportion with appendicitis in the surgical admission population was 100/300, then the proportion with appendicitis and guarding and RLQ pain in the surgical admission population would be at least $100/300 \times 55/100 = 55/300$.

If the proportion with RLQ pain and guarding with appendicitis in the surgical population was exactly 55/300, the proportion with NSAP was exactly 6/300 and the proportion with 'something else' was exactly 2/300, the proportion of those with RLQ pain and guarding who had appendicitis would be

$$55/300 \ / \ (55/300 + 6/300 + 2/300) = 55/63 = 0.873.$$

This can be simplified so that 55/300 appears only once in the equation:

$$1/\left\{1+\frac{[6/300]+[2/300]}{55/300}\right\} = 0.873$$

But as 55/300 was a minimum value and as 6/300 and 2/300 were maximum values, then the proportion with appendicitis must be greater than or equal to:

$$1/\left\{1+\frac{[6/300]+[2/300]}{55/300}\right\} = 0.873$$

The actual proportion in the example data was $76/80 = 0.95$.

Summarizing the reasoning

The original reasoning said that

$$2/300 = 200/300 \times 2/200$$

and that

$$6/300 = 150/300 \times 6/150$$

and that

$$55/300 = 100/300 \times [75/100 + 80/100 - 100/100]$$

Therefore, the original reasoning can be put into one equation as follows:

$$1/\left\{1+\frac{[150/300 \times 6/150]+[200/300 \times 2/200]}{100/300 \times [75/100 + 80/100 - 100/100]}\right\} = 55/63 = 0.873$$

This is the equation that we set out to prove was correct on 📖p.762.

The reasoning process that led to this equation can also be written in a short hand. Thus if 'S' is the studied patients admitted to a surgical ward in a month and 'N' represents NSAP, then 'the proportion with NSAP in the studied surgical population is 150/300' can be written as 'P(N/S) = 150/300' (note the capital 'P'). If 'A' represents appendicitis, 'R' represents RLQ pain, 'U' represents the 'unlisted diagnoses' linked to RLQ pain, and R∩G represents the group (or set) of patients with 'RLQ pain and guarding', then the reasoning process that led to this calculation can be written in short hand as:

$$P(A/R{\cap}G) \geq$$

$$1/\left\{1+\frac{[P(N/S){\times}P(G/N)]+[P(R/S){\times}P(U/R)]}{P(A/S){\times}[P(R/A)+P(G/A)-1]}\right\} = 55/63 = 0.873$$

Proportions and probabilities

The above expression about proportions can also be rewritten to represent probabilities. If we have a group (or set) of patients with RLQ pain and guarding and 55/63 have appendicitis, then if we choose any one of these patients and all we know is that the patient is a member of that group, then the probability of that patient having appendicitis would be 0.873. Instead of the subgroup (or subset) of patients representing the 'intersection' (written '∩') of patients with a combination of RLQ pain (R) and guarding (G), written as 'R∩G', a probability statement talks about a particular member of that group (or element of the set) with the features 'R and G' written as 'R∧G':

$$p(A/R{\wedge}G) \geq$$

$$1/\left\{1+\frac{[p(N/S){\times}p(G/N)]+[p(R/S){\times}p(U/R)]}{p(A/S){\times}[p(R/A)+p(G/A)-1]}\right\} = 55/63 = 0.873$$

Just to remind you of the various proportions used in the above reasoning which correspond to the short hand:

$$P(A/R{\cap}G) \geq$$

$$1/\left\{1+\frac{[150/300 \times 6/150]+[200/300 \times 2/200]}{100/300 \times [75/100 + 80/100 - 100/100]}\right\} = 55/63 = 0.873$$

The corresponding probability values can be written as decimals:

$$p(A/R{\wedge}G) \geq$$

$$1/\left\{1+\frac{[0.5 \times 0.04]+[0.67 \times 0.01]}{0.33 \times [0.75 + 0.80 - 1]}\right\} = 0.873$$

The formal proof of this expression when it is applied to any number of findings and diagnoses (not just two as in this case), has been published elsewhere[1, 2, 3].

The limitations of reasoning with proportions

Only two findings (RLQ pain and guarding) were used in the above example. RLQ pain and guarding occurred in a high proportion of patients with appendicitis, so that both occurred together in at least 55 patients out of 100. If 'male gender' had also been taken into account and this was present in 50/100 of patients with appendicitis, then the three findings of 'RLQ pain, guarding and being male' would only occur in a minimum of [75/100 + 80/100 + 50/100 − 100/100 + 300/100] ≥ −5/100 (minus 5/100), or zero, of patients with appendicitis. This can be written in terms of probabilities as: [0.75 + 0.8 + 0.5 − 1 + 3] ≥ −0.05 or 0.

When there are 'n' findings, then the likelihood of them occurring together is at least 'the sum of all the likelihoods minus 'n' plus 1' (or zero if the answer is 'minus something'). If there are many findings (i.e. 'n' is a large number) or if the likelihoods are low, then this rule will result in a value of 'greater than zero', which tells us very little about the probability. Furthermore, this will happen if one of the likelihoods is about a numerical value (e.g. a temperature of 37.9°) because that likelihood will be very small and almost zero. This problem can be overcome by making statistical 'dependence assumptions'.

Statistical dependence assumptions

The assumption made here is that the severity of all diseases associated with the particular combination of findings shown by the patient (e.g. RLQ pain, guarding (G) and a temperature of 37.9°) can be represented on some scale. It will also be assumed that a smaller subset of patients with a narrower interval of disease severity can be found so that the frequency of the findings shown by the patient in those with the postulated diagnostic subset (e.g. of appendicitis) will be 100%. This small subset of patients with appendicitis will be termed 'delta-appendicitis' or 'δA' so that P(R/δA) = 1, P(G/δA) = 1 and P(Temp of 37.9°/δA) = 1. It will also be assumed that there will be small subsets of other conditions in the same interval on some scale of severity e.g. 'delta-NSAP' or δN. For these subsets of diseases (e.g. delta-appendicitis or delta-NSAP) it will be assumed that the ratios of incidences, prevalences and 'likelihoods' will be the same as the ratios in the complete sets of all those with appendicitis or NSAP e.g. P(G/N) / P(G/A) = P(G/δN) / P(F/δA). However, if for some finding, e.g. 'F', P(F/N) > P(F/A) it can be assumed that P(F/δN) = 1. Thus:

$$\frac{P(\delta N/S) \times P(G/\delta N)}{P(\delta A/S) \times P(G/\delta A)} = \frac{P(N/S) \times P(G/N)}{P(A/S) \times P(G/A)} = \frac{150/300 \times 6/150}{100/300 \times 80/100}$$

But as P(G/δA) = 1

$$\frac{P(\delta N/S) \times P(G/\delta N)}{P(\delta A/S) \times 1} = \frac{P(N/S) \times P(G/N)}{P(A/S) \times P(G/A)} = \frac{150/300 \times 6/150}{100/300 \times 80/100}$$

Rearranging by moving P(δA/S) and P(δN/S) to the other side so that P(δN/S)/P(δA/S) becomes inverted to P(δA/S)/P(δN/S):

$$P(G/\delta N) = \frac{P(\delta A/S) \times P(N/S) \times P(G/N)}{P(\delta N/S) \times P(A/S) \times P(G/A)} = \frac{P(\delta A/S) \times 150/300 \times 6/150}{P(\delta N/S) \times 100/300 \times 80/100}$$

Applying the same reasoning to U (the unlisted diagnoses) instead of N for NSAP:

$$P(R/\delta U) = \frac{P(\delta A/S) \times P(U/S) \times P(R/U)}{P(\delta N/S) \times P(A/S) \times P(R/A)} = \frac{P(\delta A/S) \times 50/300 \times 2/50}{P(\delta N/S) \times 100/300 \times 75/100}$$

It has been shown already for appendicitis (A), NSAP (N), and 'unlisted' diagnoses (U) that:

$$P(A/R \cap G) \geq 1 / \left\{ 1 + \frac{[P(N/S) \times P(G/N)] + [P(U/S) \times P(R/U)]}{P(A/S) \times [P(R/A) + P(G/A) - 1]} \right\} =$$

$$1 / \left\{ 1 + \frac{[150/300 \times 6/150] + [200/300 \times 2/200]}{100/300 \times [75/100 + 80/100 - 1]} \right\}$$

The same would apply for delta-appendicitis (δA), delta-NSAP, (δN) and 'unlisted' diagnoses (δU) so that:

$$P(\delta A/R \cap G) \geq 1 / \left\{ 1 + \frac{[P(\delta N/S) \times P(\delta G/N)] + [P(\delta U/S) \times P(R/\delta U)]}{P(\delta A/S) \times [P(R/\delta A) + P(G/\delta A) - 1]} \right\}$$

But as P(R/δA) = 1 and P(G/δA) = 1 then replacing these with '1' in the above equation gives:

$$P(\delta A/R \cap G) \geq 1 / \left\{ 1 + \frac{[P(\delta N/S) \times P(\delta G/N)] + [P(\delta U/S) \times P(R/\delta U)]}{P(\delta A/S) \times [1 + 1 - 1]} \right\}$$

Simplifying the last equation by removing [1 + 1 − 1]:

$$P(\delta A/R \cap G) \geq 1 / \left\{ 1 + \frac{[P(\delta N/S) \times P(\delta G/N)]}{P(\delta A/S)} + \frac{[P(\delta U/S) \times P(R/\delta U)]}{P(\delta A/S)} \right\}$$

Substituting P(G/δN) in the above with $\dfrac{P(\delta A/S) \times P(N/S) \times P(G/N)}{P(\delta N/S) \times P(A/S) \times P(G/A)}$

from the top of this page gives:

$$1 / \left\{ 1 + \frac{\cancel{P(\delta N/S)} \times \cancel{P(\delta A/S)} \times P(N/S) \times P(G/N)}{\cancel{P(\delta A/S)} \times \cancel{P(\delta N/S)} \times P(A/S) \times P(G/A)} + \frac{[P(\delta U/S) \times P(R/\delta U)]}{P(\delta A/S)} \right\}$$

which after cancelling out $P(\delta N/S)$ and $P(\delta A/S)$ in the above gives:

$$P(\delta A/R \cap G) \geq 1 / \left\{ 1 + \frac{P(N/S) \times P(G/N)}{P(A/S) \times P(G/A)} + \frac{[P(\delta U/S) \times P(R/\delta U)]}{P(\delta A/S)} \right\}$$

Substituting $P(R/\delta U)$ in the above with $\dfrac{P(\delta N/S) \times P(U/S) \times P(R/U)}{P(\delta A/S) \times P(A/S) \times P(R/A)}$

gives:

$$1 / \left\{ 1 + \frac{P(N/S) \times P(G/N)}{P(A/S) \times P(G/A)} + \frac{P(\delta U/S) \times P(\delta A/S) \times P(U/S) \times P(R/U)}{P(\delta A/S) \times P(\delta U/S) \times P(A/S) \times P(R/A)} \right\}$$

which after cancelling out $P(\delta U/S)$ and $P(\delta A/S)$ in the above gives:

$$P(\delta A/R \cap G) \geq 1 / \left\{ 1 + \frac{P(N/S) \times P(G/N)}{P(A/S) \times P(G/A)} + \frac{P(U/S) \times P(R/U)}{P(A/S) \times P(R/A)} \right\}$$

But as $P(U/S) \times P(R/U) = P(R) \times P(U/R)$ (see Bayes theorem, 📖p.763)
And as $P(A/S) \times P(R/A) = P(R) \times P(A/R)$ (Bayes theorem again)
Then:

$$P(\delta A/R \cap G) \geq 1 / \left\{ 1 + \frac{P(N/S) \times P(G/N)}{P(A/S) \times P(G/A)} + \frac{P(R) \times P(R/U)}{P(R) \times P(A/R)} \right\}$$

But cancelling out $p(R)$ in the above equation gives:

$$P(\delta A/R \cap G) \geq 1 / \left\{ 1 + \frac{P(N/S) \times P(G/N)}{P(A/S) \times P(G/A)} + \frac{P(U/R)}{P(A/R)} \right\}$$

But as $P(N/S) \times P(G/N) = P(G) \times P(N/G)$ (Bayes theorem again)
And as $P(A/S) \times P(G/A) = P(G) \times P(G/A)$, (Bayes theorem again) then

$$P(A/R \cap G) \geq 1 / \left\{ 1 + \frac{P(G) \times P(N/G)}{P(G) \times P(A/G)} + \frac{P(U/R)}{P(A/R)} \right\}$$

But cancelling out $p(G)$ in the above equation gives:

$$P(A/R \cap G) \geq 1 / \left\{ 1 + \frac{P(N/G)}{P(A/G)} + \frac{P(U/R)}{P(A/R)} \right\}$$

Delta-appendicitis (δA) is a subset of appendicitis (A). It is possible that RLQ pain and guarding may also be associated with appendicitis separately from delta-appendicitis. Therefore, $P(A/R \cap G) \geq P(\delta A/R \cap G)$ and so:

$$P(A/R \cap G) \geq 1 / \left\{ 1 + \frac{P(N/S) \times P(G/N)}{P(A/S) \times P(G/A)} + \frac{P(U/R)}{P(A/R)} \right\}$$

The proportions from our original reasoning were

$$1/\left\{1+\frac{150/300 \times 6/150}{100/300 \times 80/100}+\frac{2/200}{75/200}\right\}=0.908$$

and also

$$P(A/R \cap G) \geq 1/\left\{1+\frac{P(N/G)}{P(A/G)}+\frac{P(U/R)}{P(A/R)}\right\}$$

The proportions form our original reasoning being

$$1/\left\{1+\frac{6/120}{80/120}+\frac{2/200}{75/200}\right\}=0.908$$

The value of $P(A/R \cap G)$ in the above two equations are based on a 'statistical dependence' assumption regarding the patient's findings in appendicitis and the other diagnoses. You will recall in the original reasoning on 📖pp.763–764 that the frequency of RLQ pain and guarding in those with NSAP could be no more than 6/150. (This was the frequency of guarding in NSAP). However, if there was statistical dependence between RLQ pain and guarding in those with NSAP, then the actual frequency of these findings in NSAP would also be 6/150. If the same applied to the unlisted diagnoses, and if we could assume that none of the differential diagnoses could occur together, then instead of using '≥' (at least) in the equation, we could use '=' (equals). However, as these are assumptions, we should treat the result as an approximation and use '≈' (approximately equal to) instead of '=' to give:

$$P(A/R \cap G) \approx 1/\left\{1+\frac{P(N/S) \times P(G/N)}{P(A/S) \times P(G/A)}+\frac{P(U/R)}{P(A/R)}\right\}$$

and

$$P(A/R \cap G) \approx 1/\left\{1+\frac{P(N/G)}{P(A/G)}+\frac{P(U/R)}{P(A/R)}\right\}$$

These above two expressions are approximations and therefore, differ from the rigorously derived expression that states that

$$P(A/R \cap G) \geq 1/\left\{1+\frac{[P(N/S) \times P(G/N)]+[P(R/S) \times P(U/R)]}{P(A/S) \times [P(R/A)+P(G/A)-1]}\right\}$$

Reasoning with diagnoses in general

In general terms, we can represent the list of 'm' diagnoses provided by a diagnostic lead by D1, D2, Dm (e.g. D1 = appendicitis, D2 = NSAP, so that m = 2), and D0 is the group of unlisted diagnoses. We can represent the postulated diagnosis (appendicitis in the above examples) by Dx (when for example Dx = D1 so that × = 1). Dj represents any one of the list of diagnoses (e.g. when j = 2 then Dj = D2, represents NSAP).

We can represent the list of 'n' findings by F1, F2, Fn (e.g. F1 = RLQ pain, F2 = guarding, etc so that n = 2). The finding chosen as the diagnostic lead can be referred to as FL (if FL represents F1, then L = 1). Fi can be used to represent any one of the list of findings (e.g. when i = 2, then Fi = F2, representing guarding).

$\sum_{i=1}^{n} P(Fi/D1)$ means 'the sum of the list $P(F1/D1) + P(F2/D1) + P(F3/D1)$, $P(Fn/D1)$ starting with $P(F1/D1)$'. The intersection of all the findings F1, F2, Fn can be represented by $F1 \cap F2 \uparrow \cap Fn$.

$\sum_{j \neq 1}^{m} P(Dj/F1)$ means the sum of the list $P(D2/F1) + P(D3/F1)$, Dm/F1) but omitting $P(D1/F1)$ because it states that this applies to each 'j' in Dj but not 1 in D1 (it says at the bottom of the symbol '$\sum$' that $j \neq 1$).

By using this short hand, we can write the above equations in terms that apply to any number of findings and any number of differential diagnoses. Therefore, the expression

$$P(A/R \cap G) \approx 1 / \left\{ 1 + \frac{P(N/G)}{P(A/G)} + \frac{P(U/R)}{P(A/R)} \right\}$$

can be written in general terms as expression (a):

$$P(Dx_{any\,j} / F1 \cap F2 \ldots \cap Fn) \approx 1 / \left\{ 1 + \frac{\sum_{j \neq x}^{m} P(Dj/Fi)_{min}}{P(Dx/Fi)} + \frac{P(D0/FL)_{L=any\,i}}{P(D1/FL)} \right\} \quad (a)$$

The expression

$$P(A/R \cap G) \approx 1 / \left\{ 1 + \frac{P(N/S) \times P(G/N)}{P(A/S) \times P(G/A)} + \frac{P(U/R)}{P(A/R)} \right\}$$

can be written in general terms as expression (b):

$$P(Dx_{any\,j} / F1 \cap F2 \ldots \cap Fn) \approx 1 / \left\{ 1 + \frac{\sum_{j \neq x}^{m} P(Dj).P(Fi/Dj)_{min}}{P(Dx).P(Fi/Dx)} + \frac{P(D0/FL)_{L=any\,i}}{P(D1/FL)} \right\} \quad (b)$$

The expression

$$P(A/R \cap G) \geq 1 / \left\{ 1 + \frac{[P(N/S) \times P(G/N)] + [P(R/S) \times P(U/R)]}{P(A/S) \times [P(R/A) \times P(G/A) - 1]} \right\}$$

can be written in general terms as expression (c) on the next page.

Expression (c) is:

$$P(Dx_{any\,j} / F1 \cap F2 \ldots \cap Fn) \approx$$
$$1 / \left\{ 1 + \frac{\sum_{j \neq x}^{m} P(Dj).P(Fi/Dj)_{min} \times P(FL).P(D0/FL)_{aL=any\,i}}{P(Dx)[\sum_{j=1}^{n} P(Fi/Dx - n + 1)]} \right\} \quad (c)$$

The derivation of equations (a)[1], (b)[1] and (c)[1, 2] are also published elsewhere.

Assuming statistical independence

Expression (b) was:

$$P(Dx_{any\,j}/F1 \cap F2 \ldots \cap Fn) \approx 1/\left\{1 + \frac{\sum_{j \neq x}^{m} P(Dj).P(Fi/Dj)_{min}}{P(Dx).P(Fi/Dx)} + \frac{P(D0/FL)_{L=any\,i}}{P(D1/FL)}\right\}$$

Expression (b) can be used with an assumption of statistical independence. When expression (b) is applied to estimating the proportion of patients with RLQ pain and guarding who turn out to have appendicitis, it is written as:

$$P(A/R \cap G) \approx 1/\left\{1 + \frac{P(N/S) \times P(G/N)}{P(A/S) \times P(G/A)} + \frac{P(U/R)}{P(A/R)}\right\}$$

The proportions used in the original reasoning in this chapter were:

$$1/\left\{1 + \frac{150/300 \times 6/150}{100/300 \times 80/100} + \frac{2/200}{75/200}\right\} = 0.908$$

The corresponding probabilities were:

$$1/\left\{1 + \frac{0.5 \times 0.04}{0.33 \times 0.8} + \frac{0.01}{0.375}\right\} = 0.908$$

The proportion with RLQ pain in those with NSAP was $123/150 = 0.82$ and the proportion with RLQ pain in those with appendicitis was $75/100 = 0.75$. If we use the assumption of statistical independence, the estimated proportion with RLQ pain and guarding in those with NSAP is $0.82 \times 0.04 = 0.328$ (i.e. $P(R/N) \times P(G/N) = 0.328$). The estimated proportion with RLQ pain and guarding in those with appendicitis is $0.75 \times 0.8 = 0.6$ (i.e. $P(R/A) \times P(G/A) = 0.6$.

If we replace $P(G/N)$ by $P(R/N) \times P(G/N)$ and if we replace $P(G/A)$ by $P(R/A) \times P(G/A)$ in the above equations, we get:

$$P(A/R \cap G) \approx 1/\left\{1 + \frac{P(N/S) \times P(R/N) + P(G/N)}{P(A/S) \times P(R/A) + P(G/A)} + \frac{P(U/R)}{P(A/R)}\right\}$$

The corresponding calculation is

$$1/\left\{1 + \frac{0.5 \times 0.04 \times 0.82}{0.33 \times 0.75 \times 0.8} + \frac{0.01}{0.375}\right\} = 0.902$$

The estimated proportion with appendicitis in those with RLQ pain and guarding is very similar when the assumption of statistical independence is made (0.902) and the statistical dependence (0.908). The actual value was $76/80 = 0.95$. This does not mean to say of course that such estimates will always be similar. If more than two findings are used, then the estimate using statistical independence would tend to be higher.

The overall likelihood ratio

Bayes theorem states that:

$$P(A/R \cap G) = \frac{P(A) \times P(R \cap G/A)}{P(R \cap G)}$$

This can be rearranged to give:

$$P(A/R \cap G) \approx 1/\left\{1 + \frac{P(Not\ A) \times P(R \cap G/Not\ A)}{P(A) \times P(R \cap G/A)}\right\}$$

The diagnostic lead is not represented in this equation at all and neither are the differential diagnoses of appendicitis, e.g. NSAP or the unlisted diagnoses. However, Bayes theorem can be used with the statistical independence assumption. According to this assumption, $P(R \cap G/A) = P(R/A) \times P(G/A) = 0.75 \times 0.8 = 0.6$. Also from the original example data, the proportion with guarding in those without appendicitis was $40/200 = 0.2$ and the proportion with RLQ pain in those without appendicitis was $125/200 = 0.625$. The proportion of patients without appendicitis is $(300-100)/300 = 200/300 = 0.667$. Bayes theorem with the assumption of statistical independence is that

$$P(A/R \cap G) \approx 1/\left\{1 + \frac{P(Not\ A) \times P(R/Not\ A) \times P(G/Not\ A)}{P(A) \times P(R/A) \times P(G/A)}\right\}$$

The corresponding calculation is:

$$1/\left\{1 + \frac{0.67 \times 0.625 \times 0.2}{0.33 \times 0.75 \times 0.8}\right\} = 0.706$$

This estimate is a little low (the actual value was $76/80 = 0.95$). Much of the available detailed information about differential diagnoses has not been used in this calculation (e.g. the low frequency of guarding in NSAP). This does not mean to say, of course, that estimates based on this approach will always be low. However, this approach does not represent the differential diagnostic thought process described in this book, which uses diagnostic leads (e.g. RLQ pain) and diagnostic differentiators (e.g. guarding).

References

1. Llewelyn, DEH (1988). Assessing the validity of diagnostic tests and clinical decisions. In: MD thesis. University of London.

2. Llewelyn, DEH (1979). Mathematical analysis of the diagnostic relevance of clinical findings. Clin Sci 57, 477–9.

3. Llewelyn, DEH (1981). Applying the principle of logical elimination to probabilistic diagnosis. Med Inform 6, 25–32.

Index

F

H

Reference values

Please note that the values and ranges vary among laboratories. Conventional units are used in some medical/scientific journals, and laboratories in some countries. Therefore both SI and conventional units are given.

Measurement	SI unit	Conventional unit	Conversion factor CF x C = SI
5- Hydroxyindole Acetic Acid (5-HIAA), urine	9.4–31.4 µmol/day	1.8–6.0 mg/day	5.230
Alanine amino-transferase (ALT)	0–41 U/L	0–41 U/L	–
Albumin	35–50 g/l	3.5–5.0 g/dL	10
Alpha-fetoprotein	0–15 µg/L	0–15 ng/mL	1.0
Aspartate amino-transferase (AST)	10–40 U/L	10–40 U/L	–
Adrenocorticotrophin			
8 a.m.	2–11.5 pmol/L	9–52 pg/mL	0.2202
4 p.m.	1.1–8.2 pmol/L	5–37 pg/mL	
Aldosterone, serum			
Supine	50–250 pmol/L	2–9 ng/dL	27.74
Upright	80–970 pmol/L	3–35 ng/dL	
Alkaline phosphatase	40–129 U/L	40–129 U/L	–
Amylase	0.33–1.83 nkat/L	20–110 U/L	0.0167
Bicarbonate	22–30 mmol/L	22–30 mEq/L	1.0
Bilirubin, total	<17.1 µmol/l	<1.0 mg/dL	17.1
Calcitonin	<2.9 pmol/L	<10 pg/mL	0.29
Calcium, serum	2.23–2.63 mmol/L	8.9–10.5 mg/dL	0.2495
Ceruloplasmin	250–650 mg/L	25–65 mg/dL	10
Chloride	98–108 mmol/l	98–108 mEq/L	1.0
Cholesterol, total desirable	< 5.2 mmol/l	< 200 mg/dL	0.02586
Chorionic Gonado-trophin, human			
Non-pregnant	<5 IU/L	<5 mIU/mL	1.0
Pregnant	<100,000 IU/L	<100,000 mIU/mL	
Copper			
Serum	11–24 µmol/L	70–155 µg/dL	0.157
Urine	<0.94 µmol/day	<60 µg/day	0.0157
Cortisol, serum			
a.m.	140–700 nmol/L	5–25 µg/dL	27.59
4 p.m	96–280 nmol/L	4–10 µg/dL	
Cortisol, urine free	28–250 nmol/day	10–90 µg/day	2.8
C-peptide, serum	0.1–1.23 nmol/L	0.3–3.7 µg/L	0.331
Creatinine	62-106 µmol/l	0.70–1.20 mg/dL	88.40
Creatinine phosphokinase	25–145 U/L	25–145 mU/mL	1.0
Estradiol			
Male & postmeno-pausal F	37–220 pmol/L	10–60 ng/L	3.671
Menstruating F	<1.45 nmol/L	< 400 ng/L	0.0037
Ferritin	20–300 µg/L	20–300 ng/mL	1.0
Folate,			
Serum	6.4–49.5 nmol/L	2.8–21.8 ng/mL	2.27
Red blood cell	272–1530 nmol/L	120–674 ng/mL	
Follicle stimulating hormone			
Male	0.6–8.6 IU/L	0.6–8.6 mIU/mL	1.0
Female	4–13 IU/L	4–13 mIU/mL	
Postmenopausal F	20–138 IU/l	20–138 mIU/mL	